Faith Community Nursing

MW00843799

P. Ann Solari-Twadell
Deborah Jean Ziebarth
Editors

Faith Community Nursing

An International Specialty Practice
Changing the Understanding of Health

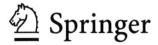 Springer

Editors
P. Ann Solari-Twadell
Marcella Niehoff School of Nursing
Loyola University Chicago
Chicago
Illinois, USA

Deborah Jean Ziebarth
Herzing University
Nursing Program Chair
Brookfield
Wisconsin, USA

ISBN 978-3-030-16128-6   ISBN 978-3-030-16126-2   (eBook)
https://doi.org/10.1007/978-3-030-16126-2

© Springer Nature Switzerland AG 2020
This work is subject to copyright. All rights are reserved by the Publisher, whether the whole or part of the material is concerned, specifically the rights of translation, reprinting, reuse of illustrations, recitation, broadcasting, reproduction on microfilms or in any other physical way, and transmission or information storage and retrieval, electronic adaptation, computer software, or by similar or dissimilar methodology now known or hereafter developed.
The use of general descriptive names, registered names, trademarks, service marks, etc. in this publication does not imply, even in the absence of a specific statement, that such names are exempt from the relevant protective laws and regulations and therefore free for general use.
The publisher, the authors, and the editors are safe to assume that the advice and information in this book are believed to be true and accurate at the date of publication. Neither the publisher nor the authors or the editors give a warranty, expressed or implied, with respect to the material contained herein or for any errors or omissions that may have been made. The publisher remains neutral with regard to jurisdictional claims in published maps and institutional affiliations.

This Springer imprint is published by the registered company Springer Nature Switzerland AG
The registered company address is: Gewerbestrasse 11, 6330 Cham, Switzerland

Foreword

Dad, throughout his life, had interesting ways to get his ideas or points across. He would listen to your thoughts whether you agreed with him or not. He would then discuss both sides with you, and somehow you would end up agreeing with him.

Case in Point

In third grade, some of my friends wore glasses, so I decided that wearing glasses would help me see better and fit in with the others. I thought I had convinced Dad that this was a good idea. Even though he disagreed with me, he said we would go to the eye doctor. The day after my appointment, Dad brought home my new glasses and put them on me. He asked if I could see better, and I said "yes." Then, he removed the glasses and put his fingers through where the lenses should have been. Dad had a way to help people see better.

All faith communities have a mission of health and salvation. This "calls" the faith community to reach out, not only to the local community, but worldwide community. A most important mission of the faith community, however, is reaching in and being supportive in creating a healthy environment for all of its members within in order to insure their health and well-being from a whole-person perspective. This "call" can be contagious and will spread outside of the church and into the community at large.

This book, like the previous ones, is an update on faith community nursing and how it is continually growing and maturing with new people, new ideas, and new concepts. The ideas for parish nursing were sown 35 years ago. Many churches, individuals, and even parish nurses have benefitted from these ideas. And more ideas continue to flourish beyond expectations by the thousands of parish nurses in 31 countries from A (Australia) to Z (Zimbabwe).

So who should be reading this informative book other than nurses, pastors, and medical doctors? The answer is simple—all congregants of any faith community. These writings of over two dozen authors and two very dedicated editors are a must-read to fully understand and appreciate the benefits and values of this mission—past, present, and future. And to the "Doubting Thomas's" (aka Finance Committees) and others who have been in the business community? The answer as aptly stated by Dr. Maria Neira, Director of the Department of Public Health and Environment at the World Health Organization, is "The wealth of a business depends on the health of its workers." I believe that the health of a church depends on the health of its members. How often do people say "my health and my family's health are the most important concern in my life"?

Dad said he never understood why churches did not have a line item in the budget for "risk-taking." He said churches should be open to testing out new ways of ministering to people. Is risk involved after 35 years of growing, learning, and educating thousands of people on a new understanding of health and the value of a faith community nurse ministry that can foster members of the faith community to make better decisions regarding their health from a whole-person perspective? It is probably a lot less of a risk than when a new pastor is called or is assigned to a church. My "A" attitude, not "B" attitude, is "Blessed are the risk takers for they shall have a faith community nurse."

These 25 chapters give the reader a better understanding of the resources offered through the Westberg Institute, formerly the International Parish Nurse Resource Center, and they show how the parish nurse evolved into the faith community nurse. Based on the contributions of these knowledgeable and determined authors, there are no limitations on what and where faith community nursing will be throughout the world for generations to come.

As you read this book, you will find out why the only time you will regret not having a parish nurse is when your parish nurse retires.

Preach Teach and **Heal**

    Or is it

P reach T each and **Heal**

John G. Westberg

Preface

This book is the work of many. The contributors, each with their own rich experiences in the practice and ministry of faith community nursing, have generously taken the time to work with the editors in making this book a reality. The chapter authors have all practiced or continue to contribute to the specialty of faith community nursing.

The title of this book, *Faith Community Nursing: An International Specialty Practice Changing the Understanding of Health*, reflects the intent to provide the reader with foundational understanding of the significant historical perspectives significant to faith community nursing, the importance of education, perspectives of faith community nursing from the nurse and other collaborating professionals, faith community and public health, organizations promoting the ongoing maturation of the practice, and, finally, issues that are integral to this specialty practice continuing the change of the understanding of health locally, nationally, organizationally, and internationally. In this book, the authors affirm and push beyond the current practices by exploring and examining contributions, education, development, professional organizations, and trends encouraging key stakeholders to begin to see faith community nursing as significant to increasing prevention and access while insuring provision of quality care.

The aims of this book are to review historical background, affirm best practices, identify and wrestle with current issues, present multiple perceptions of the practice, and share significant contributions as well as future integration of this specialty nursing practice into health care delivery. Twenty-five chapters take the reader from a foundational understanding of this historic grassroots movement to the more contemporary, present-day issues of this international professional specialty nursing practice. This specialty nursing practice is continuously evolving with multiple stakeholders invested in supporting the maturation of faith community nursing to contribute to contemporary reform of health care.

The structure of the book is presented in five parts. Part I investigates the contributions of faith community nursing to changing the understanding of health globally. This part includes four chapters describing faith community nursing as a professional specialty nursing practice, a review of theoretical applications in faith community nursing to date, key contributions being made by faith community nurses to the health of the client, as well as related cost implications. Application of wholistic and holistic nursing care is discussed as it pertains not only to faith community nursing, but to overall spiritual care of individuals. Part II of the book includes four chapters which review the importance of education in the development, standardization, and ongoing maturation of the specialty practice. Initial educational preparation, the value of ongoing continuing education, education from the perspective of different organizational models, and discussion of the role of the advanced practice nurse who is a faith community nurse are explored. Part III presents five chapters identifying different perspectives of faith community nursing and how the understanding of health and faith community nursing is seen through the eyes of the faith community leadership, nurse, physician, health care system, and public health. Part IV undertakes a review of the significant organizations that are supporting the ongoing development and integration of faith community nursing. It includes five chapters that discuss the practice through the involvement of key stakeholders to support the recognition of this specialty practice into making health care more accessible, cost-effective, and community-based while focusing on the care of the whole person. Part V includes seven chapters reviewing current issues and trends in faith community nursing with suggestions for current application to health care practices and continued integration into the delivery of health care services; sustainability of faith community nursing and the faith community nurse is addressed with suggestions for contemporary strategies that will contribute to longevity and integration of the faith community more fully into the administration of current health care services.

The benefits of this book are that it is intended for a mixed audience including faith community leaders, individuals, academic, or health care executives. By informing the reader, and in some cases challenging their mindset to integrate a more whole-person perspective of health, the benefits of faith community are explicated. The intent is to have the readers see the nurse as more than providing illness care, the faith community as more than the place that one goes to on Sunday, and health as more than physical, creating alternatives for promoting health through a deep exploration of faith community nursing.

Chicago, IL, USA   P. Ann Solari-Twadell
Brookfield, WI, USA   Deborah Jean Ziebarth

Acknowledgments

A project of this nature does not come to completion without the efforts of many individuals and organizations. The editors would like to thank both Dr. Susan Dyess and Dr. Susan Chase for their early role as coeditors for this text. Both made substantial contributions to the development of content and organization of the book. The editors would like to express their gratitude to Dr. Scott Morris, risk-taker, visionary, and key supporter of faith community nursing. He continues to lead the acceptance and modification of the *Church Health Center* in Memphis, Tennessee, to integrate the original *International Parish Nurse Resource Center*. His generosity extended to embrace all the organizational challenges and resource allocation necessary to insure the successful transition of this resource to the *Westberg Institute for Faith Community Nursing*.

Gratitude needs to be extended to faith community nurses and internationally, parish nurses, pastors, and health care executives who on a day-to-day basis work to influence people to understand health from a whole-person perspective, make lifestyle modification, and sustaining these changes over time. They create bridges for those that need access to specialized care and encourage individuals to sustain wellness at the end of life. The work of these professionals is foundational to demonstrating a whole-person understanding of health, innovation, and cost-effective and quality care for the individual, faith community, and at times the community at large.

Health care systems that have the vision of continuing to collaborate with faith communities and support the faith community nurse ministry also need to be acknowledged. Persisting to find the support and weave faith community nursing into payment mechanisms is heroic at a time when every penny is being challenged in financing ongoing care of people.

Individual acknowledgments are important to the editors. Phyllis Ann Solari-Twadell is grateful to Dr. Mary Ann McDermott for coediting three parish nursing books with her previous to this text. In addition, Ann is appreciative of all the coaching and mentoring Dr. McDermott provided to her throughout her involvement in faith community nursing. This gratitude is also extended to the Marcella Niehoff School of Nursing and the nursing faculty who support this level of scholarship. In addition, Ann is grateful for her family including her deceased husband, Stephen Twadell, who supported her through many years of school and work locally, nationally, and internationally. Also, Ann is appreciative of the continual support and understanding of her brother, Robert Solari, and his wife, Patricia; her daughter, Kim Kuhlman, and her husband, David; her stepson, Eric Twadell, and his wife, Anne; and her nephew, Joseph Solari, and his wife, Suze. The joy in life for Ann is being "Grandma" to Nathan, Clara, Stephen, and Hannah Kuhlman and Kaitlyn and Lauren Twadell as well as "Nonna" to Rowan and Vincent Solari. Each grandchild is seen as a gift from God and a blessing to enjoy.

Deborah Jean Ziebarth is thankful to her coeditor, Phyllis Ann Solari-Twadell, for her commitment and encouragement in the completion of this text. Besides being an inspirational leader in the profession of parish nursing, referred to as faith community nursing, Ann served as one of the major impetus for Deborah's completion of her PhD at the University of Wisconsin, Milwaukee. Ann served on Deborah's dissertation committee, along with her chair, Dr. Sally Lundeen.

There are many individuals along the way that have provided crucial mentoring to Deborah in her professional journey. When she was the parish nurse at Ascension Lutheran Church, Pastor Frank Janzow and Pastor Jim Bickel provided both inspirational guidance and encouragement. When she was the faith community nurse coordinator at Waukesha Memorial Hospital, Mary Lodes, as manager/director of nursing, was one of the main supporters insuring that the parish nursing program remained one of the community benefit strategies for so long. Mary also encouraged Deborah to continue on with her education. Deborah would also like to thank the team at Church Health Center for hiring her as a consultant and supporting her passion of research in faith community nursing. And finally, thank you to the Herzing University leadership, Jarvis Racine and Steve McEvoy, for seeing Deborah's potential as a leader to manage nursing programs at the Brookfield, Wisconsin Campus, as well as supporting her area of research—faith community nursing.

It goes without saying that if it was not for the love of her Lord and the support of her family, Deborah would not be where she is today. A personal thank you to Darrell Ziebarth, a loving husband, shelter, and protector, for his patience and support during the completion of this book project. Much pride and gratitude to her daughter, Kellie Knapp, and her husband, Jason Knapp; her son, Jonathan Ziebarth, and his wife, Kristin Ziebarth; and her daughter, Whitney Tang, and her husband, Gary Tang. Nothing gives Deborah more joy in life than being a "Grandma" to Micah Knapp, Sophia Knapp, Malachi Knapp, and Hezekiah Knapp and "Mimi" to Mila and Ronan Ziebarth, and Chase, Michaela, and Riley Tang.

Finally, both editors recognize those deceased leaders that have gone before them: Reverend Granger Westberg, Helen Westberg, Anne Marie Djupe, Jan Sharkey, Sheryl Cross, and other seminal leaders on whose shoulders they stand. Recognition of the early contributions of Advocate Lutheran General Hospital is also gratefully acknowledged.

Contents

Part I

Changing the Understanding of Health: Foundational Implications for Faith Community Nursing

Faith Community Nursing: A Professional Specialty Nursing Practice

1

Susan Chase and P. Ann Solari-Twadell

1.1 Faith Community as a Profession

Faith community nursing, which began as parish nursing, has evolved over the past 40 years from local groups of nurses bringing nursing care activities into a faith community setting, to the development of national meetings, a recognized curriculum, development of a scope and standards, global connections, and organizations that continue to support the further development of the practice. However, before examining the growth of faith community nursing as a recognized specialty that is part of the nursing profession, it is important to understand the significance of the designation "profession."

1.2 Characteristics of a Profession

Defining a "profession" is an evolving work that began in the 1900s with the Carnegie Foundation and a groundbreaking series of papers about professional schools. Abraham Flexner, a sociologist who was instrumental in the development of this series of papers, authored the *Flexner Report*. This report included a list of criteria that he felt were generic to any professional group (Flexner, 1915). The criteria included: (a) is basically intellectual (as opposed to physical) and is accompanied by a high degree of individual responsibility; (b) is based in a body

S. Chase (✉)
Nursing Practice Department, College of Nursing, University of Central Florida, Orlando, FL, USA

All Saints Episcopal Church, Winter Park, FL, USA
e-mail: susan.chase@ucf.edu

P. A. Solari-Twadell
Marcella Niehoff School of Nursing, Loyola University Chicago, Chicago, IL, USA
e-mail: psolari@luc.edu

© Springer Nature Switzerland AG 2020
P. A. Solari-Twadell, D. J. Ziebarth (eds.), *Faith Community Nursing*,
https://doi.org/10.1007/978-3-030-16126-2_1

of knowledge that can be learned and is developed and refined through research; (c) is practical, in addition to theoretical; (d) can be taught through a process of highly specialized professional education; (e) has a strong internal organization of members and a well-developed group consciousness; and, (f) has practitioners who are motivated by altruism (the desire to help others) and are responsible to public interests. These criteria have been benchmarks for more contemporary work on continuing to refine what it means to be a profession (Black, 2017, p. 52). Multiple health disciplines have clarified the characteristics of a profession. A White paper on pharmacy student professionalism by the American Pharmaceutical Association (2000) has recommended the following ten characteristics of a profession:

- Prolonged specialized training in a body of abstract knowledge.
- A service orientation.
- An ideology based on the original faith professed by members.
- An ethic that is binding on the practitioners.
- A body of knowledge unique to the members.
- A set of skills that forms the technique of the profession.
- A guild of those entitled to practice the profession.
- Authority granted by society in the form of licensure or certification.
- A recognized setting in which the profession is practiced.
- A theory of societal benefits derived from the ideology.

Nursing is a profession that is self-determining and recognized by society. As a professional practice, nursing has evolved over the years to bring a new focus on human health and illness and to develop and refine skills related to care of individuals, families, and communities across the health-illness spectrum and in a variety of settings (ANA, 2003). Thinking of faith community nursing as a specialty practice that is grounded in the profession of nursing, will serve to deepen the understanding of the discipline itself with its focus on the body, mind, and spirit care of human beings as they gather in communities with a wide range of health and illness concerns.

1.3   Specialization in Nursing

Specialization within the nursing profession began as early as 1880s with the development of Nurse Anesthetists. With the discovery of anesthesia techniques, it was often the nurse with special training who delivered anesthesia during procedures being conducted by surgeons. The Nurse anesthetists were followed shortly in 1891 by Public Health Nurses whose practice was developed by Lillian Wald. This was extended by the first industrial nursing service originated by Vermont Marble Company. The idea of an industrial nursing service spread quickly once the statistics gathered by the occupational health nurse documented the value and contribution of this specialty practice.

As early as 1909, nurses with specialized knowledge and skill in community-based care were in demand. They were paid for their specialty work by the Metropolitan Life Insurance Company, which had set up policies whereby the insured would receive home nursing care when needed (Hamilton, 2007). The company was motivated by two factors: recent bad publicity on deceptive practices of the insurance industry and statistical analysis that a large number of insured deaths were due to tuberculosis. In response, Lillian Wald, who had founded the Henry Street Settlement, suggested that nurses who received training in community-based nursing might be an answer to both issues (Hamilton, 2007). From the beginning, nursing specialty care was built on a unique body of knowledge and skill. Nursing specialties needed to carve out their practice territory and to find economic support for their models.

The forces that encouraged this early specialization are: the appearance of social activists who believed that the social ills of society could be ameliorated if men and women of intelligence and good will devoted themselves to correcting these ills and, the advancement in the basic sciences and technology that transformed what was known about disease and their treatment (Brodie, 1989, p. 181)

In the late 1970s and early 1980s, given the ongoing complexity of health care, the profession of nursing expanded the idea of specialization. Some specialties, including operating room nurses, infection control nurses, and school nurses, developed membership organizations. Furthermore, some of these, such as the American Association of Critical Care Nurses, developed certification programs to standardize the practice and to promote a level of care that was recognized. These efforts increased the demand for the specialty. Other practice roles developed expanded scopes of practice and responsibilities that required advanced educational degrees and certification. This expansion of the scope resulted in a designation on the nurse's license as to the responsibilities of the advanced practice nurse specialties. The advanced practice included family nurse practitioners, psychiatric nurse practitioner, and adult/gerontology clinical nurse specialists. Some have argued that to develop nursing as a profession that nursing specialties have the potential to take the focus away from the central features of the discipline, particularly if these are based in medical specialty work (Murphy & Hoeffler, 1994). However, because nursing has the responsibility for whole person health, there is room for specialization that does not align narrowly with medical specialties. Multiple terms including "specialist," "specialty nurse," "expert," and "advanced practitioner" are all terms that can cause confusion for the health care consumer (Turris, Binns, Kennedy, Finamore, & Gillrie, 2007). Faith community nurses may also need to explain the nature of their practice as a specialty to multiple audiences, including faith community leaders and members, physicians, payers, and other nurses, given the uniqueness of the practice and its setting. This chapter provides a background for these conversations.

Just as other nursing specialties developed to respond to societal need or to translate new research and technology, faith community nursing arose from a desire to promote whole person health with the focus on prevention to spiritual, physical, mental, social, occupational, and financial dimensions of individuals living in communities in order to avoid the high cost of developing preventable illness. Faith community nurses also provide expertise, guidance, and support in the spiritual care of patients. This is an area of nursing practice that is often not well developed or integral to nursing care in acute settings.

Are the conditions noted in the 1800s much different than today? Are there people, even with coverage of health care services, that are "falling through the cracks" in any health care system, not just in the U.S.A.? Could quality of life be better or improved from a whole person perspective? Would people benefit from having spiritual care more fully incorporated in their care as patients both outside and inside the hospital? Were these conditions not motivators for the development of faith community nursing as a specialty practice? At a time when there continues to be fast-paced advancement in the basic sciences and technology, faith community nursing insures that care is patient centered, whole person, individualized, prevention focused, interdisciplinary, and delivered on a continuum.

1.4   Faith Community Nursing as a Specialty Practice

Faith Community Nursing defines itself as a

> specialized practice of the profession of nursing that focuses in the intentional care of the spirit as well as the promotion of whole-person health and the prevention or minimization of illness within the context of a faith community and the wider community. A faith community nurse is a registered professional nurse who is actively licensed in a given state and who serves as a member of the staff of a faith community. The faith community nurse promotes health as wholeness of the faith community, its groups, families and individual members through the practice of nursing as defined by that state's nurse practice act in jurisdiction in which the faith community nurse practices and the documented scope and standards for this specialty practice (ANA and HMA, 2017, p. 1).

Basic to the work of the faith community nurse is to assist individuals, families, groups, faith communities, and communities at large to come to an understanding of health and illness as more than "being sick" and not only as "physical." There is no universal definition of health. It is important, if individuals are going to be more informed, more active, and involved stewards of their personal health resources that work needs to be done to help individuals to develop a personal definition of health. This definition of health includes a perspective of the whole person—spiritual, physical, mental, social, occupational, and financial. There cannot be an assumption that one person values health in the same way as another. Health is personal. Only through the individual's work of determining how they value, and define health will there be a true revolution and investment in a person making better decisions regarding health on a daily basis (Holst & Solari-Twadell, n.d., p. 5) (See Appendix A). This is some of the basic, but more difficult work of the faith community nurse.

Holst and Solari-Twadell (n.d.) speak to changing one's understanding of health, making a commitment to initiate and working at maintaining a healthier lifestyle. "We do know something about the person who will make a commitment to initiate and maintain a healthier life style. That person: Values health and well-being, genuinely believes that one's behavior can make a difference in one's health and well-being and is convinced that the benefits derived from intended health behaviors exceed the burdens of sustained efforts (p. 10)."

1.5 Looking at Health

Beginning in the late 1990s, in the U.S.A., overarching goals for the health of the country were established. This work occurred in the context of overall health outcomes for the U.S.A. ranking much lower than other industrialized nations. This has continued with the more recent health plan being set forth in *Healthy People 2020*, and work has begun for developing goals for *Healthy People 2030*. In addition to developing recommendations for reduction of death and disability due to specific disease, the Office of Disease Prevention and Health Promotion (Office of Disease Prevention and Health Promotion, n.d.) which developed Healthy People included the following objectives:

- Eliminating health disparities.
- Addressing social determinants of health.
- Improving access to quality health care.
- Strengthening public health services.
- Improving the availability and dissemination of health-related information.

Faith community nursing is consistent with the overarching goals of *Healthy People 2020*. Faith community nurses working in faith communities advocate for people to gain access to health care services; address through individual or programmatic work the aspects of health that may be socially determined; that is they include healthy eating, promoting exercise, mental health as well as supporting the health of families. They provide referrals for appropriate health care services, and coordinate with public health offices as they work in the community. They also provide health-related information in a variety of ways including health education programs, posting literature on health risk reduction and supporting individuals and families in increasing their health literacy. Faith community nurses work in collaboration with other health professionals in the faith community and community at large and strive to create environments that can assist people of all ages to develop a clearer understanding of what health means to them. This includes what interventions they can utilize, bolstered by their faith beliefs and resulting personal values, to "promote whole person health care across the life span using the skills of the professional nurse as a provider of spiritual care (ANA, 2016)."

1.6 Specialty Knowledge and Specialty Practice

Nursing specialties are based in specialty knowledge. When parish nursing first began, Reverend Granger Westberg, who at one time, had been a hospital chaplain at Augustana Hospital in Chicago, was driven to develop health services that included body, mind, and spirit to people who were outside the hospital (Westberg,

1999). In 1985, he obtained funding and secured support for a group of faith communities in the service area of the Lutheran General Hospital in Park Ridge, Illinois to participate in a pilot project placing a nurse as part of the staff of the local faith community. The nurses themselves were all registered nurses, with no specific educational background required. The knowledge and skills that these nurses would need had not yet been determined. Allowing the practice to evolve, Reverend Westberg met regularly with the nurses, hospital chaplains, and physicians responding to their suggestions for learning and enrichment. Over the years of the project, Westberg identified the following roles that parish nurses took on in developing parish nursing: Health Educator, Personal Health Counselor, Referral Agent, Integrator of Faith and Health, and Serving as a Health Advocate (Westberg, p. 38). The focus of all this work was to think of members of faith communities in a "wholistic" way using Westberg's understanding of health.

Over the years as the faith community nursing movement grew, educational workshops were offered. The Parish Nurse Resource Center was established, annual conferences were held, a curriculum for preparing new faith community nurses was developed and endorsed, and special training for faith community educators was developed and held in Chicago. These structures and activities all supported the development of the knowledge base of faith community nurses. All these developments served to build up the unique knowledge and skills of this specialty practice. Note that what started as building the knowledge of individual faith community nurses also served to expand the uniqueness of this specialty practice. Over the years this specialty became more and more based in research, as are other specialties and disciplines. As faith community nursing grew in the U.S.A., leaders were never far from remembering that modern nursing as developed and promoted by Nightingale, had its roots in a religious order in Germany, where Nightingale had studied. There are now faith community nurses practicing in many countries outside the U.S.A. Some of the interventions may be different, for example, in countries with a national health system, some of the access issues that U.S.A. faith community nurses must address with their clients are not necessary. At the core, basing health concepts in a perspective of the human as having a body, a mind, and a spirit is central to the practice. The understanding of health is from that of the whole person—spiritual, physical, mental, social, occupational, and financial.

As the numbers of faith community nurses grew, the knowledge and diversity of the practice increased, contributing to the unique knowledge and skills required to operationalize and advance this specialty nursing practice. Presentations at annual conferences shared approaches and resources that faith community nurses had developed in their local faith communities. Some of the presentations shared information and others were basic research presentations. As the knowledge base of faith community nursing grew, the information included in the preparation of the faith community nurse also matured and expanded. It became apparent over time that faith community nurses are situated to explore important areas of nursing knowledge. For example, as we know, many chronic and life-threatening health conditions can be prevented or managed in part through changing health behaviors such as exercise and transitioning to a healthy diet. It is also known that these changes do not come easily to individuals in most settings. Faith community nurses, however, are able to support people living in the community to find meaning in their health choices, to get personal support in making changes and to celebrate together when milestones are reached. Faith community nurses in most faith communities are able to work with people across the lifespan and to be present to families as they are formed, face challenges, take on responsibility for caring for elders, and ultimately, make choices about end of life care. What other nurse has the opportunity to work with such a wide range of client and family situations, engage deeply in assisting individuals and groups to discern their beliefs and values related to health across the continuum of care? The opportunities to do research through faith community nursing regarding healthy family development and support are unending.

The Nursing Social Policy Statement which addresses the profession's contract with society includes the following information which is consistent with faith community nursing:

- Humans manifest an essential unity of body, mind, and spirit.
- Human experience is contextually and culturally defined.
- Health and illness are human experiences. The presence of illness does not preclude health nor does optimal health preclude illness.
- The relationship between nurse and patient involves participation of both in the process of care.
- The interaction between the nurse and patient occurs within the context of the values and beliefs of the patient and the nurse.
- Public policy and the healthcare delivery system influence the health and well-being of society and professional nursing.
- These values and assumptions apply whether the recipient of professional nursing care is an individual, family, group, community, or population (ANA, 2003, p. 3).

Essential to the ongoing development and integration of faith community nursing into any health care system is the commitment of the faith community nurse to live out whole-person values directly in their nursing practice.

1.7   Research in Faith Community Nursing Practice Using NIC

Just as a specialty practice within the profession of nursing develops unique and specialized knowledge, there is the corresponding development of additional new nursing knowledge over time. Early research in what was then called parish nursing identified that there were not only frequently used, but also essential nursing interventions that were particular to this specialty practice. In 2001, using the Nursing Intervention Classification (NIC) 3rd Edition (McCloskey & Bulechek, 2000), Surveys (2330) were mailed as part of a larger parish nurse survey instrument to nurses that had participated in the Basic Preparation Course for Parish Nurses offered through the International Parish Nurse Resource Center. There were 1161

(54%) useable surveys returned identifying those NIC interventions that were essential and frequently used by parish nurses (Solari-Twadell, 2006, p. 19). The top ten "Essential Nursing Interventions" identified were:

1. Health Education,
2. Active Listening,
3. Spiritual Support,
4. Emotional Support,
5. Presence,
6. Spiritual Growth Facilitation,
7. Caregiver Support,
8. Grief Work Facilitation,
9. Hope Instillation,
10. Coping Enhancement.

It was recommended by the respondents in this research that "prayer," which in NIC is identified an activity, should be developed as an intervention (Solari-Twadell, 2006, p. 310).

The most frequently used interventions identified by respondents were ranked and categorized by "Used Several Times a Day/Daily," "Weekly," and/or "Monthly." There were some differences from "Several Times a Day/Daily" to "Monthly" (Solari-Twadell, 2006, pp. 23–28). The top ten "Combined Set of Interventions" most frequently used by parish nurses were identified as: (1) Learning Facilitation, (2) Learning Readiness Enhancement, (3) Active Listening, (4) Presence, (5) Touch, (6) Spiritual Support, (7) Emotional Support, (8) Spiritual Growth Facilitation, (9) Humor, and (10) Hope Instillation. The top 30 frequently used interventions employed by parish nurses identified use of interventions from six of the seven NIC Domains. The only domain not represented was "Physiologic Complex."

The value of this national research project in the U.S.A. was (1) it validated that parish nursing existed in all major religious denominations, and (2) it was active in every state in the U.S.A. In addition, the original generic functions describing what constitutes a parish nurse which was: integrator of faith and health, health educator, personal health counselor, referral agent, trainer of volunteers, developer of support groups, and health advocate was delineated to measurable interventions (Solari-Twadell, 1999, p. 3).

The ability to be able to identify the multiple interventions used and believed to be essential to the work of the parish nurse signified that this was not a simplistic specialty nursing practice, but a very complex nursing role employing interventions from six of the seven NIC Domains.

This seminal research was replicated in both the United Kingdom and Swaziland, Africa. The replication of the research was difficult to complete and make comparisons as the numbers from the original research were substantially larger than the numbers of parish nurses in both the United Kingdom and Swaziland at the time. The most substantial conclusions from this replication were that the NIC interventions employed by parish nurses in the United Kingdom were most consistent with parish nurses in the U.S.A. The most frequently used interventions by parish nurses in Swaziland were: (1) Sleep enhancement, (2) Flatulence Reduction, (3) Dying Care, (4) Teaching: Disease Process, (5) Substance Use Prevention, (6) Grief Work Facilitation, (7) Weight Gain Assistance, (8) Simple Massage, (9) Sexual Counseling, and (10) Decision Making Support. Where the interventions most frequently used in the U.S.A. were noted in the Behavioral, Health System, and Family Domains of NIC, the more frequently used interventions used by parish nurses in Swaziland were in the Physiologic Basic, Physiologic Complex, and Behavioral NIC Domains. At the time of this research in 2006, Swaziland had the highest rate of HIV/AIDS infection rate in the world with over one million people or over 40% of the population affected. The ministry of parish nursing practice in Swaziland held the beliefs that all persons are sacred and must be treated with respect and dignity and all should receive whole person care. The Swaziland parish nurses traveled miles on foot to visit their patients carrying food and resources for their patients. With most of their patients diagnosed with HIV/AIDS, these parish nurses would bathe, feed, medicate, love, and support their patients. This work was reflected in the interventions they employed and reported providing a real life reason why their interventions and the domains that these interventions represented were different than the United Kingdom and the U.S.A. (Solari-Twadell, 2011). These findings reflect the differentiation of the specialty nursing practice by culture and country while maintaining the whole person care which is a hallmark of this specialty nursing practice.

1.8 Conclusion

Professions, professionals, and professionalism must continue to evolve without losing pace with the changes in health needs, cost, payment for services, and different health systems. This means recognizing each professional's scope of practice, contribution, and adaptation to the changing health needs of society. The power to improve the current regulatory, business, and organizational conditions of health care, however, does not rest solely with nurses. Government, business, health care organizations, professional associations, and the insurance industry all must play a role. Working together, these many diverse parties can help ensure that health care systems provide seamless, affordable, quality care that is accessible to all with outcomes that demonstrate an improvement in health (Planas-Campmany, Quinto, Icart-Isern, Calvo, & Ordi, 2015, p. 58).

This chapter has introduced the concept of faith community nursing as a specialty practice within the profession of nursing. The content of the chapter reflects the development of the nursing role itself, the knowledge that is unique to the faith community nurse, the predominant nursing interventions most frequently used or understood to be essential to the specialty practice, and the importance of understanding health from a whole person perspective. Future development of the knowledge, skills, and practice of faith community nurses will occur with continued research and theory development. This specialty nursing practice will continue to contribute to the understanding of health as being based in whole person care and thus impact the future of health care delivery globally.

Appendix

Exercise 1

Personal Values Identifying What Is Important

Throughout the life you have been forming values, have actualized different values at various times in your life, and possibly changed your personal values over time. Your values formation has been influenced by your parents, teachers, friends, religious teachings as well as secular culture, beliefs, and advertising. Please take a few minutes and reflect on what some of your values are now and who or what may have influenced the formation of these values. Have your values changed over time? How have your values changed??

Values related to family
- What are my values
- Influences in the formation of those values
- Have these values changed: If so, How?

Values related to money
- What are my values
- Influences in the formation of those values
- Have these values changed: If so, How?

Values related to friends
- What are my values
- Influences in the formation of those values
- Have these values changed: If so, How?

Values related to work
- What are my values
- Influences in the formation of those values
- Have these values changed: If so, How?

Exercise 2

What Is Health????

Health is a word that has different meanings to many people. Please review the definitions of health noted below. Following the review of the following definitions, note what your personal definition of health is…

> Health is an issue of justice, of peace, of integrity, of creation and of spirituality
> —World Council of Churches (1990)

> Health is not the lack of divergent trends in our bodily or mental or spiritual life, but the power to keep them together. And healing is the act of reuniting them after the disruption of their unity.
> —Paul Tillich

Health is found in a man or woman whose living reflects a sound and liberated mind, body and spirit, freed in a healing community to have integrity, to love, and to work for good.
—Institutes of Religion and Health (1981)

Health is what we enjoy on our way to that which God is preparing for us to enjoy. It is a value and a vision word. Practically speaking health is never reached. From a faith point of view, health is an eschatological (Part of theology concerned with final destiny) idea. We seek health even as we enjoy it…it is a vision beyond the range of possibilities or failure of medicine.
—David Jenkins

Health is the absence of disease

Health is having meaning and purpose in life and living it out.

The first task in the quest of health is to understand the confusions which obscure our understanding of it. More medicine will not give us more health. Health is not something that someone else can give to someone. Health is not a human right when in fact it is a matter of personal and social responsibility.—J. C. McGilvrey

The state of being well in mind and body—Oxford Dictionary

What is your personal definition of health??????

_____
_____
_____

Exercise 3

Personal Values Related to Health: Identifying What Is Important

Please take a few minutes to reflect on these questions. Write down what your responses are to the following questions.

- What are my values related to health?
- Influences that have shaped my values related to health?
- What value related to health do I need to foster for myself?
- What health behaviors are associated with my values?
- What are the obstacles to my practicing these healthy behaviors on a regular basis?

Exercise 4

Assessing My Motivation for Change

1. Identify one behavior that if changed you believe will enhance your health and well-being.
2. How is this behavior change related to your values related to health?

3. Are there any other reasons you want to change this behavior?
4. How serious are you about making this change?
5. Are you willing to rearrange your schedule? Yes____ No ____
6. Are you willing to spend some money to accommodate this change? Yes___ No__
7. Are you willing to communicate this change to significant others in your life? Yes__ No___
8. What are the obstacles that could be I the way of making this change??

References

American Nurses Association. (2003). *Nursing's social policy statement* (2nd ed.). Silver Spring, MD: Author.

American Nurses Association (ANA). (2016). Higher education: Learning what it means to provide spiritual care. *The American Nurse*. Retrieved from http://www.theamericannurse.org/2016/11/01/higher-education/

American Nurses Association (ANA) and the Health Ministry Association (HMA). (2017). *Faith community nursing: Scope and standards*. Washington, DC: American Nurses Association.

American Pharmaceutical Association. (2000). Task force on professionalism: White paper on pharmacy student professionalism. *Journal American Pharmaceutical Association, 40*(1), 96–100.

Black, B. P. (2017). *Professional nursing: Concepts and challenges* (8th ed.). St. Louis, MO: Elsevier.

Brodie, B. (1989). A commitment to care: The development of clinical specialization in nursing. *ANNA Journal, 16*(3), 181–186.

Flexner, A. (1915). Is social work a profession? *Social Welfare History Project*. Retrieved from http://socialwelfare.library.vcu.edu/social-work/is-social-work-a-profession-1915/

Hamilton, D. (2007). The cost of caring: The Metropolitan Life Insurance Company's visiting nurse service, 1909–1953. In P. D'Antonio, E. D. Baer, S. D. Rinker, & J. Lynaugh (Eds.), *Nurses' work: Issues across time and place* (pp. 141–172). New York: Springer.

Holst, L., & Solari-Twadell, A. (n.d.). *Living life abundantly: A closer look at health values and behavior*. Park Ridge, IL: Advocate Health Care.

McCloskey, J. C., & Bulechek, G. M. (2000). *Nursing intervention classification system* (3rd ed.). St Louis, MO: Mosby.

Murphy, S. A., & Hoeffler, B. (1994). Role of the specialties in nursing science. In P. L. Chinn (Ed.), *Developing the discipline: Critical studies in nursing history and professional issues* (pp. 82–90). Gaithersburg, MD: Aspen Publications.

Office of Disease Prevention and Health Promotion. (n.d.). *History and development of health people 2020/Objective development and selection process*. Retrieved from https://www.healthypeople.gov/2020/About-Healthy-People/History-Development-Healthy-People-2020/Objective-Development-and-Selection-Process

Planas-Campmany, C., Quinto, L., Icart-Isern, M. T., Calvo, E. M., & Ordi, J. (2015). Nursing contribution to the achievement of prioritized objectives in primary health care: A cross-sectional study. *European Journal of Public Health, 26*(1), 53–59.

Solari-Twadell, P. A. (1999). The emerging practice of parish nursing. In P. A. Solari-Twadell & M. A. McDermott (Eds.), *Parish nursing: Promoting whole person health within faith communities* (pp. 3–24). Thousand Oaks, CA: Sage.

Solari-Twadell, P. A. (2006). Uncovering the intricacies of the ministry of parish nursing practice through research. In P. A. Solari-Twadell & M. A. McDermott (Eds.), *Parish nursing: Development, education and administration* (pp. 17–35). St Louis, MO: Elsevier.

Solari-Twadell, P. A. (2011). *Global perspectives on the Ministry of Parish Nursing Practice: Frequently used interventions by parish nurses in Swaziland, Africa, United Kingdom and United States.* Presented at People and Knowledge: Connecting for Global Health, Sigma Theta Tau International 41st Biennial Convention, Grapevine, TX.

Turris, S. A., Binns, D. M., Kennedy, K. J., Finamore, S., & Gillrie, C. (2007). Specialty nursing—The past, present and the future. *Journal of Emergency Nursing, 33*(5), 499–504. https://doi.org/10.1016/jen.2007.05.014

Westberg, G. (1999). A personal historical perspective on whole person health and the congregation. In P. A. Solari-Twadell & M. A. McDermott (Eds.), *Parish nursing: Promoting whole person health within faith communities* (pp. 35–41). Thousand Oaks, CA: Sage Publications.

Faith Community Nursing: As Health Ministry

2

Annette Toft Langdon and Sharon T. Hinton

2.1 Faith Community as the Center of Spiritual and Moral Development

Historically, faith communities have been found at the center of organized societies across cultures, religions, and geographical areas. Although the designs may vary, these gathering places are central to spiritual and moral development for those in attendance. Faith communities are safe places to explore beliefs, behaviors, boundaries, and life choices. Faith communities establish the sacredness of human life and the importance of whole-person-health, which is inclusive of body, mind, and spirit. Messages in the faith community provide hope, forgiveness, and healing. It is in this context that faith community nurses establish the specialty practice of faith community nursing, blending both medical and spiritual care in a manner that is compatible with the theological teachings of the faith community. The essence of the faith community nurse practice begins to inform the individuals understanding of health to be more than "not being sick."

The specialty practice of faith community nursing focuses on the intentional care of the spirit, the promotion of health from a whole person perspective, minimization of illness within the context of a faith community, or other faith-based organization (HMA and ANA, 2017). The faith community nurse practices in or with a community of faith, while integrating the faith perspective, scientific knowledge, and experiences to promote the wellness of individuals, families, and communities across generations. While this is an independent nursing role, it is operationalized in an

A. T. Langdon (✉)
Honoring Choices, Fairview Health Services, Minneapolis, MN, USA

Deacon, Evangelical Lutheran Church in America, Chicago, IL, USA

S. T. Hinton
Westberg Institute for Faith Community Nursing a Ministry of Church Health, Memphis, TN, USA
e-mail: hintons@churchhealth.org

© Springer Nature Switzerland AG 2020

17

P. A. Solari-Twadell, D. J. Ziebarth (eds.), *Faith Community Nursing*,
https://doi.org/10.1007/978-3-030-16126-2_2

interdisciplinary collaboration with clergy, staff, faith community leaders, members of the faith community, community partners, other health professionals, and institutions/agencies.

Services offered through the faith community nurse ministry are customized to match the site, beliefs, health needs, and interests of the faith community, of the larger community, as well as the skill and knowledge of the faith community nurse. Each faith community nurse brings to their role distinct gifts based on their education, experience, skills, and interests.

Although professional nursing is moving towards using nursing interventions to describe practice, early in the movement of faith community nursing the terms role and functions were frequently used. Initially, the role was conceptualized into five functions (Solari-Twadell & Westberg, 1991). Later, as more information regarding faith community nursing practice became available, the role was expanded to include seven functions (Solari-Twadell & McDermott, 1999; Jacob, 2014, p. 24) with the purpose of communicating internally to the specialty and externally regarding the practice. The initial seven basic functions of the faith community nursing role were: integrator of faith and health, personal health advisor, health educator, trainer of volunteers, developer of support groups, referral agent, and health advocate (Jacob, 2014; McDermott & Burke, 1993; Solari-Twadell & McDermott, 1999; Solari-Twadell & Westberg, 1991). As a result of seminal research on the essential and frequently used interventions, a recommendation was made to use the Nursing Intervention Classification (NIC) system to describe the faith community nursing role in order to reflect the complexity of skills and knowledge employed by the faith community nurse (Solari-Twadell & Hackbarth, 2010). In 2014, through a review of literature, the practice was also defined by six essential attributes based on what faith community nurses do (Ziebarth, 2014b). However, the simplicity of the seven functions still remains the predominant manner of describing the faith community nurse role. Thus, for this chapter, the original seven functions will be used to clarify the practice (Solari-Twadell & Westberg, 1991).

2.2 Integrator of Faith and Health

Faith community nurses integrate faith and health as they provide nursing care, always being aware of the client's faith beliefs and their own. Ongoing spiritual formation is essential for the faith community nurse's faith development. As a faith community nurse's faith matures, it encourages the nurse to not only live out personal beliefs on a day-to-day basis, but also facilitate integration of faith into nursing practice.

Faith community nurses provide spiritual care across the life span with intentionality to the role of faith and health in the life of the person being served. It is therefore important to recognize that there are developmental stages of faith. Foyer's faith development theory (1984, 1989) recognizes the underlying psychological processes that enable faith to mature. His first stage is *primal or undifferentiated faith* which emerges in the very first months of life. This is a pre-language faith based on the infant's relationship with parents. The second stage of *intuitive-projective* is in early childhood. Representations of God begin to form based on experiences with parents and other adults who are significant. In the third stage of *mythical-literal* development, the child begins to think logically and is able to discern fact from fantasy. The content of faith is formed into beliefs from a wider range of authority figures. The fourth stage of *synthetic-conventional* is when the adolescent develops interpersonal cognitions and begins to desire a personal relationship with God in which they feel loved in a deep and comprehensive way. The fifth stage of *individuative-reflective* faith development occurs in a person's early twenties, thirties, and forties when the individual assumes responsibility for their own beliefs and values. The sixth stage of *conjunctive* development occurs when the individual no longer relies on others for authority on faith values and beliefs, but has fully internalized their own faith. The seventh stage of *universalizing* is rarely attained. This individual seeks to transform the world by changing adverse social conditions from a complete identification with the perspective of God's love and justice. Assessing for faith development and being aware of these stages of faith influences the faith community nurse on appropriate spiritual interventions to choose in the care of the other.

Often integrating faith into the care of others is not obvious. Faith is personally embedded in nursing behaviors and reflected in the active listening, caring presence, spiritual support, perseverance, and ongoing engagement with the client. The mature faith of the nurse is more visible when the faith community nurse prays, shares sacred writings, and offers religious and spiritual resources or education in caring for the client.

An example of the integration of faith occurred when a faith community nurse made a home visit to an active, older member of the faith community to check her blood pressure and medication compliance. There was a conversation about family, followed by measuring blood pressure, which was within normal limits. The member shared a cup of coffee with the faith community nurse, which allowed for more conversation and storytelling. The member then asked if the faith community nurse would be open to saying a prayer for her, to which the nurse agreed. When the faith community nurse asked what the member would like included in the prayer, she had no specific request. At the close of the prayer, it was noted that the member had tears in her eyes. The member did not want to talk about those tears, but something significant had occurred during the time of prayer.

Another example of integration of faith and health occurred when a faith community nurse used a prayer of *thanksgiving* for a client moving out of her home of 40 years. The client shared how the home had been a blessing and about the difficulty of leaving this home that held so many memories. The faith community nurse created a ritual and joined the client and her family at the home. They lit a candle and the faith community nurse read scripture about God being their dwelling place from generation to generation. Together they walked through the home carrying the candle and sharing thoughts and memories as they moved from room to room. Before proceeding to the next room, they prayed, giving thanks for the gifts and memories of the room and for blessings to continue for the people who would be moving into this home. This ritual created a sense of closure and an opportunity for grieving as well as moving on for both the client and her family. The faith community nurse through this ritual facilitated recollection of significant memories, letting go of others, and beginning to look forward to a new home.

Faith community nurses may assist in a worship service, funeral, end-of-life service, or other rituals that bring meaning and comfort to others. They may participate in programming offered through the faith community such as healing services. Participation may include planning, inviting people to attend, reading scripture, or offering prayers. Being present during regular services or healing services is important as the faith community nurse is identified as part of the healing ministry of the faith community and develops relationships with those who attend and serve.

Faith community nurses develop skills that are essential to intentional care of the spirit. These skills may include spontaneous prayer, choosing scripture readings pertinent to the clients assessed problem or emotional status, and encouraging use of music to stimulate reflection, soothing the soul and relaxing the spirit. They may identify sacred writings or create meaningful rituals, while at other times meet the client's need through interventions such as listening, presence, silence, and anticipatory guidance. As faith community nurses personally address their own integration of faith and health maintenance, they model self-care for others. As they mature in their practice/ministry, their skill level in employing spiritual care tools increase. Chase-Ziolek and Iris (2002) shared that one of the benefits of practicing faith community nursing is the faith formation that occurs instinctively for the nurse.

Active listening, presence, and spiritual growth facilitation are essential nursing interventions used regularly in the practice of faith community nursing. These interventions facilitate reflection, story-telling, and problem recognition/resolution for the client. As faith community nurses are with clients, they often hear stories of disease and illness, despair and dissolution, fears and worry, guilt and shame, as well as hope and faith. The faith community nurse promotes truth telling that is the result of thoughtful reflection, which addresses health from a whole person perspective (physical, spiritual, psychosocial, behavior health, and emotional health). Questions such as what provides meaning and purpose, what is going on in the person's body, their thoughts, how they are coping, and how their spirit is impacted or impactful are all domains engaged by the faith community nurse. Faith community nurses assist others to explore where "God" is present in a situation and how personal beliefs as well as faith impacts perceptions, behaviors, and decisions. After listening, the faith community nurse may offer emotional support, spiritual support, hope instillation, coping enhancement, health education, or other resources which address wellness.

2.3 Personal Health Advisor

Faith community nurses function as a personal health advisor through the use of active listening, presence, anticipatory guidance, emotional support, spiritual support, decision-making support, coping enhancement, grief work facilitation, consultation, and health education to name a few of the nursing interventions that could be employed. The function of personal health advisor may be operationalized in conjunction with faith community educational programming, informal client conversations, or on a more personal one-to-one visit such as a blood pressure check. As the faith community nurse interacts with clients during blood pressure screening, they may ask about family, work, exercise, whether or not they have a health care directive, how they handle stress, or other areas of wellness.

An example of the health advisor function is when a regular attender at blood pressure checks talked about recent changes in his aging body and the loss of some abilities. The client reviewed parts of his life that were meaningful and he wondered how things would go in the years ahead. During the blood pressure checks, the faith community nurse not only addressed his blood pressure, medications, and lifestyle, but also supported him with interventions such as coping enhancement, age-specific education, and hope installation. These brief times together helped to develop a baseline assessment, care planning for the future, and relational trust over time.

Another example of health advisor function is when the faith community nurse visited with a client who expressed anxiety and worries about her husband, her mother, and her own health. While supporting the client through active listening, personal strength identification, spiritual support, decision-making support, self-care strategies, and referrals, the client felt empowered to take the next steps. The patient thanked the faith community nurse for listening and stated how helpful the time with the faith community nurse was and the effectiveness of the interventions employed.

The function of personal health advisor is often evident as the faith community nurse visits with clients in their home, long-term care facility, or hospital. There may be other health professionals involved in these sessions which provide an opportunity to engage the strength and expertise of an interdisciplinary team in meeting the needs of the client and/or family. "The faith community nurse collaborates … on the plan of care. As part of the health care team, the faith community nurse does not duplicate services provided by other members, but rather compliments them (Ziebarth, 2014a)." The *Faith Community Nurse and Home Health Nursing* Westberg Institute Position Statement speaks about the differences between a faith community nursing role and one of a home health nurse.

The faith community nurse has the flexibility, based on a wholistic health assessment, to visit the patient as needed to optimize wholistic health functioning. The faith community nurse may not be responding to a doctor's orders when making a home visit, but the faith community nurse engages the physician and medical home staff frequently based on assessed needs. Based on the assessment, the faith community nurse may refer the client to the physician for a clinic appointment, medication change, support services, or other services. The faith community nurse may request home health nursing services if the patient meets the criteria for the referral. In addition, the faith community nurse has the flexibility to access the faith community volunteers and services to support the patient's needs (Ziebarth, 2014a, 2014b, p. 1)

While visiting clients, a wholistic assessment is performed and a plan of care developed. The faith community nurse includes the client in developing a plan of care. As a personal health advisor, the faith community nurse may be asked to provide a plan for people seeking to adopt a healthier life style. The plan may include exercising regularly, getting adequate sleep, adequate nutrition, and reflective prayer as part of managing daily stress. The faith community nurse is often a consistent presence across the continuum of care; visiting someone at home, at the hospital or in a long-term care facility. The faith community nurse may also hear or assist in the development of a person's wishes for their end of life care.

2.4   Health Educator

As a health educator, the faith community nurse assesses the educational needs of the faith community members and often the external community. Once the assessment of learning needs is completed, the faith community nurse identifies appropriate resources and teaching strategies for informing designated target groups. Resources for educational programming can be drawn from public health sources such as *Healthy People 2020* (healthypeople2020.gov), agencies in the community, and regional resources.

In the health educator's role, healthy nutrition and weight, which is an objective from *Healthy People 2020*, is a popular topic. Events, church bulletin articles, or activities can be planned to improve healthy eating, such as developing educational programming that includes "creating a shopping list," "healthy ways to shop," "how to read nutrition labels," or "preparation of foods using less fats." Guest speakers such as licensed nutritionists from local health care organizations may be invited for one or perhaps a series of lectures and experiential learning events aimed at changing the shopping and food preparation habits of faith community members. Another important topic is exercise. An information/education table with handouts on simple every day exercises, a regular exercise group for older adults or a sign-up for a walking group can interest those that are motivated to increase or establish more regular exercise patterns.

An example of the health educator role is when the faith community nurse visited a member who lives with disabilities. The client expressed experiencing challenges when attending the faith community. These challenges were shared with a group of members who had passion for people with disabilities and had established a *Disability Awareness Committee*. Together a plan was developed to include educational events and programs to help the staff, faith community leaders, and members learn how to relate and engage people with disabilities. An experiential learning program was offered to heighten awareness. Information and education were offered for the faith community which included accessibility barriers of the building and restrooms. In collaboration with the clergy and worship leadership, a worship service was created with specific prayers, sermon, and songs that focused engaging those with disabilities and making inclusiveness a goal for the faith community.

The focus and energy of this special interest group resulted in a positive impact for the faith community. Over the course of a few years and continued advocacy, a ramp was built, automatic doors were installed, the restrooms were modified, and handicap parking was enlarged. The greater impact was that the faith community increased the support and inclusiveness of people with disabilities. The community learned that some people are "differently abled" and we all have something to share.

The activities as health educator are as varied as the needs of the faith community and sometimes the community at large. The challenge is to integrate the spiritual aspect to address whole person care.

2.5 Trainer of Volunteers

The function of training and utilizing volunteers is crucial in the development of a health ministry and to enhancing the time and effectiveness of the faith community nurse. Giving back to the community and serving others through volunteerism is at the basis of spiritual health and often an important aspect of the mission and ministry of the faith community. As more members become involved in the life of the faith community through volunteering their gifts of talent and time, they understand that God's message and "call to service" include caring for the gift of life and promoting the wellness of the whole person. The more God's people are well, the more they are able to share their gifts of love and service.

The faith community nurse can be the motivator, educator of volunteers, and the resource that helps move the entire faith community toward caring for the wellness of body, mind, and spirit. The faith community nurse often begins by encouraging the wellness of the clergy, staff, and lay-leaders. In practicing whole person health in their daily lives, the faith community nurse strives to be a role model for others on the staff and members of the faith community as a whole. Through encouraging the whole faith community to understand their role in God's healing ministry and the stewardship of personal health resources, the faith community promotes an environment of health and wholeness.

One faith community nurse developed "a ministry for busy people." The faith community nurse recruited members of the faith community for specific, time limited, volunteer experiences. These volunteer experiences did not leave the member with an ongoing time commitment that could compromise their other obligations. Yet, this short-term service created assistance to the faith community nurse, well-being for the volunteer, and engagement with the faith community.

Faith community nurses cannot practice health ministry in isolation. It takes a team. Most faith community nurses have many demands and limited hours. It can be difficult to cover the needs, whether in a small, rural, or large metro community. As the faith community nurse recruits, trains, and engages volunteers, the health ministry is multiplied. More wisdom, ideas, and energy produce creative ways to meet needs and care for people. The vitality and passion of other people bring abundant blessings through being served and by serving. Involving others creates opportunities that could not otherwise be conceived or sustained.

The most common use of volunteers by faith community nurses is through the development of a *Health Cabinet* (Westberg & McNamara, 1990) or *Health and Wellness Committee*. This committee becomes part of the organizational structure of the faith community and either works collaboratively with or under the direction of the faith community nurse. This group focuses on the promotion of wellness. Volunteers may assist in program planning, communication, recruiting others, and providing services. Some examples include planning and implementing a health fair, organizing an educational event, promoting a flu shot clinic provided by the health department, and presenting information to leadership or other established groups. The committee may also provide support and guidance for the faith community nurse; assisting with time management, prioritizing needs, making connections with people or resources in the community.

An example of collaboration between a faith community nurse and a planning committee occurred when a *Health and Wellness Committee* decided to encourage healthy eating choices by offering something besides donuts for the fellowship time. Together with the faith community nurse, they planned and implemented some changes, took the heat of "where's my donuts?" and over the course of a couple years were successful in the permanent change of offering alternative low-calorie snacks and fruit as healthier options.

Volunteers who assist with visitation or support families in crisis provide the faith community nurse with a means to expand health ministry activities. There are two types of formalized volunteer groups that often support the faith community nurse in providing on-going care. One is for listening and the other for doing. *Stephen Ministry* (stephenministries.org) or *BeFriender Ministry* (befrienderministry.org) programs train volunteers to participate in a "listening" ministry of pastoral care within the faith community. The trained volunteers learn how to actively listen without judgment, leaving room for silence and emotions. This helps the client to process their thoughts and to find their own hope and path to healing. The other group of volunteers is primarily for doing activities such as running errands, washing clothes, arranging transportation, writing cards, making calls, making meals, or providing companionship.

Both groups are dependent on the faith community nurse for education, referrals, guidance, and handling of confidential information. On-going meetings for education, inspiration, and encouragement help volunteers to maintain or grow their motivation and skills. Consistently sharing words of honest gratitude is important for these volunteers. Volunteers need to know they are valued and part of a needed, significant ministry. Regular meetings with the faith community nurse that offer time for sharing serve to deepen the trust between the faith community nurse and volunteers.

As volunteers share their gifts of time, talents, and care, they may need reminders of setting boundaries or self-care. They may also be challenged to grow in their faith as they struggle to understand God's love in the midst of suffering or tragedy. The faith community nurse can be a spiritual mentor or companion to volunteers as they learn together how to care for self and others.

2.6 Developer of Support Groups

When people are going through difficult times they may be best supported by others who know and understand because they have lived through similar experiences. The faith community nurse maintains an awareness of support group resources available in the community, offered through other faith communities or within one's own faith community. The faith community nurse might become aware of a developing need in the faith community that would be well served by the creation of a new support group. The faith community nurse may not personally know what it's like to struggle with infertility, depression, or grief and loss, but the faith community nurse can assist in finding others who do know and are willing to be a leader or co-leader in establishing a new support group. The faith community nurse may lead the support group, if that is part of their "calling" and skill-set. Or perhaps the faith community nurse will organize, market, and evaluate the progress of a new support group, recruiting others with more experience to lead or co-lead the support group. The faith community nurse may only be involved in the development of or referral to a support group.

One faith community nurse was approached after a faith community service, by a lady, who stated that she had clinical depression and wondered about starting a support group within the faith community. The faith community nurse did some research to find there were no groups available in the area, but there was a national group with resources and training to help with the development of a new support group. After conferring with the lady, the faith community nurse contacted the national group, and empowered the lady to be trained in the role of a facilitator for such a support group. The faith community nurse acted as a supportive presence for the first couple of meetings, and then stayed in contact, continuing support through listening, problem-solving, and referrals. The faith community nurse also raised awareness of depression in the faith community and greater community through education about depression and information about the group.

Support groups are created to fit a specific need. A few examples of support groups that the faith community nurse may develop, participate in, or support are: AA (Alcoholics Anonymous), AlAnon, (for friends and families of alcoholics), grief support, National Alliance on Mentally Illness (NAMI), infertility, dementia, care-givers, and spiritual support for people living with cancer. If it is not feasible to develop a support group, the faith community nurse may be instrumental in creating an informal gathering of people who have similar experiences that are willing to be mutually supportive. Support groups are another way to involve others in the ministry of health and healing.

2.7   Referral Agent and Liaison with Faith Community and Community Resources

Faith community nurses are continuous learners. They are involved in ongoing education about resources locally, regionally, and nationally. Resources may be available online, in the faith community, through the local health department, or available at community health care systems, local universities, and governmental service agencies. It is helpful for the faith community nurse to establish good working relationships with other service providers. Clarity about the faith community nurse role and availability may eliminate unrealistic expectations. Community coalitions, hospital-based community initiatives, and other community-based groups may be important connecting points for the faith community nurse. A local faith community network is an excellent source of information, support, and education for the faith community nurse.

Before referring to any resource, it is important for the faith community nurse to explore the information pertinent to that referral. Hours, providers, insurance requirements, location, and service offered are essential to know before recommending a member of the faith community to any service provider. A personal call or visit by the faith community nurse to this referring agency is important. This allows not only for the faith community nurse to get to know the provider, but also for the provider to get to know the faith community nurse. The establishment of a relationship with agencies in the community makes the faith community nurse the perfect liaison from the faith community to other sources of support for members of the faith community.

In order to properly refer to a service, requesting information and any required forms will assist in matching the service with the need. The faith community nurse may need to prepare and support the client for the referral appointment by assisting with gathering of any required documentation such as a birth certificate, pre-completing any forms, accompanying the client, and following up on the referral experience. It is important for the faith community nurse to routinely document referrals, and follow-up evaluations to assure that the requested services are being provided in a satisfactory manner.

Examples of where faith community nurses may refer to are: clinics, specialists, a counseling center, support group(s), options for senior housing, home care assistance, food pantry, clothes closet, crisis centers, hospice, or service agencies like the Area Agency on Aging. While faith community nurse confidentiality is of upmost importance while working with members of the faith community, it is also important to prevent the perception of bias by offering more than one option for referral whenever possible. This process allows the person or family requesting the referral to make the final decision.

2.8   Health Advocate

The faith community nurse is the "voice for the voiceless," especially for those who do not have caregivers or others to advocate for them. As the advocate for individuals, families, groups, and communities, the faith community nurse often educates clients on how to speak on their own behalf. However, the faith community nurse as a health professional may speak on behalf of the client, especially in the healthcare setting. Navigating any health system or resource can be complex and energy consuming. Individuals, especially the older adult, may be reluctant to ask for what they need for many reasons. There may be a lack of understanding of the diagnosis and treatment, follow-up required, or cultural norms that need to be represented. This may place medical caregivers in an authoritarian position with the client having a reluctance to disagree. The faith community nurse advocates by educating and coaching the client about what questions to ask and how to initiate a conversation.

Assisting the individual to make phone calls, requesting needed services, and accompanying the person to access services may assist in preparing that person to be a better advocate for their own personal well-being from a whole person perspective.

Advocacy includes participating at the community and organization level so that a health professional's perspective is included before decisions are made that affect the lives of others. Faith community nurses, as frontline community-based health providers, have a wealth of knowledge and experience that promotes whole person health and wellness through the advocacy role. This can be demonstrated with a wide range of opportunities. For example, one faith community nurse advocated for a member of the faith community who was experiencing difficulty discussing her end-of-life wishes with her family and physician. This experience revealed that the faith community, as a whole, had minimal knowledge of end-of-life planning. The faith community nurse advocated for an expert from a nearby hospital to offer a series of workshops. The faith community nurse also advocated for the hospital to extend hospice services into the community and as a result was asked to join the *End-of-life Coalition*, first as a member and then as a member of the Board of Directors. The faith community nurse continued to be an advocate for end-of-life education and eventually was invited to speak to the state legislature to advocate for legislation to encourage a mandated planning for end of life.

2.9 Strategies for Initiating the Practice of Faith Community Nursing

The practice of faith community nursing is a spiritual and professional "calling." At some point, a nurse becomes aware of a "call"; an inner prompting, recurring vision, or suggestion from a colleague to explore faith and nursing. Discovering faith community nursing may fulfill a desire to practice nursing in a way that is more whole person oriented with integrating faith and health. Next steps include gathering information, conducting a search of literature and websites, perhaps visiting some practicing faith community nurses in their faith communities. Conversation with clergy and faith community leaders are very important to ascertain their knowledge and interest in the development of such a ministry for the faith community.

Faith communities may also initiate the process of developing a health ministry with the possibility of having a faith community nurse. They may recognize a need or hear about health ministry, initiate gathering of information, and begin conversations with clergy, staff, leaders, and members. A faith community may start with forming a task force to study the subject and report back and/or establish a permanent committee to focus on health ministry. Over time there may be a realization that by developing a faith community program, there will be need of a health professional dedicated just to this ministry. Through the formation of a faith community nursing ministry in a congregation, the leadership and membership of the congregation are supporting a professional model of health ministry. They may consider this to be a ministry to reach out and care for the community. Ultimately, this committee serves to support and work collaboratively with the faith community nurse. It is important to recognize that faith community nursing is one form of health ministry. A *Health Ministry Committee* can offer a variety of programs through their work as a group.

The role of the clergy and the leadership of the faith community are key to the establishment and long-term sustainability of the health ministry and the position of the faith community nurse. Support and collaborative working relationships are essential for development and growth of this ministry. Education and resource allocation need to be considered. Role descriptions and understanding of responsibilities, time commitment, and accountability are also essential. Clergy and ministry leaders need to be open to share the ministry, to network and develop a positive partnership where each role dovetails with the others to provide a solid foundation for a ministry of health and wellness.

Involvement by the faith community is vital to the longevity and impact of the faith community nurse and the health ministry. Without this involvement, the ministry may generate excitement for a few people and quickly be lost if the faith community nurse or supporting leaders move or retire. With solid planning, the faith community nurse and health ministry can have a lasting impact on the understanding of health and the wellness of individuals, families, and the community as a whole.

Informing and involving the whole faith community may be done through continuous visibility and communication, by establishing a permanent place for health ministry in the organizational structure and by placing the faith community nurse position in the organizational structure regardless of their status of payment.

2.10 Visibility and Communication

It is important to introduce the faith community nurse to the faith community and to describe the role, responsibilities and functions of the faith community nurse. In addition, how the position and ministry fit into the broader mission of the faith community must be made clear to all. Often a ritual of commissioning or installation is helpful which encourages awareness and the development of trust with the faith community nurse. Some clergy may also find it important to have the faith community nurse accompany them on home visits or attend leadership meetings where there can be a clarity of responsibilities, development of trust, and encouragement of the homebound or leaders to accept and include the faith community nurse.

The visibility of a faith community nurse needs to be routine and ongoing in the faith community. Some may give a brief wellness talk during services weekly or monthly. Other faith community nurses may assist with worship in various ways or offer prayer opportunities and special healing services. Some faith community nurses may bring a wellness devotion to groups that regularly meet, like the worship and music committee or youth study. Most faith community nurses provide visibility through their presence before or after worship events when they are available for conversation, blood pressure checks, or to provide resources. Faith community publications such as websites, newsletters, and bulletins also provide communication to promote the integration of faith and health as well as add to visibility. To be visible, available, and accessible promotes trust and the success of the ministry. In the theoretic model of faith community nursing, accessible, approachable, trust, and long-term are essential elements of the core of the model (Ziebarth, 2014b).

2.11 Health Cabinet or Wellness Committee

Development of a specific committee for "health ministry" to support and promote the work of the faith community nurse is known to add longevity to the ministry. Addressing and adapting the organizational structure to accommodate the faith community nurse's position and health ministry committee gives credence through a message that this ministry is part of the whole ongoing ministry of the faith community and is not a temporary program. The *Health Ministry Committee/Cabinet* ideally has direct representation on the main council or board of authority and with that provides presence and voice to the importance of the health, healing, and wellness ministry of the faith community. This allows for greater integration of the faith community nurse/health ministry with all other areas of involvement in the faith community. For example, youth ministry or outreach events may more easily consider how the faith community nurse can support the most at-risk population in regards to health (Capuzzi & Gross, 2014; Clatts, Davis, & Sotheran, 2017; Kelly, 2006).

Westberg's model (1990) of a *Health Cabinet* has these committees of volunteers working under three aims. The first aim is to assess the overall *health* and *unhealthy* in the life of the faith community and make a plan; second, sponsor health presentations/activities in the faith community; and third, develop new health-related activities. The goal of the health cabinet is to turn the *unhealthy* around.

2.12 Staff Member

Whether the faith community nurse is paid, unpaid, and part-time or full time, their inclusion as part of the staff is essential. The presence of the faith community nurse at staff meetings invites intention, integration of the health and wellness ministry, and the practice of faith community nursing. The staff may more easily think about how they could work collaboratively with the faith community nurse. What new perspective might the faith community nurse bring to an already existing ministry? How might current ministries involve the faith community nurse and health ministry? The presence of the faith community nurse also opens the door for modeling wellness and encouraging the health and wellness of the staff. They may bring healthy treats or share a devotion of caring for the gift of health. They may also connect with staff individually to care and encourage their wellness. As they do this, the staff members further understand the role and importance of faith community nursing.

In the beginning or whenever there is a new faith community nurse, there needs to be a role orientation (Ziebarth & Miller, 2010). The faith community nurse needs to understand the organizational structure, how decisions are made, and boundaries of authority, both professional and personal within the faith community. The faith community nurse will need to know the roles of other staff or ministry leaders and what resources or supplies are available to them, such as use of a computer, printer, stamps, and paper. They may also need orientation to the faith tradition if the tradition is not their own. The faith community nurse will also need to know who will be doing their annual evaluation and by what standards will they be assessed (Ziebarth, 2006).

There are observable advantages of a paid faith community nurse. Having a paid faith community nurse may allow easier integration with the staff and ministries of the faith community, resulting in greater accountability, collaboration, and functional working relationships. One faith community nurse was unpaid for 10 years and when she transitioned to part-time paid, she said she felt she had more credibility as a leader and increased access and communications with the staff.

Some cautions about an unpaid position as a faith community nurse and the integration of that position. To build a solid health ministry in the faith community, the nurse needs to be visible and seen as part of the organizational structure. Using the phrase "unpaid" instead of "volunteer" may be helpful. "Tithing" one's salary back to the faith community may be a possibility, but leaves the future financial support for this position in question for the next faith community nurse who may need the salary. It is also important to note that some state laws prohibit the practice of volunteering additional hours in a position that is paid.

2.13   Self-Care

The health needs of the faith community and limited work hours can weigh heavy. The faith community nurse needs to maintain healthy habits to avoid burnout or compassion fatigue. Setting personal and professional boundaries early on and establishing a means of accountability will help with maintaining healthy boundaries.

Working the hours agreed upon, whether paid or unpaid, will safeguard passion and energy of the faith community nurse. It will also encourage collaboration and use of volunteers to assist or lead ministry programs. It is far easier to say "yes" than to say "no." It is very difficult to reverse course once the faith community nurse has become available 24 hours a day. It's good to be thoughtful and prayerful about saying "yes." Use the faith community nurse's position description in detailing expectations, hours, and responsibilities. Covering the nursery on Sunday morning, for example, is probably outside expected duties. Prayerfully consider requests and "listen to your gut." A faith community nurse reluctantly said "yes" to a speaking request and then went grudgingly to fulfill the request as there was little time to adequately prepare given other responsibilities of the position. From this she learned to listen to her spirit and God's leading so she could be a "cheerful giver"* and have delight in giving of her time and energy (*2 Corinthians 9:7).

Daily personal devotions or quiet time can refresh and strengthen the faith community nurse for the day. It's like driving with a full tank. Faith community nurses are no different than those they serve, all need God's love and strength for "daily bread." Paying attention to God's guidance and tending of one's heart in faith formation is important. Faith community nurses have health issues too and many times use these personal challenges as experience in caring for others. One faith community nurse struggled with grief and depression, another experienced breast cancer. Both grew in sensitivity and knowledge of practical and spiritual resources which were helpful in their care of others with similar experiences.

Self-care for spiritual growth and support can be maintained through regularly seeking the wisdom of clergy or a spiritual director or by participating in spiritual retreats. It is also helpful to join a faith community nurse network and meet regularly with others to share needs and learnings. The Westberg Institute Faith Community Nurse Knowledge Sharing Platform (www.westberginstitute.org) is an example of a free networking resource where over 1000 faith community nurses from around the world share experiences, resources, and support of each other.

An additional aspect of self-care includes lifelong learning for both nursing and spiritual care knowledge. Nursing knowledge is available through continuing education offered by mainstream nursing organizations as well as the faith community nursing specialty practice offerings through the Westberg Institute (http://www.westberginstitute.org/), Health Ministries Association (http://www.hmassoc.org/), and Faith Community Nurse International (https://www.fcninternational.org/). Spiritual care knowledge is available through faith communities, practice organizations, and other organizations such as the Spiritual Care Association (http://spiritualcareassociation.org/), schools of theology and seminaries and denominational resources. Faith community nurses also have the opportunity to take additional spiritual care courses and cross-train as chaplains through the Healthcare Chaplaincy Network (https://www.healthcarechaplaincy.org/).

Self-care also involves regular physical activity, taking time to eat well, using coping methods in reducing stress, tending to personal relationships, enjoyment of the arts, and laughter! When faith community nurses get busy (and there's always people to care for and work yet to be done), it is tempting to neglect oneself. It's good to be aware of signs or symptoms of self-neglect, such as restlessness, lack of energy, sleeplessness, irritability, and loss of creativity. As faith community nurses walk with awareness of God's presence and deep love, they will be guided in the care of self and others, making a lasting impact on health and wholeness.

2.14 Conclusion

Faith community nursing is a key to framing the meaning of health for the person over time. In working with the faith community nurse, the person can gain clarity of their personal beliefs and values related to health and how to effectively live them out supporting whole person self-care. Through engagement with a faith community that supports whole person health the individual finds a community that is engaged in similar health goals and understanding of health. The practice of faith community nursing is a gift to nurses who are "called" to serve and to those whom they serve. All faith communities can benefit from the establishment of a health ministry and the multifaceted functions of the specialty practice of faith community nursing. It cannot be overstated that the "call" to integrate faith and health is indeed a benefit to the well-being of individuals, the faith community, and the community at large.

References

American Nurses Association and Health Ministries Association. (2017). *Faith community nursing: Scope and standards of practice* (3rd ed.). Silver Spring, MD: Nursesbooks.org.

Capuzzi, D., & Gross, D. R. (Eds.). (2014). *Youth at risk: A prevention resource for counselors, teachers, and parents*. New York: Wiley.

Chase-Ziolek, M., & Iris, M. (2002). Nurses perspectives on the distinctive aspects of providing nursing care in a congregational setting. *Journal of Community Health Nursing, 19*(3), 173–186.

Clatts, M. C., Davis, W. R., & Sotheran, J. L. (2017). Correlates and distribution of HTV risk behaviors among homeless youths in New York City: Implications for prevention and policy. In G. Anderson, C. Ryan, S. Taylor-Brown, & M. White-Gray (Eds.), *Children and HIV/AIDS* (pp. 103–116). New York: Routledge.

Fowler, J. W. (1984). *Becoming adult, becoming Christian: Adult development and Christian faith*. New York: HarperCollins.

Fowler, J. W. (1989). *Faith development in early childhood*. Lanham, MD: Rowman & Littlefield.

Jacob, S. (Ed.). (2014). *Foundations of faith community nursing* (3rd ed.). Memphis, TN: Church Health Center.

Kelly, P. (2006). The entrepreneurial self and 'youth at-risk': Exploring the horizons of identity in the twenty-first century. *Journal of Youth Studies, 9*(1), 17–32.

McDermott, M. A., & Burke, J. (1993). When the population is a congregation: The emerging role of the parish nurse. *Journal of Community Health Nursing, 10*(3), 179–190.

Solari-Twadell, A., & Westberg, G. (1991). Body, mind, and soul. *Health Progress, 72*, 24–28.

Solari-Twadell, P. A., & Hackbarth, D. P. (2010). Evidence for a new paradigm of the ministry of parish nursing practice using the nursing intervention classification system. *Nursing Outlook, 58*(2), 69–75.

Solari-Twadell, P. A., & McDermott, M. A. (Eds.). (1999). *Parish nursing: Promoting whole person health within faith communities*. Thousand Oaks, CA: Sage.

Westberg, G. E., & McNamara, J. W. (1990). *The parish nurse: Providing a minister of health for your congregation*. Minneapolis, MN: Augsburg Books.

Ziebarth, D. (2006). Policies and procedures for the ministry of parish nursing practice. In P. A. Solari-Twadell & M. A. McDermott (Eds.), *Parish nursing: Development, education, and administration*. St. Louis, MO: Elsevier Health Sciences.

Ziebarth, D. (2014a). *Faith community nursing and home health nursing*. Westberg Institute Position Statement.

Ziebarth, D. (2014b). Evolutionary conceptual analysis: Faith community nursing. *Journal of Religion and Health, 53*(6), 1817–1835.

Ziebarth, D., & Miller, C. (2010). Exploring parish nurses' perceptions of parish nurse training. *Journal of Continuing Education in Nursing, 41*(6), 273–280.

Faith Community Nursing: A *Wholistic* and *Holistic* Nursing Practice

3

Deborah Jean Ziebarth and P. Ann Solari-Twadell

3.1 Wholistic or Holistic?

Historically, *wholistic* and *holistic* have often created confusion in the minds of practitioners and consumers. What does each term represent? Is there a difference in philosophy and application? Is one term more in sync with faith community nursing than the other? Westberg was often frustrated himself when errors were made in describing the Wholistic Health Centers he developed in faith communities. They were described as *holistic* instead of *wholistic*. In an article, he apologized to the public because writers were using the term *holistic* in describing the work that he was leading. In Granger Westberg Verbatim: *A Vision for Faith and Health* (Peterson, 1982). Westberg writes, "There is great ferment on the West Coast around the general subject of *holistic* medicine. Recently, some 3000 people attended a two-day conference there on holistic medicine, but I sense that they are really not talking about the same thing as we are. They show great enthusiasm for what we might consider "far out kinds of health care". I salute them for their willingness to test new ways to get to the cause and cure of illness. However, a number of people are confused by the similarity of our names. I have tried very hard to keep our project within the fold of traditional American medicine and religion. I have regularly conferred with officers or staff at the American Medical Association, the Association of American Medical Colleges, and bishops and officers of mainline Christian churches. They have all encouraged our innovative programs as long as we keep within reasonable limits" (p. 43). Westberg saw the work of the *Wholistic Health Centers* as separate and distinct from the frequently used term, *holistic* health.

D. J. Ziebarth (✉)
Department of Nursing Program Chair, Herzing University, Brookfield, WI, USA
e-mail: dziebarth@herzing.edu

P. A. Solari-Twadell
Marcella Niehoff School of Nursing, Loyola University Chicago, Chicago, IL, USA
e-mail: psolari@luc.edu

© Springer Nature Switzerland AG 2020
P. A. Solari-Twadell, D. J. Ziebarth (eds.), *Faith Community Nursing*,
https://doi.org/10.1007/978-3-030-16126-2_3

For the purposes of this chapter, a table is used to provide the reader with a comparison between these two terms (Table 3.1 in Appendix). The terms w*holistic* and *holistic* are reviewed in light of the following 12 key categories: (1) Origins; (2) Underpinnings; (3) Delivery of Care; (4) Definitions; (5) Significant Works; (6), Specialty Organizations; (7) Certification; (8) Scope of Practice and Standards; (9) Ongoing Education; (10) Ongoing Research; (11) Use by Faith Community Nurses, and (12) Medical Subject Headings (MeSH) term.

3.2 Origins

Both terms *wholistic* and *holistic* have similar beginnings as far back as the fourth century B.C. as both the works of Socrates and Hippocrates stress the whole person. *Holistic* also holds the work of Florence Nightingale to be foundational. Nightingale, known widely, as the founder of modern nursing, wrote of the "benevolent nature of God and universal law" (Calabria & Macrae, 1994, p. xxviii). She believed that Christianity provided a "moral framework for life" (p. xxix). However, Nightingale also noted that "the perfect God expresses Himself through universal laws" (p. 18). Nightingale was highly critical of the Church of England. She also had a fascination with the Roman Catholic Church, but was also well read and knowledgeable in philosophy and current day philosophical thinking.

In the Scope and Standards of Parish Nursing (American Nurses Association/Health Ministry Association, 1998), the term *wholistic* health care is described as an integrated approach to caring for the whole person including the spiritual aspects of care. It states, "The principles of *wholistic* health care arose from the understanding that human beings strive for wholeness in their relationship with God or higher power, themselves, their families, the society, and the environment in which they live" (p. 2).

In exploring both of the terms *wholistic* and *holistic*, there is a clarity regarding health as being more than physical, which is compatible with faith community nursing. However, there are clear differences in how that understanding of health is applied and practiced with each term. It is important for faith community nurses to understand what is different between the two terms and their application. In addition, if the nurse is intending to practice with a *holistic* understanding, does she/he have the education and preparation to practice according to the *Holistic Nursing: Scope and Standards of Practice* (AHNA and ANA, 2013). It is also important to determine what terminology is consistent with the manner in which the faith community nurse is interested in working with clients and how the application of whole person health will be actualized in practice.

In faith community nursing, the descriptor *wholistic* is used often in describing health or interventions delivered by the nurse (Bard, 2006; Brudenell, 2003; Burkhart & Androwich, 2004; Burkhart, Konicek, Moorhead, & Androwich, 2005; Burkhart & Solari-Twadell, 2001; Chase-Ziolek & Iris, 2002; Chase-Ziolek & Striepe, 1999; Farrell & Rigney, 2005; Hinton, 2009; King & Tessaro, 2009; Koenig, 2008; McGinnis & Zoske, 2008; O'Brien, 2003; Rethemeyer & Wehling, 2004; Rydholm, 1997; Scott & Summer, 1993; Solari-Twadell & Hackbarth, 2010;

Solari-Twadell & Westberg, 1991; Tuck, Pullen, & Wallace, 2001; Tuck & Wallace, 2000; Tuck, Wallace, & Pullen, 2001; Van Loon, 1998; Wallace, Tuck, Boland, & Witucki, 2002; Ziebarth, 2014, 2015a; Ziebarth & Miller, 2010). The term was generated through the early works of Rev. Granger Westberg (1961, 1979, 1986, 1990).

3.3   Underpinnings: Wholistic

The use of the descriptor *wholistic* has a history going back to the roots of the practice of faith community nursing. The precursor to faith community nursing is Westberg's work with *Wholistic Health Centers*. *Wholistic Health Centers* were family practice medical care facilities that were housed within faith communities. They utilized an interdisciplinary team of physicians, pastoral counselors, and nurses, who focused on all dimension of an individual's health care needs (Westberg, 1986, 1990, 2015). The *Wholistic Health Centers* were said to deliver humanistic medicine or *wholistic* medicine (Cunningham, 1974). Jane Westberg (Westberg's daughter) writes in her book *Gentle Rebel: The Life and Work of Granger Westberg* (2015) that the *Wholistic Health Center* model "took into account the whole person in providing personalized care, which was comprehensive in nature and embraced the notion of self-responsibility, health promotion, and health education and emphasized preventative medicine" (p. 199). Westberg's definition of wholistic *health care* is found in Table 3.1 in Appendix.

The theological assumptions of *wholistic health care* are identified in the book *Theological Roots of Wholistic Health Care: A Response to the Religious Questions that Have Been Raised* (Westberg, 1979). This book was written with the *Wholistic Health Centers* in mind. The assumptions answer the what and why of *wholistic health care* delivery. Abbreviated content related to "Theological Assumptions" is noted as "Underpinnings" in Table 3.1 in Appendix. The following expands the understanding of the content noted in Table 3.1 in Appendix under "underpinnings":

1. Place Matters. A building and its physical arrangement have symbolic value for all that use it. Health care delivered in a faith community symbolizes: (a) the penultimate nature of healing, (b) the need for *wholistic* health care inclusive of the spiritual realms, as well as physical and mental care, (c) the presence of God as the ultimate source of healing, (d) the kind of compassion and sacrificial concern for people that is so characteristic of the life and ministry of Jesus Christ, and (e) the congregation with a mission and mandate to heal (pp. 33–36).
2. The Nature of Persons. The nature and destiny of man begin and end with God. The value that of each person is derived from the value, which God bestows upon persons, and is not dependent upon productivity or usefulness. Each person is a unity of body, mind, spirit, and soul and is responsible for their own health, for other persons, and the world (p. 38).
3. Sickness and Health. The brokenness and disintegration which penetrates every level of life are all aspects of the same sickness. A person can be sick mentally, emotionally, and spiritually. Sickness can either be constructive or destructive. Sickness leads to death.

4. Health and salvation are twin expressions of a wholeness, which has its source in God. Healing can be broadly defined as constructive forces, which are at work at each level of an individual's life, within human relationships. All healing is inseparable related to and dependent upon the cross and the resurrection of Christ (pp. 40–44).
5. Healing Agents. An agent is one that has the power to affect change. The job of healing calls for a multidisciplinary team. Different professional providers bring special expertise. The focus of responsibility for health must be kept with the patient as the healing agent. Every person is a healing agent. The primary healing agent is God. Healing agents discover a unity in the service of Christ (pp. 45–47).

3.4   Delivery of Care: Wholistic

There were two interventions that were practiced in the *Wholistic Health Centers*: (1) an *Initial Health Planning Conference* and (2) programming developed in response to the "Five Needs of the Health Care Delivery System" (Tubesing, Holinger, Westberg, & Lighter, 1977). The inventory was used to guide the *Initial Health Planning Conference* (IHPC) to teach patients to focus on the wholeness of his/her health rather than just the diagnosis and assessment. The three underlying assumptions for the IHPC inventory's use were that: (1) stress is a causal factor in disease; (2) identifying both needs and resources is in itself therapeutic for the patient; and (3) the process of identifying recent life stresses teaches the patient a method for analyzing his/her personal disease in the future. Tubesing et al. (1977), describe the IHPC: This content is noted as "Delivery of Care" on Table 3.1 in Appendix.

The detailed description of the *Wholistic Health Care Centers* developed by Westberg is important as it explained the early use of the term *wholistic*. Parish nursing, now known as faith community nursing, was piloted in Arizona when Pastor Kettle from *"Our Savior's Lutheran Church"* asked if their small church could just try to place a nurse in their faith community rather than a team of providers. Westberg was in support and defined four main roles of the nurse. This nurse working in the faith community was considered to be: (a) health educator for the faith community and community, (b) personal health counselor, (c) facilitator and teacher of volunteers, and (d) a liaison person as well as an organizer of support groups. It was expected that the nurse would integrate faith into all expects of the role. Westberg stated that his goal was to "…place one nurse in every church as a minister of health on the parish staff" (p. 230). Thus, the term parish nurse was born to describe the nurse practicing *wholistic health care*.

Solari-Twadell and McDermott (1999) shared the philosophical principles of parish nursing in their second textbook titled: *Parish Nursing: Promoting Whole Person Health within Faith Communities*. The four philosophical principles of parish nursing mirrored the work of the nurses in the *Wholistic Health Care Centers*. They are:

1. The spiritual dimension is central to the practice and encompasses the physical, psychological, and social dimensions of nursing practice.

2. The parish nurse balances knowledge with skill, the sciences with theology and humanities, service with worship, and nursing care functions with pastoral care functions.
3. The focus of the practice is the faith community and its ministry. The parish nurse, in collaboration with pastoral staff and members, participates in the ongoing transformation of the faith community into a setting of healing. Through partnership with other community health resources, fosters new and creative responses to health concerns. Parish nursing interventions are designed to build on and strengthen the capacities of the individual(s), to understand and care for one another in the light of their relationship to God, faith traditions, themselves, and the broader community. The practice holds that all persons are sacred and must be treated with respect and dignity. In response to this belief, the parish nurse assists and empowers individuals to become more active partners in the management of their personal health resources.
4. The parish nurse understands health to be a dynamic process that embodies the spiritual, psychological, physical, and social dimensions of the person. Spiritual health is central to well-being and influences a person's entire being. Therefore, a sense of well-being and illness may occur simultaneously. Healing may occur in the absence of cure (Ryan et al., 1994, cited in Solari-Twadell, 1999).

These principles were developed by the Philosophy Work Group at the First Invitational Educational Colloquium held in Mundelein, Illinois in June 1994. The members of this work group were Dr. Judith Ryan, Ruth Berry, Janet Griffin, and Dr. Jean Reeves (Solari-Twadell, 1999, pp. 15–16). This work was ultimately endorsed by all participants of the colloquium.

Wordsworth (2015) in her book, *Rediscovering a Ministry of Health*, states that "…in the last of these principles, cure is understood as complete absence of the physical or mental disease, whereas healing is seen as a *wholistic* and dynamic concept that may bring remission of symptoms and shalom but not necessarily cure" (p. 22). There is a general understanding around the world that parish nurses predominantly provide *wholistic health care.*

In the Scope and Standards of Parish Nursing (American Nurses Association/ Health Ministry Association [ANA/HMA], 1998), the term *wholistic health care* is described as an integrated approach to caring for the whole person including the spiritual aspects of care. It states, "The principles of *wholistic* health care arose from the understanding that human beings strive for wholeness in their relationship with God or higher power, themselves, their families, the society, and the environment in which they live" (p. 2).

3.5 Recent Exploration of Wholistic Health Care

In a recent analysis of *wholistic health care*, Ziebarth (2016) used the Rodgers' Evolutionary Method of discovery to identify antecedents, attributes, and consequences of *wholistic* as a descriptor of health care. A total of 63 sources of literature in the realms of literature included Medical (6), Psychosocial (4), Spiritual (9), and Nursing (29) (21 parish/faith community nursing) was used. Additionally, 15 books were used. The definition of *Wholistic* Care was developed and can be found in Table 3.1 in Appendix. The following definitions were also created through this exploration providing more clarification of related terms:

- *Wholistic* Health: *Wholistic* health is the human experience of optimal harmony, balance, and function of the interconnected and interdependent unity of the spiritual, physical, mental, and social dimensions. The quality of wholistic health is influenced by human development at a given age and an individual's genetic endowments, which operate in and through one's environments, experiences, and relationships (p. 1820).
- *Wholistic* Health Care: *Wholistic* health care is the assessment, diagnosis, treatment, and prevention of *wholistic* illness in human beings to maintain *wholistic* health or enhance *wholistic* healing. Identified *wholistic* health needs are addressed simultaneously by one or a team of allied health professionals in the provision of primary care, secondary care, and tertiary care. *Wholistic* health care is patient centered and considers the totality of the person (e.g., human development at a given age, genetic endowments, disease processes, environment, culture, experiences, relationships, communication, assets, attitudes, beliefs, and lifestyle behaviors). Patient centered refers to the patient as active participant in deciding the course of care. Essential attributes of *wholistic* health care are faith integrating, health promoting, disease managing, coordinating, empowering, and accessing health care. *Wholistic* health care may occur in collaboration with a faith-based organization to mobilize volunteers to support and promote individual, family, and community health (p. 1820).
- *Wholistic* Illness: *Wholistic* illness is the human experience of declining harmony, balance, and/or function of the interconnected and interdependent unity of the spiritual, physical, mental, and social dimensions. *Wholistic* illness occurring in one dimension impacts other dimensions. Severity of *wholistic* illness is influenced by human development at a given age and an individual's genetic endowments, which operate in and through one's environments, experiences, and relationships (p. 1820).
- *Wholistic* Healing: *Wholistic* healing is the human experience of movement toward optimal harmony, balance, and function of the interconnected and interdependent unity of spiritual, physical, mental, and social dimensions. *Wholistic* healing occurring in one dimension impacts other dimensions. *Wholistic* healing is influenced by human development at a given age and an individual's genetic endowments, which operate in and through one's environments, experiences, and relationships (p. 1820).
- *Wholistic* Health Care Provider(s): *Wholistic* health care providers are knowledgeable and skillful in the essential attributes (i.e., faith integrating, health promoting, disease managing, coordinating, empowering, and accessing health care). They possess personal character traits that allow them to deliver ethically sound, unbiased care. They are attentive, responsive, and intentional in providing

services that encompasses the interconnected and interdependent unity of spiritual, physical, mental, and social dimensions of every patient. The relationship to the patient (i.e., person, family, or community) is of central importance. They are accessible, approachable, available, and accountable to patients. They are mindful of self, patient, and context in the provision of care (p. 1821).

- Patient: A patient is an interconnected and interdependent unity of spiritual, physical, mental, and social dimensions. The quality of the unity is influenced by human development at a given age and genetic endowments, which operate in and through one's environments, experiences, and relationships (p. 1821).
- Consequence of *Wholistic* Health Care: Consequences of *wholistic* health care is the maintenance of *wholistic* health or the enhancement of *wholistic* healing (p. 1821).

Just like the practice of faith community nursing, the evolution of *wholistic* as a descriptor of health care is not static, and it will continue to change. This work may be beneficial to study the effectiveness of *wholistic health care* and to create a conceptual model-based application for practice.

3.6 Underpinnings: Holistic

The specialty practice of *holistic* nursing identifies five core values. These core values are listed in Table 3.1 in the Appendix. The following will expand on the understanding of these five core values.

3.7 Core Values

3.7.1 Core Value One: Holistic Philosophy, Theory, and Ethics

Holistic nursing employs various nursing theories in addition to other theories that represent perspectives of wholeness and healing. Some of these theories include: Theory of Consciousness, Systems Theory, complexity science, Chaos Theory, Energy Field Theory, C. Pibram's Holographic Universe, D. Bohm's Implicit/Explicate Order, Psychoneuroimmunology, K. Weber's Integral Theory of consciousness, Spirituality, Alternative Medical Systems such as Traditional Oriental Medicine, Ayurveda, Native American, indigenous healing, Eastern Contemplative orientation such as Zen Buddhism and Taoism (Mariano, 2016, p. 60). *Holism* supports that all things are connected, under-girded by human ethics and dignity through use of the *Patient's Bill of Rights*.

3.7.2 Core Value Two: Holistic Caring Process

Holistic nurses encourage the implementation of interventions that will result in healing, peace, comfort, and a subjective sense of well-being for the person. Different modalities may be employed with the client such as cognitive restructuring, stress management, visualization, aromatherapy, and therapeutic touch (Mariano, 2016, p. 63). In addition to different modalities of caring, there are different credentials that a *holistic* nurse may obtain through completion of a certification process. The levels of certification that are available through the *American Holistic Nurses Credentialing Corporation* (AHNCC) advance "*Holistic* Nursing" and "Nurse Coaching." The certification examinations are accredited by the Accreditation Board for Specialty Nursing Certification [ABSNC] and are recognized by the American Nurses Credentialing Center [ANCC] Magnet Program. The six certification credentials that are currently in use are:

- Holistic Nurse-Board Certified (HN-BC).
- Holistic Nurse Baccalaureate-Board Certified (HNB-BC).
- Advanced Holistic Nurse-Board Certified (AHN-BC).
- Advanced Practice Holistic Nurse-Board Certified (APHN-BC).
- Nurse Coach-Board Certified (NC-BC).
- Health and Wellness Nurse Coach-Board Certified (HWNC-BC)" (AHNA, 2018).

3.7.3 Core Value Three: Holistic Communication, Therapeutic Healing Environment, and Cultural Diversity

Holistic nursing holds that the nurse has an obligation to create a therapeutic healing environment. The nurse is seen as "the healing environment and as an instrument of healing," while the human spirit is understood as a major force in the healing of the person. *Holistic* communication is a vehicle for assisting the person to find meaning in their experience. Significant to the nurse is always to be authentic, caring, compassionate, and sincere using reflective listening in working with another. The *holistic* nurse recognizes that the understanding of health and healing is bound in the culture of the other. The nurse always values the understanding of the person which is often reflected in the person's culture.

The larger environment is in the forefront of the *holistic* nurse's mind. The nurse recognizes the significance of environmental issues as integral to the creation of stressors with an effect not only on the person's well-being, but the plant itself.

3.7.4 Core Value Four: Holistic Education and Research

Holistic education and guidance of individuals and families through the process of making health care decisions especially with the use of allopathic and complementary/alternative practices is inherent in the practice of *holistic* nursing. Important to the ongoing development of this specialty practice, *holistic* nurses conduct and evaluate research. The focus of the research in *holistic* nursing can include studies on *holistic* therapies such as therapeutic touch, prayer, and aromatherapy. In addition, instrument development that can measure caring behaviors, cultural competence, or client's responses to *holistic* interventions is also predominant. The *American Association of Holistic Nurses* has an active research agenda for the specialty practice with the goal of documenting and advancing the specialty (Mariano, 2016, p. 66).

3.7.5   Core Value Five: Holistic Nurse Self-Reflection and Self-Care

Baseline to the practice of *holistic* nursing is self-care. The holistic nurse engages in self-assessment seeking harmony, peace, and balance in their own personal life so that they are in a better position to assist another is doing the same. Self-reflection is a key to this personal self-care process. In order to be a role model for others, the *holistic* nurse employs personal awareness including knowledge of one's own values, feelings, perceptions, and judgments. This includes creating a personal healing environment which supports self-healing and ongoing use of yoga, good nutrition, energy therapies, and lifelong learning (Mariano, 2016, p. 66).

3.8   Delivery of Care: Holistic Nursing

Holistic nursing is used to define patient centered care in which the nursing focus is on the patient as a unified whole being (Cordeau, 2010). The "active practice of *holistic* nursing is defined as all nursing practice that cares for the person as an integrated, *holistic* human being, inseparable and integral with the environment and employs an iterative and integrative process that involves six steps (Table 3.1 in Appendix). *Holistic* practice draws on holistic nursing knowledge, theories, expertise, and intuition to guide nurses in becoming therapeutic partners with clients in a mutually evolving process toward healing and holism. *Holistic* nursing is universal in nature and may be practiced in any clinical setting, community, private practice, hospital, educational institution or research foundation" (AHNA, 2018). The view of holism is not focused as much on what a provider does, but more as a philosophy or attitude as well as a way of living life which includes integration of self-care, self-responsibility, spirituality, and inclusion of reflection in everyday life. The inclusion of the practice of reflection is intended to support greater awareness of the interconnectedness of self with others, nature and spirit, as well as the relationship with the global community (AHNA, 2018). *Holistic* nursing is intended to address not only the manner in which care of the person is perceived-mind, body spirit, but also how the caregiver perceives care of self, environment, and the world.

The practice of *holistic* nursing upholds the belief that individuals seek healing from health professionals; however, the individuals carry the healing with them. The intervention of presence has a very significant place in the education of the *holistic* nurse. The use of presence within the practice of *holistic* nursing is a skill that nurses work to develop through ongoing education, breathing and relaxation, reflection, self-understanding, and practice. Through working with a client with this level of insight *holistic* nursing is believed to create an environment for the client that supports the client's ability to use their energy to facilitate their personal healing. Care delivery within *holism* is defined as being both patient centered and person centered.

3.9 Synopsis (Table 3.1 in Appendix)

The terms *wholistic* and *holistic* are defined as part of Table 3.1 in the Appendix. These terms are often used in describing patient care. However, the essence of the definitions as pertaining to *holism* is more detailed specifying principles and values that are integral to the theories and beliefs related to this specialty nursing practice. The definition for *holism* notes the significance of interconnectedness and use of alternative and complementary therapies.

It is difficult to address the term *holistic* without acknowledging the professional societies dedicated to this purpose. They are the *American Holistic Health Association*, the *American Holistic Medical Association*, and the *American Holistic Nurses Association*. For the purposes of this chapter the *American Holistic Nurses Association* is the primary focus. This professional nursing organization was founded in January 17, 1981 in Houston, Texas with 33 nurses from eight states in attendance. It took over 20 years for this unique practice to be acknowledged as a specialty nursing practice in December 2006. This specialty nursing organization is dedicated to continual development of a distinct body of knowledge that continues to be refined through research and which guides this nursing practice. The current mission of this specialty nursing organization is to "illuminate holism in nursing practice, community, advocacy, research and education." The vision statement of the organization is that "every nurse be a holistic nurse" (AHNA, 2018).

3.10 Significant Works

Important written works support both *wholistic* and *holistic terms* and are noted in Table 3.1 in appendix. Except for the recent evolutionary concept analysis (Ziebarth, 2015a, 2015b), there is little to advance the understanding, application, or integration of the term *wholistic*. The term *wholistic* was not used to describe a specialty nursing practice. Whereas, historically, the *American Association of Holistic Nurses* with over 5000 members, multiple chapters, several levels of certification, and a Scope and Standards of Nursing Practice continues to advance the understanding, practice, and research on the term *holistic* for the profession of nursing.

3.11 Specialty Nursing Organization

As noted previously, there is no specialty organization, nursing dedicated to the advancement in the understanding and application of the term *wholistic*. Faith community nurses will use the term given the affiliation with Reverend Granger

Westberg and the *Wholistic Health Centers*, but the specialty practice of faith community nursing is not dedicated to the advancement of this term. The *American Holistic Nurses Association,* along with the *American Holistic Health Association* and the *American Holistic Medical Association*, support regular press releases and position papers that support the ongoing integration and advancement of the term *holism*. Examples of position papers published by the *American Holistic Nurses Association* are:

- Position on the Role of Nurses in the Practice of Complementary & Integrative Health Approaches (CIHA) .
- White Paper on Holistic Nursing Research.

This membership organization also sponsors a regularly published professional journal—*Journal of Holistic Nursing* along with press releases to keep membership updated and informed of best practices and current information. There is no such membership structure supporting the use of *wholistic* nursing practice.

3.12   Certification, Scope of Nursing Practice, Ongoing Education, and Research

As described earlier, with no specialty organization or special interested group supporting the continuous, in-depth exploration of the use, application, and outcomes of the use of the term *wholistic*, the word remains an occasionally used descriptor. There is no scope of practice ongoing education and little research that defines the integration and application of this term. Both "*holistic* care"(p. 88) and "*wholistic*" (p. 90) are defined in the *Faith Community Nursing (3rd Ed) Scope and Standards* (2017).

3.13   Medical Subject Heading: MeSh Term

Wholistic is not a recognized descriptor. Whenever the word is entered into the computer as text, it is immediately identified as a spelling error and corrects to the word *holistic*. This is because the term *wholistic* is not a recognized descriptor in standard dictionaries or the National Library of Medicine's controlled vocabulary thesaurus (MeSH). There are 27,883 descriptors in the 2016 MeSH with over 87,000 entry terms that assist in finding the most appropriate MeSH descriptor. An effort is underway through the Westberg Institute (formerly the International Parish Nurse Resource Center for faith community nursing) to add the descriptor *wholistic* to the MeSH list. Because of this current and frequent inconvenience, many faith community nursing authors and researchers have confessed to using the MeSH corrected descriptor, *holistic* (Ziebarth, 2016).

3.14 Implications and Conclusion

This is a brief insight into the use of the terms *wholistic* and *holistic* as it pertains to nursing practice today. A faith community nurse may be a member of the *American Association of Holistic Nurses*, complete one or all six of the certifications offered through this specialty nursing organization, and employ the skills developed through ongoing education to care for the clients served, or a faith community nurse may not belong to the *American Association of Holistic Nurses*, but holds the beliefs and philosophy at the basis of this specialty practice as significant to their own faith community nursing practice. *Holistic* nursing practice can be consistent with the practice of faith community nursing. However, specialized education and preparation are needed to practice holism as defined by this specialty nursing organization.

What is important in choosing to use the term *wholistic or holistic* is not so much which term is used, but how and why one term is chosen over the other. Use of the term "whole person" may be the clearest description which does not carry with it any particular philosophical or practice prescription except to acknowledge that people are more than physical beings.

So what is important for a faith community nurse to discern regarding their nursing practice? It is important to be clear what your personal philosophy of nursing care is, what do you believe to be at the heart of nursing practice for you? What is your personal mission statement? What are your professional beliefs and values as a nurse? How do these beliefs transfer to one's personal life? What skills do you believe are consistent with the way you would like to practice faith community nursing? How are you going to develop yourself as a faith community nurse? What ongoing educational opportunities will you seek to develop and improve your nursing skills in providing whole person care? What spiritual direction, mentoring, or coaching will you seek to insure that you have the necessary support to achieve excellence in faith community nursing practice?

One's personal philosophy, faith, beliefs, values, and experience will assist in identifying a personal nursing practice philosophy. The nurses' personal beliefs and values regarding one's individual nursing practice will provide the personal underpinnings to discern clearly how to deliver whole person care. This is a process that each faith community nurse must reflect upon as it will provide guidance for ongoing personal and professional development. The terminology that is used in describing faith community nursing is personal, distinct, and inherent in how each faith community nurse defines their beliefs, values, and professional nursing practice.

The bottom line is that whether you choose to use the expression *wholistic or holistic,* the choice should reflect the faith community nurse's personal philosophy and philosophy of nursing practice as well as the beliefs and values related to faith community nursing practice. The choice is for each to make, what is important is that there is a clear understanding what each faith community nurse is communicating about themselves, their beliefs, and the manner in which you chose to practice faith community nursing. Whether it is *holistic, wholistic,* or whole person, one thing is clear. Faith community nursing is about changing the understanding of health to include the care of the whole person.

Appendix

Table 3.1 Comparison of Wholism and Holism

Spelling	Wholistic	Holistic
1. Origins	Socrates (fourth century B.C.) stressed the importance of looking at the whole in healing a part Granger Westberg—Wholistic Health Centers and Parish Nursing Parish Nurse Literature	Socrates (fourth century B.C.) stated, "Curing the soul that is the first thing." In holism, symptoms are believed to be an expression of the body's wisdom as it reacts to curing its own disease Hippocrates, the father of Western Medicine, espoused a holistic orientation teaching doctors to observe their patients' life circumstances and emotional states Florence Nightingale who believed in care that focused on unity, wellness, and the interrelationship of human beings, events, and environments (Dossey, 2016, p. 57)
2. Underpinnings	1. Place matters: A faith community has a symbolic value 2. The nature and destiny of a person begins and ends with God 3. Health—Health and salvation are twin expressions of a wholeness 4. Sickness–Brokenness and disintegration penetrate the whole person 5. Healing agents have the power to affect change	Holistic nursing emanates from five core values: 1. Holistic Philosophy, Theory, and Ethics 2. Holistic Caring Process 3. Holistic Communication, Therapeutic Healing Environment, and Cultural Diversity 4. Holistic Education and Research 5. Holistic Nurse Self-Reflection and Self-Care (Mariano, 2016, pp. 59–66)
3. Delivery of care	Traditional, humanistic comprehensive in nature embracing the notion of self-responsibility and prevention The patient taught to focus on the wholeness of his/her health rather the diagnosis Three underlying assumptions: (1) stress is a causal factor in disease; (2) identifying both needs and resources is in itself therapeutic for the patient; and (3) the process of identifying recent life stresses teaches the patient a method for analyzing his/her personal disease in the future (Tubesing et al., 1977)	*Holistic Nursing Practice Process*: An iterative and integrative process that involves six steps that can occur simultaneously: (1) assessing, (2) diagnosing and identifying patterns, challenges, needs, and health issues; (3) identifying outcomes, (4) Planning care, (5) Implementing the plan, (6) Evaluating (Mariano, 2016, p. 55) *Patient Centered Care*: Care that is respectful of and responsive to individual patient preferences, needs, and values, and that insures that patient values guide all clinical decisions. Patient centered care encompasses identifying, respecting, and caring about patient differences, values, preferences, and expressed needs; relieving pain and suffering; coordinating continuous care/listening to; clearly informing, communicating with, and educating patients; sharing decision making and management; continually advocating disease prevention, wellness, and promotion of healthy lifestyles including a focus on population health (Mariano, 2016, p. 55) *Person Centered Care*: The human caring process in which the holistic nurse gives full attention and intention to the whole self of a person not merely the current presenting symptoms, illness, crisis, or tasks to be accomplished and that also includes reinforcing the person's meaning and experience of oneness and unity; the condition of trust that is created in which holistic care can be given and received (Mariano, 2016, p. 55)

(continued)

Table 3.1 (continued)

Spelling	Wholistic	Holistic
4. Definitions	Westberg defined wholistic health care as "...the metaphysical affirmation of body, mind, and spirit integrated in a whole, independent of and greater than the sum of its parts. In practice, wholistic health care means actively searching with a patient all dimensions of his/her life (physical, emotional, intellectual, spiritual, interpersonal) for causes and symptoms of disease, then creatively exploring these same modalities for treatment strategies to restore or maintain health" (Tubesing et al., 1977, p. 219) Wholistic health is the human experience of optimal harmony, balance, and function of the interconnected and interdependent unity of the spiritual, physical, mental, and social dimensions. The quality of wholistic health is influenced by human development at a given age and an individual's genetic endowments, which operate in and through one's environments, experiences, and relationships (Ziebarth, 2016, p. 1820)	A theory that the universe and especially nature is correctly seen in terms of interacting wholes (as of living organisms) that are more than the mere sum of elementary particles (Merriam-Webster, 2006) *Holistic Nursing*: All nursing practice that has healing the whole person as its goal and honors relationship-centered care and the interconnectedness of self, others, nature, and spirituality; focuses on protecting, promoting, and optimizing health and wellness; incorporating integrative modalities/complementary and alternative (CAM) as appropriate (Mariano, 2016, p. 3)

	Wholistic	Holistic
5. Significant works	Westberg, G. E. (1961). Minister and Doctor Meet. Academic Medicine. Westberg, G. E. (1979). Theological roots of Wholistic Health Care: A response to the religious questions that have been raised. Tubesing, D. A., Holinger, P. C., Westberg, G. E., & Lighter, E. A. (1977). The Wholistic Health Center Project: An action-research model for providing preventive, whole-person health care at the primary level. Solari-Twadell, P. A. (1999). The emerging practice of parish nursing. Ziebarth, D. (2015). Wholistic Health Care: Evolutional Conceptual Analysis	L. Bertalanffly. 1928. Modern theories of development: An introduction to theoretical biology. New York: Oxford University Press. Dossey, L. Recovering the soul: A scientific and spiritual search. 1989. New York: Bantam New Age Books. Dossey, B.M., Keegan, L. Guzzetta, C.E., Kolkmeier, L.G. 1993. Holistic Nursing: A handbook for practice. New York: Aspen Publishers. Barrere, C., Blaszko Helming, M.A., Sheilds, D.A & Avino, K.M. 2016. Holistic nursing: A handbook for practice (7th Ed). Massachusetts: Jones and Bartlett Learning
6. Specialty organizations	None	American Holistic Health Association. American Holistic Medical Association. American Holistic Nurses Association
7. Certification	No	Yes
8. Scope of practice and standards of practice	No	Yes
9. Ongoing education	No	Yes
10. Ongoing research	Yes	Yes
11. Used by faith community nurses	Yes	Yes
12. Medical subject headings (MeSH) term	No	Yes

References

American Holistic Nurse Association and the American Nurses Association. (2013). *Holistic nursing: Scope and standards of practice*. Silver Spring, MD: Nursebooks.

American Holistic Nurses Association. (2018). Retrieved July 18, 2018, from http://www.ahna.org

American Nursing Association and Health Ministries Association. (1998). *Parish nursing scope and standards of practice*. Silver Spring, MD: Nursesbooks.

Bard, J. (2006). Faith community nurses and the prevention and management of addiction problems. *Journal of Addictions Nursing, 17*, 115–120.

Brudenell, I. (2003). Parish nursing: Nurturing body, mind, spirit, and community. *Public Health Nursing, 20*, 85–94.

Burkhart, L., & Androwich, I. (2004). Measuring the domain completeness of the nursing interventions classification in parish nurse documentation. *CIN Computers, Informatics, Nursing, 22*, 72–82.

Burkhart, L., Konicek, D., Moorhead, S., & Androwich, I. (2005). Mapping parish nurse documentation into the nursing interventions classifications: A research method. *CIN Computers, Informatics, Nursing, 23*, 220–229.

Burkhart, L., & Solari-Twadell, A. (2001). Spirituality and religiousness: Differentiating the diagnoses through a review of the nursing literature. *International Journal of Nursing Terminologies and Classifications, 12*(2), 45–54.

Calabria, M. D., & Macrae, J. A. (Eds.). (1994). *Suggestions for thought by Florence Nightingale: Selections and commentaries*. Philadelphia: University of Pennsylvania Press.

Chase-Ziolek, M., & Iris, M. (2002). Nurses perspectives on the distinctive aspects of providing nursing care in a congregational setting. *Journal of Community Health Nursing, 19*, 173–186.

Chase-Ziolek, M., & Striepe, J. (1999). A comparison of urban versus rural experiences of nurses volunteering to promote health in churches. *Public Health Nursing, 16*, 270–279.

Cordeau, M. A. (2010). The lived experience of clinical simulation of novice nursing students. *International Journal of Human Caring, 14*, 9–15.

Cunningham, R. J. (1974). From holiness to healing: The faith cure in America 1872–1892. *Church History, 43*(04), 499–513.

Dictionary, M. W. (2006). *The Merriam-Webster Dictionary*. Merriam-Webster, Incorporated.

Dossey, B. M. (2016). Nursing: Holistic, integral, and integrative—local to global. In *Holistic nursing: A handbook for practice* (pp. 3–52). Boston: Jones and Bartlett Publishers.

Farrell, S. P., & Rigney, D. B. (2005). From dream to reality: How a parish nurse program was born. *Journal of Christian Nursing, 22*, 34–37.

Hinton, S. T. (2009). Nursing in the church: Insights. *Journal of Christian Nursing, 26*, 175.

King, M. A., & Tessaro, I. (2009). Parish nursing: Promoting healthy lifestyles in the church. *Journal of Christian Nursing, 26*, 22–24.

Koenig, H. G. (2008). Concerns about measuring "spirituality" in research. *The Journal of Nervous and Mental Disease, 196*(5), 349–355.

Mariano, C. (2016). Holistic nursing scope and standards of practice. In C. C. Barrere, M. A. Blaszko Helming, D. A. Sheilds, & K. M. Avino (Eds.), *Holistic nursing: A handbook for practice* (7th ed.). Gaithersburg, MA: Jones and Bartlett Publishers. Retrieved July 18, 2018, from http://www.thinksforumusablog.org

McGinnis, S. L., & Zoske, F. M. (2008). The emerging role of faith community nurses in prevention and management of chronic disease. *Policy, Politics and Nursing Practice, 9*, 173–180.

O'Brien, M. E. (2003). Conceptual models of parish nursing practice: A middle-range theory of spiritual well-being in illness. In *Parish nursing: Healthcare ministry within the church* (pp. 99–115). Sudbury, MA: Jones and Bartlett.

Peterson, W. (1982). *Granger Westberg Verbatim: A vision for faith and health*. St. Louis, MO: Westberg Institute.

Rethemeyer, A., & Wehling, B. A. (2004). How are we doing? Measuring the effectiveness of parish nursing. *Journal of Christian Nursing, 21*(2), 10–12.

Rydholm, L. (1997). Patient-focused care in parish nursing. *Holistic Nursing Practice, 11*(3), 47–60.

Scott, L., & Summer, J. (1993). How do parish nurses help people? A research perspective. *Journal of Christian Nursing, 10*(1), 16–18.

Solari-Twadell, A., & Westberg, G. (1991). Body, mind, and soul. *Health Progress, 72*, 24–28.

Solari-Twadell, P. A. (1999). The emerging practice of parish nursing. In *Parish nursing: Promoting whole person health within faith communities* (pp. 3–24). Thousand Oaks, CA: Sage.

Solari-Twadell, P. A., & Hackbarth, D. P. (2010). Evidence for a new paradigm of the ministry of parish nursing practice using the nursing intervention classification system. *Nursing Outlook, 58*, 69–75.

Solari-Twadell, P. A., & McDermott, M. A. (Eds.). (1999). *Parish nursing: Promoting whole person health within faith communities*. Thousand Oaks, CA: Sage.

Tubesing, D. A., Holinger, P. C., Westberg, G. E., & Lighter, E. A. (1977). The Wholistic Health Center Project: An action-research model for providing preventive, whole-person health care at the primary level. *Medical Care, 15*(3), 217–227.

Tuck, I., Pullen, L., & Wallace, D. (2001). A comparative study of the spiritual perspectives and interventions of mental health and parish nurses. *Issues in Mental Health Nursing, 22*, 593–605.

Tuck, I., Wallace, D., & Pullen, L. (2001). Spirituality and spiritual care provided by parish nurses. *Western Journal of Nursing Research, 23*, 441–453.

Tuck, I., & Wallace, D. C. (2000). Exploring parish nursing from an ethnographic perspective. *Journal of Transcultural Nursing, 11*, 290–299.

Van Loon, A. (1998). The development of faith community nursing programs as a response to changing Australian health policy. *Health Education and Behavior, 25*, 790–799.

Wallace, D. C., Tuck, I., Boland, C. S., & Witucki, J. M. (2002). Client perceptions of parish nursing. *Public Health Nursing, 19*, 128–135.

Westberg, G. (1986). The role of congregations in preventive medicine. *Journal of Religion and Health, 25*, 193–197.

Westberg, G. (1990). *The parish nurse: Providing a ministry of health for your congregation*. Minneapolis, MN: Augsburg.

Westberg, G. E. (1961). Minister and doctor meet. *Academic Medicine, 36*(9), xxiv.

Westberg, G. E. (1979). *Theological roots of Wholistic Health Care: A response to the religious questions that have been raised*. Hinsdale, IL: Wholistic Health Centers.

Westberg, J. (2015). *The gentle rebel: The life and work of Granger Westberg. Pioneer in whole person health*. Memphis, TN: Church Health Center.

Wordsworth, H. A. (2015). *Rediscovering a Ministry of Health: Parish nursing as a mission of the local church*. Eugene, OR: Wipf and Stock Publishers.

Ziebarth, D. (2014). Evolutionary conceptual analysis: Faith community nursing. *Journal of Religion and Health, 53*(6), 1817–1835.

Ziebarth, D. (2015a). Why a faith community nurse program: A five finger response. *Journal of Christian Nursing, 32*(2), 88–93.

Ziebarth, D. (2015b). *International Parish Nurse Resource Center position paper: How is faith community nursing the same or different than other nursing specialties*. Memphis, TN: Church Health Center.

Ziebarth, D., & Miller, C. (2010). Exploring parish nurses' perceptions of parish nurse training. *Journal of Continuing Education in Nursing, 41*(6), 273–280.

Ziebarth, D. J. (2016). Wholistic health care: Evolutionary conceptual analysis. *Journal of Religion and Health, 55*(5), 1800–1823.

Advancing Nursing Theory Within Faith Community Nursing

4

Deborah Jean Ziebarth and P. Ann Solari-Twadell

4.1 Advancing Nursing Theory Within Faith Community Nursing

Nursing conceptual frameworks and nursing theory-based practice models can be used as a guide to faith community nursing practice and establish a foundation for the evolution of this specialty nursing practice (Bunkers, 1999, p. 205). Theories are the identification of unique concepts that are linked by statements of relationships. These linking statements are called propositions and describe relationships between phenomena (Meleis, 1991, 1992, 2010, 2011; Meleis & Trangenstein, 1994). Every specialty nursing practice has certain phenomena that are of interest and identified as significant and unique to practice. A paradigm identifies and explains how that specialty practice relates with the identified concepts or phenomena. In nursing, there are four recognized components of a paradigm: nursing, health, person, and environment (Fawcett, 2000, 2005; Flaming, 2004). These are also referred to as the essential elements of any nursing theory (Pearson, Vaughan, & FitzGerald, 2005). There are 104 specialties in the profession of nursing (Discover Nursing, 2018). Faith community nursing is one of them and has beginnings of theory development (Hickman, 2011). This chapter intends to explore faith community nursing theory development and how these works have the potential to impact the understanding of health, nursing, person, and environment. Faith community nursing theory development has continued over the last 30 years. It is important to recognize these beginnings in order for further development to take place.

D. J. Ziebarth (✉)
Nursing Program Chair, Herzing University, Brookfield, WI, USA
e-mail: dziebarth@herzing.edu

P. A. Solari-Twadell
Marcella Niehoff School of Nursing, Loyola University Chicago, Chicago, IL, USA
e-mail: psolari@luc.edu

© Springer Nature Switzerland AG 2020   51
P. A. Solari-Twadell, D. J. Ziebarth (eds.), *Faith Community Nursing*,
https://doi.org/10.1007/978-3-030-16126-2_4

It is important to distinguish between models and theories. Theories and models have much in common and are both composed of concepts and propositions. Both theory and model development are valued in faith community nursing. An exploration of both is important for recognizing contributions over time.

4.2   Models

Models are described as a simple representation of reality (Alligood, 2013; Anderson, McFarlane, & Helton, 1986; Fawcett, 2000) or a simplified way of organizing a complex phenomenon. Models are considered a tool that can be used to represent an idea, process, or object in logical terms in order to visualize both structure and relationships. Models come in various forms. For example, a one-dimensional model of the heart would be a verbal outline of its structure and function. A two-dimensional model would take the form of a diagram of the heart showing the various structures and how they relate to each other. This two-dimensional model will provide more information than the one-dimensional model. A three-dimensional model may take the form of a plastic teaching replica of the heart that could be taken apart and the internal structures removed and examined. This three-dimensional model gives even more information about the structure, relationship, and function of the heart than the previous one. All three model forms are helpful for clarification and elucidation.

4.3   Theories

Since nursing focuses on human beings, and nursing science is human science, predicting how a person is cared for by a nurse will respond to a health challenge with an absolute degree of certainty in each situation, is difficult, if not, impossible. The only thing that can be done is to generate different theories to assist in describing, explaining, predicting, or anticipating human behaviors. Theories can offer ways of portraying human responses to health issues that can be recognized as a pattern. One definition of theory is "…a set of concepts, definitions and propositions that project a systematic view of particular or controlling phenomena" (Chinn & Jacobs, 1978, p. 70). Chinn and Jacobs-Kramer later formulated a more qualitative definition with theory being a rigorous structuring of ideas that is a purposeful and systematic view of phenomena (1988). In practical terms, as nurses come to know patients in their care and the sources of illness or distress, it can be helpful to refer to theories of how people respond and experience health issues. For example, if a person, because of recent surgery, has an arm in a brace, then basic self-care activities will be compromised. The nurse can predict the need for human or structural support to allow the person to complete basic activities of daily living. Theories of self-care, wound healing, and possible fear of future loss of capacity may be useful in this scenario.

Nursing theories exist at several levels. Grand theories tend to account for all four metaparadigm concepts: humans, health, nursing, and environment. They tend to offer overarching and general statements about the nature of the relationship among those concepts. Other theories are more specific and are often referred to as middle-range theories. A mid-range nursing theory presents concepts at a lower level of abstraction. Mid-range theories are more tangible and can be verified through testing. An example of a mid-range theory is Mishel's Theory of Uncertainty (1990) which noted that one source of distress for patients and families is often not knowing the diagnosis or not knowing what a diagnosis will mean for their future.

4.4   The Argument: Why Utilize Nursing Theory in Practice?

So why is this chapter even included in this text? This chapter acknowledges work that has been done by faith community nurses to explicate their understanding of faith community nursing practice. Furthermore, this work has the capacity to assist all faith community nurses to more fully understand the care provided to clients served. In addition, the work completed thus far on more clearly identifying the uniqueness of faith community nursing practice through model and theory development is also very important to communicating to the nursing profession at large the significance and uniqueness of faith community nursing as a specialty nursing practice. Most important is the significance this model development can have for the practice and research of faith community nursing.

4.5   Faith Community Nursing Theoretical Works

Before delving into faith community nursing model development, it is important to acknowledge the grand theorists of nursing. Grand theorists such as: Neuman—Systems Theory (1980), Parse—The Science of Human Becoming (1981), Orem—Self-Care Deficit Theory (1983), King—Open Systems Theory (1983), Benner—Humanistic Model (1984), Watson—Theory of Care/Caring Science (1988), Newman—Health as Expanding Consciousness (1990), Rogers-The Science of Unitary Human Beings (1990), and Roy and Andrews—Adaptation Theory (1999) among others, all have a contribution to make to the care of clients by faith community nurses. Many of these nursing theorist's works, especially those grand nursing theorists who are concerned with the concept of transformation, have unique contributions to make to the nursing practice of faith community nurses. In addition, the early work of these grand nursing theorists provides a foundation for the further development of models and theories particular to faith community nursing.

Over the last 30 years several authors have contributed to theoretical models for faith community nursing. The following theoretical works will be explored in a chronological sequence and explicate further information noted on the attached Table 4.1. The following is a list of the reviewed theories

1. Circle Model of Spiritual Care (Schnorr, 1990).
2. Parish Nursing: A Conceptual Framework (Bergquist & King, 1994).

Table 4.1 Conceptual Theory Matrix

Conceptual model	Nursing	Health	Person	Environment	Based on experience or/and EBP	Peer-reviewed journal	Tested	Citations
Spiritual caregiving: a key component of Parish nursing	Not noted in this writing	Not noted in this writing	Not noted in this writing	Not noted in this writing	Grounded Theory and unstructured interviews to collect data from 46 nurses in 12 states, 1 territory, and 2 foreign countries	No	Cannot find	Schnorr (1990)
Parish nursing: a conceptual framework	Parish nursing practice includes the roles of health educator, health counselor, leader of groups, and community liaison. The goal of nursing in this model is to enhance the holistic health and well-being of the faith community members	Health is defined as optimal wellness and wholeness. Emotional well-being, an integral part of health, is reduced when unity and harmony are missing, insufficient, or disrupted	Concept of person as the client/patient of the parish nurse and described as individual, family, or group, the client has spiritual qualities and is usually a faith community participant but can also be a member of the broader community	Faith community	Experience	Yes	Cannot find	Bergquist and King (1994)

Human becoming as parish nursing	Theory-based health ministry based on Parse's theory of human becoming. The central focus of this nursing theory-based health model is quality of life in the parish community. Central to parish nursing practice is living true presence with those in the parish	Health is viewed as a personal commitment to a lived value system	Viewed as an individual, as a family, as a community, or as a country. The person is a unitary, indivisible whole and interrelates with others in the environment while experiencing the past, present, and future all at once. At an abstract level, person denotes humankind	People and communities will define what is important to them and what is desired for quality of life	Experience	Yes	Cannot find	Bunkers et al. (1997) and Bunkers (1998, 1999)
The parish nursing continuity of care model	The nurse is the focal point of the model who connects individuals and families with resources to provide care to a congregation over life's continuum. The goal of nursing is to promote holistic health and well-being by enhancing the sense of harmony with the mind, body, and spirit within the faith community	Health is described as an evolving process with physical, emotional, and spiritual properties. Wellness is holistically promoted by addressing the physical, emotional, and spiritual needs	The person is a complex entity. Physical, mental, cultural, social, emotional, and spiritual aspects are interrelated. The person is a whole being with body, mind, and spirit facets that interact with each other to maintain optimal physical, emotional, and spiritual health, respectively	Faith community	Experience	Yes	Cannot find	Wilson (1997)

(continued)

Table 4.1 (continued)

Conceptual model	Nursing	Health	Person	Environment	Based on experience or/ and EBP	Peer-reviewed journal	Tested	Citations
The Miller model of parish nursing	Nursing is conceptualized as a mission and a ministry. The major integrating concepts are: person/parishioner, health, parish nurse, and community/parish. The core integrating concept of the Miller Model is the Triune God	Health and healing are integral to a Christian church's mission and ministry. Health is defined with the two overlapping concepts of shalom-wholeness and stewardship	The client is depicted as being a complex entity with physical, mental, cultural, social, emotional, and spiritual aspects that are all interrelated. The individuals and families within the congregation come from a variety of cultural and social backgrounds and include aspects of family, friends, and the faith community	The environment is made up of contexts viewed from the nurse's perspective. The local congregation and church-related activities form the primary context	Experience	Yes	Cannot find	Miller (1997)
Circle of Christian caring	Nursing is an opportunity to combine the spiritual and physical dimensions of caregiving and to affirm the church as a place for disease prevention and health promotion. Parish nurse roles are health educator, health counselor, referral/ resource/client advocate, facilitator/leader, and home visitor. There are focused nursing activities or responsibilities related to each role	Descriptors for the concept of health include medical conditions, end-of-life processes, and recovering from illness or striving for holistic healing	The person has equal body, mind, and spirit components	The environment has a social quality and is composed of the faith community or congregation, and the broader geographic community	Experience	Yes	Cannot find	Maddox (2001)

Spiritual well-being in illness framework	Health	The person as client	Environment	Experience	Yes	Further	O'Brien (2003)
Nursing is referred to as ministry. The primary ministry of the nurse is to assess and support the spiritual well-being of the member through caring interactions and interventions. The nurse functions in the roles as advocate, counselor, educator, and referral agent giving necessary attention to the client's physical, emotional, and social well-being	Health is not specifically defined but can be interpreted from the model as functionality and finding or having spiritual meaning. Illness is based on the degree of functional impairment and one's inability to find spiritual meaning	The person as client has a physical, psychosocial, and spiritual nature, and the ability to find meaning in and to accept pain, suffering, and illness. The person is capable of accepting and transcending pain and suffering in light of higher powers	Environment is not specifically defined but can be interpreted from the model as both the congregation and the client's ever-changing life events	Experience	Yes	explored and evolved to spiritual care: Parish nursing: Healthcare ministry within the church (O'Brien, 2003). Parish nursing: meeting spiritual needs of elders near the end of life. (O'Brien, 2006) The Spiritual Assessment Scale (SAS) contains 21 items of 3 subscales: personal faith, religious practice, and spiritual contentment Spirituality in nursing: Standing on holy ground. (2008, 2011)	

(continued)

Table 4.1 (continued)

Conceptual model	Nursing	Health	Person	Environment	Based on experience or/ and EBP	Peer-reviewed journal	Tested	Citations
Emerging processes that support development of a middle-range theory	Not identified in this writing. Based on Margaret Newman's philosophy of unitary transformative nursing	Not identified in this writing. Based on Margaret Newman's philosophy of unitary transformative nursing	Not identified in this writing. Based on Margaret Newman's philosophy of unitary transformative nursing	Not identified in this writing. Based on Margaret Newman's philosophy of unitary transformative nursing	Grounded Theory guided the data collection. A paid institutional faith community nursing model that was based in a health care system and partnered with communities of faith was employed to enable identification of basic social processes that form the foundation of the developed model. Three part-time, seasoned faith community nurses submitted stories that were de-identified. These stories were the data that provided the foundation for this research	Yes	No	Dyess and Chase (2012)

Faith community nursing theoretical definition and model							Ziebarth (2014)
The nurse/client (client as person, family, group, or community) relationship is central. This relationship occurs when the client seeks or is targeted by the nurse for wholistic health care interventions. Essential attributes and interventions surround this relationship and occur in an iterative motion over time with intentionality. The essential attributes are faith integrating, health promoting, disease managing, coordinating, empowering, and accessing health care. Essential attributes are defined by interventions in the theory	Health is wholistic in nature and is defined as "... the human experience of optimal harmony, balance, and function of the interconnected and interdependent unity of the spiritual, physical, mental, and social dimensions. The quality of wholistic health is influenced by human development at a given age and an individual's genetic endowments, which operate in and through one's environments, experiences, and relationships" (Ziebarth, 2016b, p. 123)	The person, family, group, or community seeking or receiving wholistic care from the faith community nurse. The client is seen as complex with different aspects related to the whole totality of being. Components of being include physical, health characteristics, emotional, social, mental, cultural, and spiritual aspects. Clients live with chronic illness, have medical conditions, end-of-life processes, and are recovering from illness. They desire all levels of prevention, symptom management, wholistic approaches, support, and coping strategies	The environment is a faith community, home, health institution, or other community setting as part of a community, national, or global health initiative. The nurse works in or with a faith community	EBP The author analyzed 124 research and theoretical articles from multiple disciplines (nursing, education, religion, and international health) to understand the historical and social nature of the practice of faith community nursing and how it has changed over time	Yes	Yes, theory has been tested at least twice. Transitional Care Interventions as Implemented By Faith Community Nurses (Ziebarth, 2016a) The theory was used to align transitional care interventions to the essential attributes of faith community nursing Wholistic health care: evolutionary conceptual analysis (Ziebarth, 2016a). The theory was used to compare wholistic health essential attributes

3. Nursing Theory Guided Model of Health Ministry (Bunkers, 1999; Bunkers, Michaels, & Ethridge, 1997).
4. The Parish Nursing Continuity of Care Model (Wilson, 1997).
5. The Miller Model of Parish Nursing (Miller, 1997).
6. The Circle of Christian Caring Theory (Maddox, 2001).
7. Spiritual Well-Being in Illness framework (O'Brien, 1982, 2003).
8. Emerging Processes that Support Development of a Middle-Range Theory (Dyess & Chase, 2012)
9. Faith Community Nursing Theory and Model (Ziebarth, 2014).

Many of the early theories will have the label "parish nursing." The name of this specialty practice changed from parish nursing to faith community nursing with the second printing of the Scope and Standards (American Nurses Association/Health Ministry Association, 2005) and remained the label of choice on the second revision (2010) and third edition (2017). The Faith Community Nursing: Scope and Standards of Practice states that the name was chosen for the guidelines "…to have one label inclusive of all faith traditions and to accurately label the location and focus of practice" (ANA and HMA, 2005, p. 2). Furthermore, the faith community nurse "…may still be referred to as a parish nurse, congregational nurse, health ministry nurse, crescent nurse, or health and wellness nurse to fit a community's culture and faith tradition" (ANA and HMA, 2005, p. 2). Other labels are also used such as health minister, health pastor, spiritual nurse, and church nurse (IPNRC, 2010; Jacob, 2014; Patterson & Slutz, 2011). As we explore faith community nursing theories in a chronological sequenced manner, the name of the practice will change.

4.6   CIRCLE Model: Spiritual Nursing Care

Dr. Marcia Schnorr noted that most research on spiritual care had previously been completed in a "hospital setting" (Schnorr, 1990, p. 205). The CIRCLE Model was developed for use by a nurse in any setting, thus, the importance to parish nursing.

Grounded theory was used to complete 46 unstructured interviews representing nurses from 12 states, one territory, and two foreign countries. This sample included nurses working in both paid and unpaid positions representing different specialty nursing practices, the nurse participants represented three basic educational programs with the participants having from one to 42 years of nursing experience. Forty-four of the participants identified themselves as Christian (Schnorr, 1990, p. 205).

As a result of this research the CIRCLE model of spiritual care was developed. The model consists of a large circle which represents the setting. Within the larger circle are two overlapping circles. One of the circles represents the recipient of spiritual nursing care and the other circle the provider of nursing care. In the overlapping section of the intersecting circles is the Nursing Process. The word CIRCLE represents: C = Caring, I = intuition, R = respect for religion beliefs and practices, C = caution, L = listening, and E = emotional support. In this model "Assessment" has three main tools: religious cues, emotional cues, and assessment guides (p. 207). Planning and Intervention has six specific concepts. They are caring, intuition, respect for religious beliefs and practices, caution, listening, and emotional support. Evaluation was noted through the use of case studies (pp. 213–215).

4.7   Summary

Dr. Schnorr distinguishes in her work the difference between religion and spirituality. Spirituality is defined as the "life principle that pervades the entire being, integrating and transcending all other dimensions of life," while religion is "an organized system of beliefs and practices" (Schnorr, 1990, p. 202). Noted is the discomfort that parish nurses may have in providing spiritual care; however, the importance of the setting and emphasis of the importance of spiritual care as "the essence" of this specialty practice make the use of a model for spiritual care most important.

4.8   Parish Nursing: A Conceptual Framework

Bergquist and King (1994) published the first conceptual model directed to the specialty of parish nursing. They grounded their model in the historical view of nursing as caring for the whole person: body, mind, and spirit. Based on a literature review on "parish" nursing, they grouped major ideas into "client, health, the nurse, the environment and the nursing process (p. 155)." They developed a graphic model with intersecting circles of Client and Nurse both within the larger circle of faith community and larger community. Important concepts related to the client included individuals, families with a range of ages and social groups. The larger community was seen as client as well, because the faith community connected to wider community services and resources. The parish nurse was defined by Westberg (2015) as able to work in faith and health arenas and to bring out the spiritual aspects of care. The goal of parish nursing in this model is to "enhance the holistic health and well-being of individual, families and groups within the faith community" (Bergquist & King, 1994, p. 161). Physical, emotional, and spiritual interventions and outcomes reflect the cohesion of the body, mind, and spirit. The parish nurse's commitment to wholeness involves activities in several domains: physical health and wellness, emotional health and wellness, and spiritual health and wellness. Each domain lists specific nursing activities and expected client outcomes. For example, physical health and well-being includes activities of health promotion and promotion of self-care activities. Outcomes for this domain include engagement in health-related practices and increased feelings of well-being. In the emotional health and well-being domain, activities include caring and social support and outcomes include decreased feelings of loneliness and raised consciousness. Finally, in the spiritual health and well-being domain, activities include prayer and facilitation of spiritual activities with outcomes of meaning to life and death and mended relationships. All these activities and outcomes are based in the literature sources.

The nurse is characterized as a spiritually mature person who (a) continually grows in personal faith, (b) remains sensitive to the relationship between faith and health, (c) applies spiritual features to health care, and (d) counsels individuals, families, and groups about spiritual concerns.

4.9   Summary

In Bergquist and King (1994), nursing is described as offering a clear opportunity to include spirituality and religious beliefs into nursing care. This theory describes the unique features of the client as including families, groups, and the faith community itself. The authors provide clear examples of specialized care activities and expected outcomes appropriate to the environmental setting and suggest the possibility of the faith community engaging the larger community with outreach and development of clinics in collaboration with universities and community agencies. Testing of this model could not be found in the literature.

4.10   Nursing Theory Guided Model of Health Ministry

Bunkers work of a nursing theory-based health ministry is based on Parse's Theory of Human Becoming interwoven with Christian beliefs based on the Eight Beatitudes (Bunkers, 1999, p. 209). This congregational model which includes the health cabinet, pastor, parish nurse, and community as four components of a circle surrounding the parishioner and parish community is surrounded by the Eight Beatitudes. The model is subtitled as a "Christ Centered Covenant" with a subtitle of "Co-creating Health in a Parish Community." This model notes the "richness of interweaving nursing beliefs and values with faith values of a parish community" (Bunkers, 1999, p. 213).

This model was developed through months of study and dialogue with the central focus of the theory-based health model being quality of life in the parish community (Bunkers, 1999, p. 209).

4.11   Summary

Although this theory-based model was not tested, it offers a conceptual model for theory-based practice which melds nursing theory with Christian beliefs directed toward quality of life of the congregation and its members. Testing and application of this model could not be found.

4.12   The Parish Nursing Continuity of Care Model

The Parish Nursing Continuity of Care Model (Wilson, 1997), model emphasizes harmony in mind, body, and spirit. "The nurse is the focal point of the model. As caregiver, the nurse connects individuals and families with resources. In addition, the nurse provides care to a congregation over life's continuum. This continuum is described as: physical birth; new life—being born again in Christ; suffering—the pains and sorrows of life; surrender—to God's grace and mercy; and, physical death and resurrection—everlasting life in glory with Christ" (p. 94). The nurse functions from a broad, general knowledge base and must be able to offer in-depth spiritual care and foster the spiritual growth of the client. The nurse is (a) an agent of love and caring, and (b) the focal point that connects people and their needs with social resources. The goal of nursing is to promote holistic health and well-being by enhancing the sense of harmony with the mind, body, and spirit within the faith community. One role of the nurse is to provide education for individuals, families, groups, and the community. Educational activities vary based on needs of the faith community, support of the organization, and strengths and expertise of the nurse. Nursing roles vary based on the cultural needs of the faith community. Health is described as an evolving process with physical, emotional, and spiritual properties that (a) work to maintain balance, and (b) strive to achieve an optimal level of wellness. Wellness is holistically promoted by addressing the physical, emotional, and spiritual needs of an individual. Health is referred to as holistic. Holistic health has physical and emotional properties, needs, and self-care. Optimal emotional health is one element of total health, and meeting emotional needs is one factor of total wellness. The person is a complex entity. Physical, mental, cultural, social, emotional, and spiritual aspects are interrelated. The person is a whole being with body, mind, and spirit facets that interact with each other. The goal is to maintain optimal physical, emotional, and spiritual health, respectively. Individuals and families have a variety of physical and mental health characteristics. The person exists and functions within the social context of a congregation. As individuals or groups, clients have the social characteristics of different ages, backgrounds, socioeconomic levels, and developmental stages. The person, as individuals or families within a congregation, is a whole being with body, mind, and spirit facets that interact with each other to maintain optimal physical, emotional, and spiritual health. The faith community is the larger environment. The congregation is a feature in the environment, and community services surround the person. One feature of the environment has a birth to death component. The faith community environment itself can promote health by sponsoring health related activities.

4.13 Summary

The Parish Nursing Continuity of Care Model (Wilson, 1997) describes the nurse as having a general knowledge base. In addition, the nurse must be able to offer in-depth spiritual care. The nurse specifically connects people with social resources and provides education for individuals, families, groups, and the community. Health is holistic with an evolving process with physical, emotional, and spiritual, properties that interact with each other to maintain balance and strive to achieve an optimal level of wellness. The person is a complex entity with physical, mental, cultural, social, emotional, and spiritual aspects that are interrelated and interact to maintain optimal physical, emotional, and spiritual health, respectively. The environment is the faith community. Testing of this model could not be found.

4.14   The Miller Model of Parish Nursing

The Miller Model of Parish Nursing (Miller, 1997) is underpinned by the philosophical foundations of Evangelical Christianity. The major integrating concepts are: person/parishioner, health, parish nurse, and community/parish. The core integrating concept of the Miller Model is the Triune God. Miller (1997) explains that God is personal, sovereign, good, just, merciful, and has loving relationships with people. Everyone and everything were created good by God, and God intended for people to have harmonious relationships with Him, others, and nature. Nursing is conceptualized as a mission and a ministry with philosophical and pragmatic features. The philosophies of the Evangelical Christian faith support the "why" aspect of the mission. Nursing practice is the pragmatic "what" and "how" of the ministry. Love, gracious compassion, co-participation, and spiritual care contribute to the roles and functions of the nurse. Health and healing are integral to a Christian church's mission and ministry. Health is defined with the two overlapping concepts of shalom-wholeness and stewardship. Shalom-wholeness refers to dwelling at peace and in harmony with oneself, God, other people, and the created world. Stewardship means being entrusted with something valuable and accountable for all gifts, resources, education, including those of a financial nature received from God. A person's vocation and ability to earn money are considered health promoting resources. Health promoting resources include God, family, friends, the faith community, health care services, social services, vocation, and recreation. It also includes personal knowledge, learning abilities, and educational activities. The client is depicted as being a complex entity with physical, mental, cultural, social, emotional, and spiritual aspects that are all interrelated. The individuals and families within the congregation come from a variety of cultural and social backgrounds and include aspects of family, friends, and the faith community. The spiritual component of the person is central and the person is transformed by a spiritual relationship with the triune God. The person uses the power of God to be a responsible participant in personal health promotion. The environment is made up of contexts viewed from the nurse's perspective. The local congregation and church-related activities form the primary context. The socio-cultural community, health care community, and Christian community are other context components. The faith community environment can promote health by nurturing spiritual values.

4.15   Summary

Nursing is conceptualized as an Evangelical Christian mission and a ministry with philosophical and pragmatic features of love, gracious compassion, co-participation, and spiritual care. Health is defined with the two overlapping concepts of shalom-wholeness and stewardship. The client is depicted as being a complex entity with physical, mental, cultural, social, emotional, and spiritual aspects that are all interrelated. The environment is made up of contexts viewed from the nurse's perspective and includes local congregation and church-related activities. Testing of this model could not be found.

4.16 The Circle of Christian Caring Theory

Maddox (2001) developed the *Circle of Christian Caring*. This model was created specifically for the practice of parish nursing. The pictorial model of the Circle of Christian Caring (Maddox, 2001) is a circle with spokes that represent major ministries of the congregation. The "Parish Nurse" is one of those spokes. The inner ring of Congregation and Community encircles the mind, body, and spirit in a Venn Diagram shape. The person is clearly presented as having mind/body/spirit concerns and strengths. The environment is largely seen as the faith community, but also the larger community in which the congregation is situated as programming was open to anyone who was interested. The realm of nursing practice is an ongoing and integrative process. Nursing is envisioned as "…an opportunity to combine the spiritual and physical dimensions of care-giving and to affirm the church as a place for disease prevention and health promotion" (p. 12). Descriptors for the concept of health include medical conditions, end-of-life processes, and recovering from illness or striving for holistic healing. Holistic healing is interpreted as addressing the spiritual dimension. The person is referred to as client. Based on examination of the pictorial model, three inner, overlapping circles represent the person as having equal body, mind, and spirit components. Descriptors for the client's needs are medical conditions, end-of-life processes, and recovering from illness. The environment has a social quality and it is composed of the faith community or congregation, and the broader geographic community.

4.17 Summary

Nursing combines the spiritual and physical dimensions of caregiving in a Christian faith community. Nursing focused activities relate to roles in disease prevention and health promotion. Descriptors for the concept of health include medical conditions, end-of-life processes, and recovering from illness or striving for holistic healing or the spiritual dimension. The model focuses primarily on the actions of nursing care and not as much on person, environment, or health. Testing of the theory could not be found.

4.18 Spiritual Well-Being in Illness Framework

O'Brien (1982) originally created the framework for all nursing in response to studying long-term hemodialysis patients ($N = 126$) (*Religious Faith and Adjustment to Long-term Hemodialysis*). She found an empirical relationship between social support and well-being. In 2003, *The Spiritual Well-Being in Illness framework* was published to guide the parish nurse in providing care for seriously ill or disabled clients. That was followed by *Parish nursing: meeting spiritual needs of elders near the end of life.* O'Brien (2006); the *Spiritual Assessment Scale: Personal Faith, Religious Practice, and Spiritual Contentment; Spirituality in nursing: Standing on Holy Ground* (2008, 2011). Most recently (2017) the book, *Spirituality in nursing* was published. Nursing is referred to as ministry. The primary ministry of the nurse is to assess and support the spiritual well-being of the client through caring interactions and interventions. Health is not specifically defined, but can be interpreted from the model as functionality and discovering or having spiritual meaning in life. Illness is based on the degree of functional impairment and one's inability to find spiritual meaning. Ill and disabled persons have physical or psychosocial deficits that contribute to their functional impairment. Stressful life events and positive social support influence the person's ability to find spiritual meaning in the experience of illness. Social support comes from family, friends, congregation, and caregivers.

The person as client has a physical, psychosocial, and spiritual nature, and the ability to find meaning in and to accept pain, suffering, and illness. The person is capable of accepting and transcending pain and suffering in light of higher powers. Spiritual resources, attitudes, and behaviors affect the individual's ability to accept or embrace pain, suffering, and illness. Personal faith, spiritual contentment, and religious practices form the category of spiritual resources. Environment is not specifically defined but can be interpreted from the model as both the client's ever-changing life events and faith community. These events, which can be stressful in nature, can surround and overtake the person at any given time.

4.19 Summary

This model supports the primary ministry of the nurse to be assessment and support of the spiritual well-being of the client through caring interactions and interventions. Health is functionality or finding spiritual meaning in the midst of illness. According to this framework, the person has a physical, psychosocial, and spiritual nature, and the ability to find spiritual meaning in the experience of illness. The environment includes the client's ever-changing life events and congregation. O'Brien has developed instruments to test assumptions of the model.

4.20 Emerging Processes that Support Development of a Middle-Range Theory

Dyess and Chase (2012) focused their work on the processes that support theoretical development for holistic nursing in the context of a faith community (Dyess & Chase, 2012, p. 221). The research was based on the philosophy of unitary transformative nursing developed by Margaret Newman and often used by holistic nurses.

A paid institutional faith community nursing model that was based in a health care system and partnered with communities of faith was employed to enable identification of basic social processes that form the foundation of the developed model. Three part-time, seasoned faith community nurses submitted stories that were de-identified. These stories were the data that provided the foundation for this research. Grounded Theory guided the data collection and analysis resulting in theory generation. Grounded Theory methodology was chosen due to the ability to identify "basic social processes" that facilitated model development (Dyess & Chase, 2012, p. 223).

The model presented as a result of their research is non-linear, at times recursive, and a simultaneous process describing nursing practice for the faith community nurse to be: *"Entering a Private World*—faith community nurses enter the private world of the other and through authentic presence seek to come to know and understand caring for the unique individual in the concept of his or her life, *Connecting to Faith*—linking to denominational traditions and congregational mores, *Mutually Transforming*—experiences of profound transformation that is mutually experienced by the client and the nurse acknowledging the work of the Divine, and *Sustaining Health*—recognition of gaps in health care that create fear and anxiety can be addressed supporting health of the client (Dyess & Chase, 2012, p. 224). These core processes are aligned with sustaining health in a faith community nursing practice.

The findings from this research "represent an articulation for development of a middle-range theoretical basis for the holistic practice of the faith community nurse". Middle-range theory "seeks to define more clearly concepts related to a narrow dimension of actual nursing practice" (Dyess & Chase, 2012, p. 224).

4.21 Summary

This study was associated with Judeo Christian denominations (Dyess & Chase, 2012, p. 226). The results of this research provided new knowledge related to the processes of faith community nursing practice. This work has not been tested.

4.22 The Faith Community Nursing Theory

Ziebarth (2014) developed the conceptual model, *Faith Community Nursing*, visually presenting the practice in a bullseye overlay of six enlarging circles with the nurse/client (client as person, family, group, or community) relationship central.

This relationship occurs when the clients seek or are targeted by the nurse for wholistic health care interventions. Essential attributes and interventions surround this relationship and occur in an iterative motion over time with intentionality. The essential attributes are faith integrating, health promoting, disease managing, coordinating, empowering, and accessing health care. Faith integrating is a core and continuous occurring attribute. The practice occurs in a faith community, home, health institution, and other community settings with fluidity as part of a community, national, or global health initiative (See Figure 22.1, p. 301). The theory was created using a Rodgers' Evolutionary methodology, which looks at the antecedents, attributes, and consequences of a concept. The concept was faith community nursing. The theory has been tested at least twice in light of wholistic care and transitional care (Ziebarth, 2016a, 2016b). The first time was in alignment of transitional care interventions to the essential attributes of faith community nursing (Ziebarth, 2016a). The second time was when wholistic health essential attributes were compared with those from the faith community nursing theory (Ziebarth, 2016b). Both times the essential attributes of faith integrating, health promoting, disease managing, coordinating, empowering, and accessing health care were able to be used to describe transitional care as provided by faith community nurses and wholistic health interventions. Other nurses from other disciplines have also requested use of the faith community nurse model, which permission was given.

4.23 Nursing Practice

The nurse is a registered nurse, who works in or with a faith community. The practice of nursing is referred to as faith community nursing and is a method of healthcare delivery that is centered in a relationship between the nurse and client (client as person, family, group, or community). The relationship between the client and nurse occurs in a circular motion over time when the client either seeks or is targeted for wholistic health care. Faith integrating is a continuous occurring attribute with intentional interventions. Health promoting, disease managing, coordinating, empowering, and accessing health care are other essential attributes that occur with intentionality based on the assessment of the nurse.

Nurse/Client Relationship. Faith community nurses are easily accessible and approachable and offer services in a personal nurse/client relationship. Nurses appreciate the benefits of long-term relationships with clients, which create trust. Nurses have less control in the relationship with the client as contrasted with practicing in a hospital work setting. The six essential attributes occur in the nurse/client relationship.

1. *Faith Integrating.* Integrating faith is seen as nursing interventions such as religious rituals (readings, songs, music, communion, and healing service), spiritual assessments, and spiritual and religious care interventions such as presence, touch, spiritual and emotional support, prayer and meditations, spiritual growth facilitation, hope and forgiveness instillation, humor, resources and referrals, and showing compassion.
2. *Health Promoting.* Health promoting is made operational as health-focused programing (screenings and education), health counseling, health resources, advocacy, end-of-life planning, assessments, surveys, policy development, research, and primary and secondary levels of prevention activities.
3. *Disease Managing.* Disease managing is made operational as symptom management, care planning, disease resources or referrals, disease support services, management or surveillance of therapeutic regime, visits, disease-focused education, disease counseling, advocacy, and tertiary level of prevention activities.

4. *Coordinating.* Coordinating is made operational as planning and facilitating ongoing activities (screenings, community health events, education, support groups), recurring meetings (health committee, social concerns, volunteer training), support services (meals, transportation, calls, visits, cards), media (newsletters, bulletins, health displays), and case management. Coordinating is also seen in organizing the health record, data collection, and reports.

5. *Empowering.* Empowering is made operational by helping people to be better partners in the management of their health. Empowering is seen in faith community nursing as capacity building, supporting, encouraging, health support services, surveillance, counseling, self-efficacy activities such as education on how to use the healthcare system, and education techniques such as return demonstration and motivation interviewing. Empowering is also seen in serving as preceptors for students.

6. *Accessing Health Care.* Accessing health care is operationalized in assisting individuals to access health care by decreasing barriers and navigating healthcare systems. It is also seen through the multidisciplinary and interdisciplinary practice within a healthcare team. On a national level, faith community nurses have been involved with health policy development and research that increased healthcare access.

4.24   Consequences of Faith Community Nursing

Participants have reported many physical, psychosocial, spiritual, and educational benefits after interactions with a faith community nurse. They have increased: (a) empowerment and skills to make decisions, coping, follow through, and to access health resources; (b) knowledge and understanding related to disease and treatment options, the relationship between health and faith; (c) effective and regular access to medical home and support from the faith community; and (d) increased quality of life and healthier lifestyles. The greatest impact on the health of the congregation is regular blood pressure screenings, education about heart disease, eating healthier, exercise programs, and overall health-focused programs.

Health is wholistic in nature. Health care is delivered with the goal of wholistic health functioning. The definition of wholistic health is found in Chapter 3.

This theory used previous practice theories to describe the person as an antecedent to faith community nursing. They define the client as the person, family, group, or community seeking or receiving wholistic care from the faith community nurse. The client is seen as complex with different aspects related to the whole totality of being. Components of being include physical, health characteristics, emotional, social, mental, cultural, and spiritual aspects. Clients live in a community which is part of a global society. Clients live with chronic illness, have medical conditions, end-of-life processes, and are recovering from illness. They desire all levels of prevention, symptom management, wholistic approaches, support, and coping strategies (Bergquist & King, 1994; Dyess & Chase, 2010; Maddox, 2001; Miller, 1997; O'Brien, 2003).

The environment is a faith community, home, health institution, or other community setting as part of a community, national, or global health initiative. The nurse works in or with a faith community.

4.25   Summary

Faith integrating, health promoting, disease managing, coordinating, empowering, and accessing health care are continuous occurring attributes through intentional interventions. Health is the human experience of optimal harmony, balance, and function of the interconnected and interdependent unity of the spiritual, physical, mental, and social dimensions. It is influenced by human development at a given age and an individual's genetic endowments, which operate in and through one's environments, experiences, and relationships. The client is the person, family, group, or community seeking or receiving wholistic care from the faith community nurse. The environment is a faith community, home, health institution, or other community setting as part of a community, national, or global health initiative. The registered nurse practices in partnership in or with a faith community.

4.26   Discussion

A descriptive matrix (Marsh, 1990) reduces the totality of findings in this chapter into columns to compare and contrast the work. See Table 4.1 Conceptual Theory Matrix. The content of Table 4.1 is based on the examination of parish nursing, faith community nursing literature to extrapolate conceptual theoretical frameworks from a historical, evolution perspective. All of the identified works have value and provide a foundation for further research and development. However, the purpose is not just to theoretically define, but ultimately to provide guidance for faith community nursing practice.

The environments vary slightly but all agree that the faith community is a partner in the provision of care and offers certain attributing characteristics. All theories used descriptive words such as whole person, wholistic or holistic in describing interventions of the nurse, health, and the person. This use of a broad and overarching concept such as "whole person" attempts to capture the totality of the being. The spiritual, physical, mental, cultural, social, and emotional dimensions of a person are interrelated and represent a person's health and needs. In faith community nursing, the nurse provides care to each dimension of the person, with special focus on the spiritual dimension.

4.26.1   Spirituality and Faith Community Nursing

In the Scope and Standards of Faith Community Nursing (2010) two processes are mentioned in the definition of the practice: promoting wholistic health, wherein intentionally caring for the spirit, and preventing or minimizing illness. It goes on to say that there are five assumptions of faith community nursing: (1) health and illness are human experiences; (2) health is the integration of the spiritual, physical, psychological, and social aspects of the [patient] to create a sense of harmony with self, others, the environment, and a higher power; (3) health may be experienced in the presence of disease or injury; (4) the presence of illness does not preclude health nor does optimal health preclude illness; and (5) healing is a process of integrating the body, mind, and spirit to create wholeness, health, and a sense of well-being, even when the [patient's] illness is not cured] (p. 8).

All explored faith community nursing theories have the tenets of whole person health in describing a unity of more than a physical component of health. They include spiritual, physical, psychological/mental, emotional, cultural, and social components of health that must be cared for together. The spiritual component is of central importance. Asking a patient about meaning, forgiveness, guilt, or shame may be just as important as listening to their lung sounds. Getting to the origin of illnesses may be just as important as the illness itself.

Many of conceptual frameworks presented heavily represent a Judeo-Christian foundation. Faith community nursing, although developed through the lens of Christianity, is intended to be inter-faith and ecumenical. Future conceptual models and theory development need to reflect that understanding or the findings will continue to be limited to Christian faith communities and faith community nursing practices.

In summary, faith community nursing conceptual model development continues to guide the metaparadigm concepts of nursing. Humans are seen as whole persons with aspects that represent body, mind, and spirit. Faith community nursing is particularly strong in elucidating the spiritual aspects of the person. Environment is well developed with respect to the faith community itself. Faith community nursing involves care not just of a person, but for the community as a whole. Health is perceived as a balance of body, mind, and spirit and includes all health states including freedom from symptoms, the experience of short-term illness or chronic debilitating conditions, as well as aging and death. Health for faith community nursing can be present in all these situations. Finally, nursing itself is shown in a unique light with emphasis on health promotion and prevention, and spiritual care. Faith community nursing is called to continue advancing this specialty nursing practice through promoting the continuing evolution of nursing theory.

References

Alligood, M. R. (2013). *Nursing theory-E-book: Utilization & application.* St. Louis, MO: Elsevier Health Sciences.

American Nurses Association and Health Ministries Association. (2010). *Faith community nursing: Scope and standards of practice* (2nd ed.). Silver Spring, MD: Nursesbooks.org.

American Nursing Association & Health Ministries Association. (2005). *Faith community nursing scope & standards of practice.* Silver Spring, MD: Nursesbooks.

Anderson, E., McFarlane, J., & Helton, A. (1986). Community-as-client: A model for practice. *Nursing Outlook, 34*(5), 220–224.

Benner, P. (1984). *From novice to expert: Power and excellence in nursing practice.* Palo Alto, CA: Addison-Wesely.

Bergquist, S., & King, J. (1994). Parish nursing: A conceptual framework. *Journal of Holistic Nursing, 12*, 155–170. https://doi.org/10.1177/089801019401200206

Bunkers, S. S. (1998). Practice applications a nursing theory guided model of health ministry: Human becoming in parish nursing. *Nursing Science Quarterly, 11*(1), 7–8.

Bunkers, S. S. (1999). Translating nursing conceptual frameworks and theory for nursing practice. In P. A. Solari-Twadell & M. A. McDermott (Eds.), *Parish nursing: Promoting whole person health within faith communitie* (pp. 205–213). Thousand Oaks, CA: Sage.

Bunkers, S. S., Michaels, C., & Ethridge, P. (1997). Advanced practice nursing in community: Nursing's opportunity. *Advanced Practice Nursing Quarterly, 2*(4), 79–84.

Chinn, P. L., & Jacobs, M. K. (1978). A model for theory development in nursing. *Advances in Nursing Science, 1*(1), 1–12.

Discover Nursing. (2018). Found at https://www.discovernursing.com/explore-specialties

Dyess, S., & Chase, S. K. (2010). Caring for adults living with a chronic illness through communities of faith. *International Journal of Human Caring, 14*(4), 38–44.

Dyess, S., & Chase, S. K. (2012). Sustaining health in faith community nursing practice: Emerging processes that support the development of a middle-range theory. *Holistic Nursing Practice, 26*(4), 221–227. https://doi.org/10.1097/HNP.0b013e318258527cS

Fawcett, J. (2000). *Analysis and evaluation of contemporary nursing knowledge: Nursing models and theories*. Philadelphia: FA Davis.

Fawcett, J. (2005). Criteria for evaluation of theory. *Nursing Science Quarterly, 18*(2), 131–135.

Flaming, D. (2004). Nursing theories as nursing ontologies. *Nursing Philosophy, 5*(3), 224–229.

Hickman, J. (2011). *Fast facts for the faith community nurse: Implementing faith community nursing/parish nursing in a nutshell*. New York: Springer Publishing Co.

International Parish Nurse Resource Center. (2010). *International parish nursing*. http://www.parishnurses.org/InternationalParishNursing_229.aspx

Jacob, S. (Ed.). (2014). *Foundations of faith community nursing* (3rd ed.). Memphis, TN: Church Health Center.

Jacobs-Kramer, M. K., & Chinn, P. L. (1988). Perspectives on knowing: A model of nursing knowledge. *Research and Theory for Nursing Practice, 2*(2), 129.

King, I. M. (1983). *King's theory of nursing. Family health: A theoretical approach to nursing care* (pp. 177–188). New York: Wiley.

Maddox, M. (2001). Circle of Christian caring: A model for parish nursing practice. *Journal of Christian Nursing, 18*(3), 11–13. https://journals.lww.com/journalofchristiannursing/Citation/2001/18030/Circle_of_Christian_Caring__A_Model_for_Parish.4.aspx

Marsh, G. W. (1990). Refining an emergent life-style: Change theory through matrix analysis. *Advances in Nursing Science, 12*, 41–52.

Meleis, A. I. (1991). Between two cultures: Identity, roles, and health. *Health Care for Women International, 12*(4), 365–377.

Meleis, A. I. (1992). Directions for nursing theory development in the 21st century. *Nursing Science Quarterly, 5*(3), 112–117.

Meleis, A. I. (2010). *Transitions theory: Middle range and situation specific theories in nursing research and practice*. New York: Springer Publishing Company.

Meleis, A. I. (2011). *Theoretical nursing: Development and progress*. Philadelphia: Lippincott Williams & Wilkins.

Meleis, A. I., & Trangenstein, P. A. (1994). Facilitating transitions: Redefinition of the nursing mission. *Nursing Outlook, 42*(6), 255–259.

Miller, L. W. (1997). Nursing through the lens of faith: A conceptual model. *Journal of Christian Nursing, 14*(1), 17–21. https://journals.lww.com/journalofchristiannursing/Citation/1997/14010/NURSING_Through_the_Lens_of_Faith__A_Conceptual.8.aspx

Mishel, M. H. (1990). Reconceptualization of the uncertainty in illness theory. *Image: The Journal of Nursing Scholarship, 22*(4), 256–262.

Neuman, B. (1980). The Betty Neuman health-care systems model: A total person approach to patient problems. In *Conceptual models for nursing practice* (2nd ed.). New York: Appleton-Century–Crofts.

Newman, M. A. (1990). Newman's theory of health as praxis. *Nursing Science Quarterly, 3*(1), 37–41.

O'Brien, M. E. (1982). Religious faith and adjustment to long-term hemodialysis. *Journal of Religion and Health, 21*(1), 68–80.

O'Brien, M. E. (2003). Conceptual models of parish nursing practice: A middle-range theory of spiritual well-being in illness. In *Parish nursing: Healthcare ministry within the church* (pp. 99–115). Sudbury: Jones and Bartlett.

O'Brien, M. E. (2006). Parish nursing: Meeting spiritual needs of elders near the end of life. *Journal of Christian Nursing, 23*(1), 28–33.

O'Brien, M. E. (2017). *Spirituality in nursing*. Burlington, VT: Jones & Bartlett Learning.

Orem, D. E. (1983). The self-care deficit theory of nursing: A general theory. In *Family health: A theoretical approach to nursing care*. New York: Willey Medical Publications.

Parse, R. R. (1981). *Man-living-health: A theory of nursing*. New York: Wiley.

Patterson, D., & Slutz, M. (2011). Faith community/parish nursing: What's in a name? *Journal of Christian Nursing, 28*(1), 31–33.

Pearson, A., Vaughan, B., & FitzGerald, M. (2005). *Nursing models for practice*. Oxford: Elsevier Health Sciences.

Rogers, M. E. (1990). Nursing: Science of unitary, irreducible, human beings: Update 1990. *NLN Publications* 15-2285, New York, pp. 5–11.

Roy, C., & Andrews, H. A. (1999). *The Roy adaptation model* (2nd ed.). Stamford, CT: Appleton & Lange.

Schnorr, M. A. (1990). Spiritual caregiving: A key component of parish nursing. In P. A. Solari-Twadell, A. M. Djupe, & M. A. McDemott (Eds.), *Parish nursing: The developing practice* (pp. 201–219). Park Ridge, IL: National Parish Nurse Resource Center, Lutheran General Health Care System.

Watson, M. J. (1988). New dimensions of human caring theory. *Nursing Science Quarterly, 1*(4), 175–181.

Westberg, J. (2015). *The gentle rebel: The life and work of granger Westberg*. Memphis, TN: Pioneer in whole person health. Church Health Center.

Wilson, R. P. (1997). What does the parish nurse do? *Journal of Christian Nursing, 14*(1), 13–16. https://journals.lww.com/journalofchristiannursing/Citation/1997/14010/What_Does_a_Parish_Nurse_Do_.6.aspx

Ziebarth, D. (2014). Evolutionary conceptual analysis: Faith community nursing. *Journal of Religion and Health, 53*(6), 1817–1835.

Ziebarth, D. J. (2016a). Wholistic health care: Evolutionary conceptual analysis. *Journal of Religion and Health, 55*(5), 1800–1823.

Ziebarth, D. J. (2016b). Transitional care interventions as implemented by faith community nurses. *Journal of Christian Nursing, 33*(2), 112–118.

Part II

Changing the Understanding of Health: Education and Faith Community Nursing

Standardization of Educational Preparation of Faith Community Nurses

5

Susan Jacob and P. Ann Solari-Twadell

5.1 Evolution of Faith Community Nursing Education

The well-being of the professional practice and ministry of faith community nursing requires comprehensive education programs to prepare the "cadre" of providers in the specialty to meet societal needs. The rapid growth of faith community nursing from a modern day start in Park Ridge, Illinois in 1984 to international locations mandated that educational programs be developed which would: (a) provide the faith community nurse with a basic understanding of the functions of this role and role definition consistent with the Faith Community Nursing: Scope and Standards of Practice (ANA and HMA, 2017); (b) prepare the faith community nurse with an understanding of the significance of the faith community as a practice setting; (c) ensure that the understanding of health was consistent with care of the whole person; (d) stress the importance of working as part of an interprofessional team and the value of collaboration; (e) establish norms for the practice and ministry of faith community nursing in consideration of denominational differences; (f) promote an understanding of the most frequently used and essential interventions employed in the care of the whole person; (g) integrate the intentional care of the spirit as the essence of a nursing role; (h) appreciate the importance of process; (i) encourage intentional self-care; (j) emphasize the importance of knowing community resources and their payment requirements; and (k) stimulate networking among faith community nurses.

S. Jacob (✉)
Westberg Institute for Faith Community Nursing (Formerly IPNRC) a Ministry of Church Health, Memphis, TN, USA
e-mail: Jacobs@churchhealthcenter.org

P. A. Solari-Twadell
Marcella Niehoff School of Nursing, Loyola University Chicago, Chicago, IL, USA
e-mail: psolari@luc.edu

© Springer Nature Switzerland AG 2020
P. A. Solari-Twadell, D. J. Ziebarth (eds.), *Faith Community Nursing*,
https://doi.org/10.1007/978-3-030-16126-2_5

The *International Parish Nurse Resource Center* (IPNRC) was developed to provide assistance to those interested in faith community nursing. The beginning of an educational program for the then "parish" nurses was in 1987 with a one-day educational conference. This one-day conference grew into what is known today as the *Annual Westberg Symposium*. In 1989, an *Orientation to Parish Nursing* program was initiated. The structure of this educational offering was a two and one-half day program offering continuing education units which included spending a half-day with a parish nurse from Lutheran General Hospital. This programming was discontinued in 1996 when a "lengthier, evidence-based curriculum for basic preparation" was developed (McDermott & Solari-Twadell, 2006, p. 122).

In the early 1990s, educational programs flourished in parish nursing. The IPNRC documented 52 parish nurse educational programs. Collaboration was present from the beginning with 32 parish nursing programs being sponsored by health care systems, 12 that were university based, one in a seminary, and the remainder through parish nurse networks (McDermott, Solari-Twadell, & Matheus, 1998). However, the length, content, and outcomes for the programs were somewhat different. There seemed to be a difference according to region, denomination, and understanding of the role. This presented a potential problem for this innovative, community-based, spiritually oriented model of care presenting different understandings with the potential of confusing the public, particularly members of faith communities.

Faith community nursing, being part of the profession of nursing, has an inherent responsibility to be judicious in ensuring the quality of the practitioners representing the practice. Accordingly, in 1994 the IPNRC used an extended two and one-half day colloquium to engage 26 experts in parish nursing and parish nursing education, as well as clergy, to create guidelines for parish nurse education. The outcome was a document that described and differentiated parish nurse orientation, basic preparation, continuing education, and degree granting educational offerings (Solari-Twadell, McDermott, Ryan, & Djupe, 1994). Following this effort, work began with two higher education organizations: Marquette University, Milwaukee, Wisconsin and Loyola University, Chicago, Illinois. These universities served as collaborators with the IPNRC in the development of a core curriculum. The then 3000 readers of Perspectives—the quarterly newsletter published by the IPNRC—served as a source of identifying content experts for participation in the development of the core curriculum.

Once a draft of the core curriculum was developed, it was peer reviewed, and then in more detail studied, as part of another two and one-half day colloquium in April, 1997, by a panel of experts which represented ministerial leaders, parish nurses, educators, and the nursing deans of Loyola University and Marquette University. In addition, representatives of the National League for Nursing (NLN) and the American Nurses Association (ANA) participated in this meeting. Similar processes have been used to revise the core curriculum in 2004, 2009, and 2014. Revisions are currently underway for a revised curriculum that will be released in 2019.

The development of education for faith community nurses was international from the beginning with representation from Canada and Australia. Due to this involvement, Anne Van Loon from University of South Australia developed a modification of the US version in 1996. Today the "core curriculum" offered through the Westberg Institute, formerly the IPNRC, has been modified for approximately 30 countries across the world including Canada, Germany, Pakistan, South Africa, South Korea, Swaziland, UK, and Ukraine. Due to the diverse settings represented, these basic curriculum modules are adapted to match regional professional nursing standards of practice and regulations, cultural norms, geographic area, and the faith traditions of the particular location. The *Westberg Institute Foundations Course* materials now include *Guidelines for Teaching the Foundations of Faith Community Nursing Course* internationally.

5.2   Process as Content

Process dynamics are integral to the delivery and success of any faith community nurse offering. The emphasis on "process" enhances the spiritual dimension of faith community nursing. This provides an opportunity for educators to model "process" with participants. Allowing participants to experience the ministry aspects of faith community nursing practice, while affirming the integration of whole person health, supports the inclusion of experiential learning. It is important for the educator to know the faith traditions and culture of each of the participants. Inclusion of texts, rituals, prayers, music, and references from various faith traditions and cultures emphasizes sensitivity and valuing of each person's unique needs and perspectives. Also, participants can be asked to include items, experiences, or stories from their background (IPNRC, 2014).

What sets faith community nursing education apart from other continuing nursing education programs is the integration of spirituality in the curriculum. This is not just content to be assimilated in a traditional course format, but an actual "call" to serve in a ministry role for a faith community or faith-based organization. With that in mind, process dynamics include methods that help create a safe, sacred milieu for the participants. From the first greeting, to the closing or shared worship of a dedication service, process dynamics help make the Foundation's course unique and faith-filled. Classroom teaching techniques overlap closely with process dynamics, but there are distinctions. Process dynamics consciously includes humor, play time, and spiritual sharing on a personal level that often transcends commonly held beliefs about how participants learn. Outcomes related to process dynamics include: experiencing the impact of intentional hospitality for creation of a safe and inviting space; exploring the impact of hospitality in creating a safe space; revealing personal qualities through a variety of sharing exercises; and experiencing communal bonding with other participants (Church Health Center, 2019).

5.3 Standardization of Educational Preparation of Faith Community Nurses

In an attempt to maintain the integrity of the educational preparation of faith community nurses, and to distinguish the educational program development and process as inclusive of peer, national and international review, and not just another parish nurse educational offering, the terms "standardized" and "endorsed" were used to title the curricula developed through the IPNRC. The use of this language created controversy and questions within the parish nurse community. Following the development of the early curriculum, the first edition of the Parish Nursing Scope and Standards of Practice (ANA and HMA, 1998) was developed and approved by the American Nurses Association (ANA) and the Health Ministries Association (HMA). This effort headed by Norma Small from Georgetown University School of Nursing provided leadership to the declaration of "parish" nursing as a specialty nursing practice (Small, 1990). In addition to the development of standardized education for faith community nurses, as new roles emerged, new curricula were developed. In 1996, a course for parish nurse coordinators was developed, and in 1998, a course for parish nurse educators was developed through a similar developmental process to that which produced the original curriculum for parish nurses.

Foundations for Faith Community Nursing (2019) is the most recent comprehensive, evidence-based curriculum preparing licensed registered nurses for the specialized practice of faith community nursing. This curriculum focuses on the intentional care of the spirit, as well as, promotion of whole-person health and the prevention or minimization of illness within the context of a faith community and the wider community. Wholistic health and prevention or minimization of illness within the context of faith communities is foundational. Modules contain essential content that is aligned with the *Faith Community Nursing: Scope and Standards for Practice* (2017). Learning outcomes-based content outlines, critical thinking questions, group learning activities, case studies, and practical resources are included in the curriculum (Church Health Center, 2019).

5.4 Faith Community Nursing Curriculum Conceptual Model

Faith community nursing is recognized as a specialty nursing practice that combines professional nursing and health ministry. The curriculum is developed in accordance with the mission and goals of faith community nursing, as well as expected outcomes for nurses who practice within the specialty. The curriculum reflects professional nursing standards and guidelines, as well as faith community nursing standards and guidelines.

Faith community nursing emphasizes health and healing within the faith community as well as the larger community. The philosophy of this curriculum embraces four major concepts.

5.5   Foundations of Faith Community Nursing Curriculum (2014, p. 9)

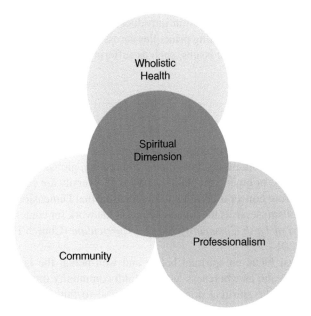

5.6   The Spiritual Dimension

The spiritual dimension is the core of faith community nursing practice. It is described as the need for meaning, purpose and fulfillment in life, the hope or will to live, and belief and faith. The spiritual dimension is important for the attainment of an overall sense of health, well-being, and quality of life. Crisis, illness, and hospitalization can affect spiritual well-being. Living out our beliefs and faith with self, others, and God or a higher power is core to faith community nursing practice.

5.7   Professionalism

Professionalism identifies parameters within which the faith community nurse practices, including *Nursing: Scope and Standards of Practice* (ANA, 2015), *Code of Ethics for Nurses with Interpretive Statements* (ANA, 2008), Faith Community Nursing: Scope and Standards of Practice (ANA and HMA, 2012, 2017), and state or country nurse practice acts. Other concepts deal with communication, collaboration, documentation, and how to begin this ministry.

5.8   Wholistic Health

The faith community nurse promotes "shalom" as a foundation for wholism, health and healing. Health promotion introduces the concepts of education, prevention, and teaching and learning principles across the life span. Wholistic health includes addressing other life issues, such as suffering, grief and loss, and family violence.

5.9   Community

A community is a group with common interests, including the faith community, professional nursing community, geographic community, global community, demographic community, or other communities. Issues of diversity are considered within this model. The four concepts (Wholistic Health, Spiritual Dimension, Community, and Professionalism) serve as the organizational framework for content units within the *Foundations of Faith Community Nursing Curriculum* (Church Health Center, 2019; IPNRC, 2014).

With a central focus on spiritual health and well-being, the faith community nurse promotes health as wholeness within a faith community through the practice of nursing. While the spiritual dimension is central to faith community nursing practice, each of the other concepts within the model (Wholistic Health, Community, and Professionalism) interacts with one or more of the other concepts, in addition to interacting with the spiritual dimension in practice.

5.10   Benefits of Standardized Curriculum

In order to ensure a minimum level of competency among faith community nurses across the U.S.A. and around the world, a standardized curriculum is essential. There is a body of common knowledge that every faith community nurse needs to know to provide nursing care with intentional care of the spirit. Standardization ensures that all faith community nurses are learning the same thing and maintain the same level of competency. At the same time, however, the curriculum administration respects educators through allowing them the flexibility, autonomy, and creativity to adapt the course to their unique participants. Standardization also provides a means of holding educators accountable for teaching specific content and using the same process dynamics. The Westberg Institute provides a peer-reviewed, outcomes-driven, evidence-based curriculum for faith community nursing with supporting resources at a reasonable cost for entities such as schools of nursing, community-based organizations, professional nursing organizations, or faith communities to become educational partners. *Foundations of Faith Community Nursing* (2014) provides learning outcomes and curriculum guidelines for educators in faith community nursing. The learning outcomes and curriculum guidelines are evidence-based and are designed to help educators meet the needs of registered nurses who work within faith communities to provide wholistic nursing with intentional care of the spirit.

5.11 Competencies and Skills

Participants in *Foundations of Faith Community Nursing* (2019) complete 36.5 hours of standardized curriculum to receive a *Certificate of Completion*. The curriculum is developed in accordance with expected outcomes for nurses who practice within the specialty. The curriculum reflects professional nursing standards and guidelines as well as faith community nursing standards and guidelines. A collection of resources that support the delivery of faith community nursing is also included in the standardized curriculum. The curriculum framework provides a set of learning outcomes that defines the content to be learned in terms of clear, definable standards and competencies of what the faith community nurse should know and be able to do. Educational partners are encouraged to establish curricular programs that support student mastery of *Foundations of Faith Community Nursing* (2019) while reflecting on their unique values which may be based in specific denominations, nations, or communities. Instructional practices should provide each participant with the best opportunity to meet these standards by supporting their specific learning needs.

There are 15 modules in the 2019 Foundations curriculum. Modules are designed to be between 2 and 4 h in length. Modules may be presented in a single group meeting, a retreat format, or online. The 2014 curriculum had a minimum of 8.5 total hours, whereas the 2019 edition is designed with 36.5 minimum total hours. The suggested order of modules (2019, pp. viii) is presented in Table 5.1.

A national Health Ministries Association (HMA) task force worked with the American Nurses Credentialing Center (ANCC) to define criteria and process for formal recognition of faith community nursing. One of the outcomes was to establish 34 contact hours of continuing education content specific to faith community nursing as the minimum course length for the preparation of this nursing specialty (ANA and HMA, 2012, p. 11).

5.12 Why a Curriculum Review?

The *Foundations for Faith Community Nursing* (IPNRC, 2014) course is on a 5-year revision cycle to reflect changes to the Scope and Standards for Faith Community Nurses, as they are periodically revised, so the nurses who receive education understand and meet the competencies and standards for the specialized practice. The revision process allows the opportunity to conduct research on how well the existing edition and content are meeting the needs of the educators who use it and considers changes in format and features. The revision process also provides the opportunity to compare the product to materials from other organizations and consider both, whether there is a need to make it more distinctive or more substantive in specific

Table 5.1 Modules

Module	Clock hours
History and philosophy	1
Health, healing, and whole-person health	2
Spiritual care	2
Prayer	2
Beginning your ministry	3
Communication and collaboration	2
Legal aspects	2
Ethical aspects	2
Documenting practice	2
Health promotion	4
Behavioral health	2.5
Violence	2
Loss, suffering, and grief	2
Assessment and accessing resources	4
Advocacy, care coordination, and transitional care	4
Total contact hours	36.5

areas. Revising the curriculum ensures that the Westberg Institute offers up-to-date materials with excellent content and presentation so nurses at the forefront of living out the "call" to care for both body and spirit have the best training possible to leverage their work in faith communities to promote whole person health. It is also important to assess the needs of faith communities based on health and illness trends affecting our society at large. The Westberg Institute solicits suggestions from faith community nurses, faith community nurse educators, and requests a comprehensive review by faith community nursing experts.

Changes in the profession based on evidence and pertinent professional documents such as white papers, position statements, and clinical guidelines need to be assessed and taken into consideration when curriculum revisions are made. Examples of important documents that are revised on a regular basis and are considered during the revision process include the Scope and Standards for Faith Community Nursing (2017), Scope and Standards of Nursing Practice (2015), Nursing Social Policy Statement (2015), Code of Ethics (2008), American Association of Colleges of Nursing (AACN) Essentials of Baccalaureate Education (2018), the Institute of Medicine Report (2011), and Healthy People 2020 Objectives (2000).

5.13   Alignment with Scope and Standards

The *Foundations of Faith Community Nursing* course (Church Health Center, 2019; IPNRC, 2014) is closely aligned with the ANA's *Scope and Standards of Professional Nursing* (2015) as well as the *Scope and Standards of Faith Community Nursing Practice* (2017). The specialty standards are integrated throughout the content and at the end of each module. Specific standards from the *Scope and Standards of Faith Community Nursing* that relate to the module content are listed at the end of each module. This listing provides clear connections between the material presented and the competencies faith community nurses should demonstrate to meet each standard.

5.14 Integrity of Curriculum

The integrity of the curriculum is maintained by educational partners who are authorized to use the material as they educate faith community nurses. Educational partner institution or organizations sign an agreement with Westberg Institute to maintain the integrity of the curriculum. Partner organizations pay fees and sign agreements to use the curriculum, so they have an investment in maintaining the standard.

Educational partners must identify a master's prepared faith community nurse to serve as lead faculty. The lead faculty must complete a *Faith Community Nursing Faculty* course before the partner organization can offer the Foundation's course. The major responsibility of the lead faculty is to provide oversight for all courses offered by the educational partner. The lead faculty ensures that the entire content is offered in a minimum of 38 contact hours. They must be present at least 80% of the time a course is offered. Educational partners may present the course material to groups of participants, whether for formal academic course credit or faith community nurse training; some partners add additional content to the basic program, but all Westberg Institute official content must be offered. Educational partners are obligated to evaluate the courses they offer and to inform participants about whether Continuing Education credit is being offered for the course. Today there are almost 150 educational partner organizations across the U.S.A. and in over 30 countries.

5.15 Collaborating for a Best Practice Education Model

The development of the educational model and curriculum for faith community nurses has been the result of collaboration with national and international faith community nurses, faculty who teach faith community nurses, and experts in the field, as well as with organizations associated with the practice. The Westberg Institute has collaborated with the Health Ministry Association, the *Healthcare Chaplaincy Network (HCCN)*, and the *Spiritual Care Association (SCA)*. Evidence and research findings have been integrated into standardized curricula that prepare faith community nurses, educators, and coordinators to provide quality evidence-based education and care in diverse settings. In April 2018, the *SCA*, an affiliate of *HCCN*, began offering faith community nurses affiliated with the Westberg Institute the following three offerings: Spiritual Care Generalist Certificate; Credentialed Chaplain (CC); and Board Certified Chaplain (BCC) training. This collaborative relationship between Westberg Institute and the SCA resulted in establishing a streamlined pathway for faith community nurses to build on their foundational knowledge to achieve additional expertise in spiritual care.

5.16   Faith Community Nurse Course for Coordinators

An evidence-based course was developed for *Faith Community Nurse Coordinators* (McDermott et al., 1998) who oversee faith community nurse programs in structured settings that are sponsored by health or community organizations. The coordinator is an individual who may also be called manager, supervisor, or director and refers to the one who is responsible for the coordination, management, networking, and/or consultation for the continuing education and spiritual development of faith community nurses within a sponsoring institution, geographic area, or region.

The success of any faith community nurse program depends on strong leadership. The coordinator role is the voice of the program and must gather support from the institution, by collecting pertinent data, reporting to administration effectively, and overseeing monetary resources wisely. To develop a quality staff, the coordinator must set standards and offer assistance, encouragement, and education while evaluating the staff for effectiveness. In the community, excellent communication skills are necessary to work with faith communities, recruit new partners, and collaborate with health professionals and community agencies. For the faith communities, the coordinator must also be available as a resource for health matters, faith concerns, and implementation (Church Health Center, 2019).

The *Faith Community Nurse Course for Coordinators* provides the knowledge and skills that are essential for leading faith community nurses in structured settings. This course includes key information that is essential for coordinators as they create, develop, and oversee faith community nursing programs. Essential knowledge includes program development, marketing, human resource management, cultural congruence and inclusion, research utilization to promote best practices, self-care, documentation, funding and grant writing, and evaluation. The course is now online and is available on demand by the Westberg Institute in partnership with the Spiritual Care Association. The curriculum is reviewed and revised on a regular basis to ensure continuity and alignment to the *Scope and Standards of Faith Community Nursing* (2017), societal changes, and best practices.

5.17   Future Trends

The *Foundations of Faith Community Nursing* (Church Health Center, 2019) courses are being offered in various modes of delivery. Face to face remains the most prevalent delivery model across the U.S.A. and around the world, but many courses are being developed as hybrid courses that are a combination of online and face to face delivery. Fewer are offered in a completely online format, but online courses are in high demand by nurses in the U.S.A. It is likely that online courses will increase in number as nurses' family and work commitments demand the flexibility afforded by online courses.

The Westberg Institute is developing *Topics in Faith Community Nursing* series that will explore a variety of subjects, issues, and themes relevant to faith community nurses and others involved in specific dimensions of health ministry. These offerings will replace the supplemental modules and draw from the dated modules as inspiration. In addition, they will serve a wider audience than the previous supplemental modules, including nurses who have not completed *Foundations* training. For faith community nurses, these books will enrich their practice by providing meaningful, engaging content around specific issues. The first two in the series are *Transitional Care* and *Advanced Spiritual Care*, both of which were presented for the first time in the 2017 *Westberg on the Road* conferences.

5.17.1 Advanced Spiritual Care

Faith community nurses bring nursing expertise along with additional education in spiritual care to their professional practice. Chaplains provide non-denominational spiritual support to those who are unable to attend organized religious services. There is an emerging blended role of the nurse chaplain using the *HCCN* guidelines for nurses to achieve a certificate as a spiritual care generalist, attend *Clinical Pastoral Education* (CPE) online courses created for nurses, and educational opportunities for nurses to become certified chaplains.

5.17.2 Transitional Care

Evidence demonstrates a critical gap in continuity of care as patients' transition to different levels of care. As the medical community focuses more and more on the importance of efficiently and effectively managing transitional care to reduce hospital readmissions, faith community nurses are being recognized for playing a vital role in transitional care. Evidence points to the effectiveness of nurse-led initiatives that focus on the individual's needs, community-based healthcare resources, and evidence-based interventions as critical to addressing this gap. Faith community nurses have the educational preparation and wholistic approach that prepares them well to provide a pivotal role in closing the gap in transitional care (Campbell, 2017).

5.18   Summary

The preparation of faith community nurses has evolved along with the role, but the early development of standards and a standardized curriculum has supported the growth of faith community nursing across the U.S.A. and globally. Having a core of knowledge and skills supports increased collaboration and cooperation across sites and denominations. As the role continues to develop, there are systems in place to allow the educational standards to include new knowledge and skill.

References

American Association of Colleges of Nursing. (2018). *The essentials of baccalaureate education for professional nursing practice* (p. 2008). Washington, DC: Author.

American Nurses Association. (2008). *Code of ethics for nurses.* Silver Spring, MD: Author.

American Nurses Association. (2015). *Nursing: Scope and standards of practice* (3rd ed.). Silver Spring, MD: Author.

American Nurses Association & Health Ministries Association. (1998). *Scope and standards of parish nursing practice.* Washington, DC: American Nurses Association.

American Nurses Association, Health Ministries Association, Inc. (2012). *Faith community nursing: Scope and standards of practice* (2nd ed.). Silver Spring, MD: Nursesbooks.org.

American Nurses Association, Health Ministries Association, Inc. (2017). *Faith community nursing: Scope and standards of practice* (3rd ed.). Silver Spring, MD: Nursesbooks.org.

Campbell, K. P. (2017). *Transitional care training guide for faith community nurses.* Memphis, TN: Church Health.

Church Health Center. (2019). *Foundations of faith community nursing curriculum, 2019 revision.* Memphis, TN: Church Health.

Institute of Medicine (US). Committee on the Robert Wood Johnson Foundation Initiative on the Future of Nursing. (2011). *The future of nursing: Leading change, advancing health.* Washington, DC: National Academies Press.

International Parish Nurse Resource Center. (2014). *Foundations of faith community nursing curriculum, 2014 revision.* Memphis, TN: Church Health.

McDermott, M. A., & Solari-Twadell, P. A. (2006). Parish nurse curricula. In P. A. Solari-Twadell & M. A. Mc Dermott (Eds.), *Parish nursing: Development, education and administration.* St. Louis, MO: Elsevier/Mosby.

McDermott, M. A., Solari-Twadell, P. A., & Matheus, R. (1998). Promoting quality education for the parish nurse and parish nurse coordinator. *Nursing Health Care Perspectives, 19*(1), 4–6.

People H, US Department of Health and Human Services. (2000). *Healthy people 2008.* Washington, DC: Office of Disease Prevention and Health Promotion, US Department of Health and Human Services.

Small, N. (1990). Curriculum development for parish nursing: An educator's perspective. In P. A. Solari-Twadell, A. M. Djupe, & M. A. McDermott (Eds.), *Parish nursing the developing practice.* Oak Brook, IL: Advocate Health Care.

Solari-Twadell, P. A., McDermott, M. A., Ryan, J., & Djupe, A. M. (1994). *Assuring the viability of for the future: Guideline development for parish nurse education programs.* Park Ridge, IL: Lutheran General Health System.

Ongoing Continuing Education and Formation of Faith Community Nurses

6

Donna Callaghan and Judy Ann Shackelford

Registered professional nurses are expected to practice according to their scope and standards of practice (ANA, 2015). Faith community nurses are also expected to practice in line with their specialty scope and standards of practice (ANA, 2017). Standard eight in Faith Community Nursing: Scope and Standards of Practice (3rd Ed) focuses on education and states "the faith community nurse attains knowledge and competence that reflect current nursing practice." Two of the competencies that are addressed in this standard are: (a) participation in ongoing educational activities related to appropriate knowledge bases, professional issues, and spiritual care and (b) demonstration of a commitment to life-long learning through self-reflection and inquiry to address learning and personal growth needs. Therefore, the nurse needs to commit to continuing their education and formation throughout their professional lives (ANA, 2017, p. 148).

Beginning with Granger Westberg's vision for wholistic health care provided by a parish nurse, the importance of ensuring current information reaches patients has always been a priority. The *International Parish Nurse Resource Center* (IPNRC), which is now known as the *Westberg Institute*, became a clearinghouse for information and the home of the foundations of parish nursing course. This preparation course became the "gold standard" for continuing education and formation of parish nurses. Currently the *Westberg Institute* is housed by the *Church Health Center* in Memphis, TN. This center provides many publications and educational programs to support faith community nurses in their quest for knowledge and spiritual formation. Since faith community nurses provide intentional care of the spirit, it is imperative that they seek both continuing education that focuses on whole person

D. Callaghan (✉)
School of Nursing, Widener University, Chester, PA, USA
e-mail: dmcallaghan@widener.edu

J. Ann Shackelford
Department of Nursing, St. John's College, Springfield, IL, USA
e-mail: judy.shackelford@sjcs.edu

© Springer Nature Switzerland AG 2020
P. A. Solari-Twadell, D. J. Ziebarth (eds.), *Faith Community Nursing*,
https://doi.org/10.1007/978-3-030-16126-2_6

health, population health and continuously attending to and nurturing their own spirituality (Westberg Institute, 2018a). The *Westberg Institute* website states the following about the importance of spiritual formation:

- The spiritual dimension is central to faith community nursing practice.
- Personal spiritual formation is an ongoing, essential component of practice for the faith community nurse and includes both self-care and hospitality, through opening the heart to self and others.
- Spiritual formation is an intentional process of intimacy with God to foster spiritual growth (WI, 2018b)

Spiritual formation opportunities may be found as face to face programs provided by the continuing education and formation resources that are identified in this chapter. However, there are numerous websites that offer free spiritual formation resources such as https://www.ignatianspirituality.com/ that can help foster a faith community nurse's journey of spiritual self-care (Ignatian Spirituality, 2018). Regional, national, and international continuing education and formation resources are accessible for the faith community nurse for ongoing continuing education. In addition, there are virtual knowledge platforms, nursing databases, and literature that are available to guide the practice of faith community nurses.

6.1   Continuing Education and Formation Resources

Demonstrating current specialized knowledge and competence takes continued professional development through continuing education and mentoring. A hallmark of faith community nursing is the spiritual context in which the nurse/patient relationship is established. In order for the faith community nurse to integrate spiritual care in a comprehensive manner into practice, personal spiritual formation is an ongoing necessity. Ongoing spiritual formation can be done on an individual basis through the relationship with a spiritual director, through faith communities, retreats or on a larger scale through local, regional, state, national, or international continuing education activities. Such activities may be free or require funding. Financial support for continuing education for faith community nurses varies. It can be self-supported or sponsored by a faith community, place of employment, partnering health care organizations, or available grants. Discounts for various continuing education activities may come as a benefit of membership from specific professional organizations.

6.2   Regional

Continuing Education (CE) may be earned through a variety of ways including but not limited to in-person classes or seminars, academic classes, teaching CE courses, or publications. CE may be offered though nursing or through participation in Clinical Pastoral Education (CPE) programs. States may vary regarding continuing education requirements for nurses in general. Each state may require and designate approved CE sponsors under the Nurse Practice Act of each State. Approved CE sponsors include several organizations and sponsors. The benefit of approved CE sponsors is that they have been vetted and meet established standards of the specified state. Approved CE sponsors are a mark of excellence when looking for CE programs because such sponsors are committed to established standards which ensure quality CE programming. The mission, vision, and/or goals of the approved CE sponsor may limit the type of CE programs offered. Dependent upon the mission or goals, CE sponsors may not provide the spiritual formation or view nursing through the lens of spiritual care. The following are a few examples of approved nursing CE sponsors:

- American Nurses Credentialing Center (ANCC) accreditors or providers
- American College of Nurse Practitioners
- American Academy of Nurse Practitioners
- Nurse Practitioner Association for Continuing Education (NPACE)
- American Association of Nurse Anesthetists
- National Association of Clinical Nurse Specialists (NACNS)
- American College of Nurse Midwives
- Providers approved by a state board of nursing
- Professional associations that provide CE in a form and manner consistent with the administrative code of the Nurse Practice Act for specific states
- Approved nursing education programs, other accredited schools, colleges, or universities, or state agencies that provide CE in a form and manner consistent with the administrative code of the Nurse Practice Act for specific states
- Programs that provide continuing medical education (CME)
- Licensed hospital employers

Additionally, academic credits may be used to fulfill CE requirements. It may be necessary for specific state administrative codes to be referenced for designated courses and conversion of academic credits to CE contact hours. The importance of seeking approved CE sponsors ensures the quality and standard of programs. Approved CE sponsor programs:

- contribute to the advancement, extension, and enhancement of professional skills and scientific knowledge in the practice of nursing;
- foster the enhancement of general or specialized nursing practice and values;
- are developed and presented by persons with education and/or experience in the subject matter of the program;
- specify the program objectives, content, and teaching methods to be used; and
- specify the number of CE hours that may be applied to fulfilling CE requirement for state licensure (Illinois Nurse Practice Act Administrative Code 2016).

The purpose of pursuing CE will assist in deciding the program that will best suit the learner's needs. If it is to maintain certification, an accredited CE sponsor or provider may be required. Seeking approved CE sponsors or providers will help guarantee the quality of the program. The faith community nurse will benefit from CE for professional development, knowledge enhancement, and skill development.

Topics pertinent to faith community nursing are those that reflect the essential knowledge for practice. Since faith community nurse's work with patients across the lifespan, they should have knowledge of the most essential and frequently used nursing interventions for practice. In addition, faith community nurses work collaboratively with clergy and health organization administrators. Topics such as professional collaboration and communication will help to promote successful inter-professional relationships.

Health System Offerings Hospitals are a source of CE for nurses in general. The CE process and focus will depend on the needs assessment of the nurses and priorities of the organization. Disease-specific topics such as obesity, diabetes, hypertension, addictions, and asthma are routinely offered. Palliative care and transitional care are growing areas in hospitals and outpatient settings, which sustains and enhances the practice of faith community nursing. Faith community nurses are considered to be a support for home-based services (Lentz, 2018). CE is commonly offered in such instances with the more contemporary expansion of the faith community nursing role. The faith community nurse may not have access as an employee but may be invited as a nurse working in the community.

University Offerings There are schools of nursing that offer the *Foundations of Faith Community Nursing* curriculum as CE and/or academic credit. The *Westberg Institute* provides current listings of schools and organizations with location, times, and contact information for *Foundations of Faith Community Nursing and Health Courses* (https://westberginstitute.org/foundations-of-faith-community-nursing/). Curriculum for these courses is specifically designed to educate and prepare nurses in the practice of faith community nursing (Westberg Institute, 2018c).

There are other universities and seminaries that offer a postmaster's graduate certificate in parish nursing. The Advanced Parish Nursing Certificate includes courses such as: Introduction to Theological Study, Research & Writing, Parish I, II, Advanced Parish Nursing, Medical Ethics, Pastoral and Spiritual Care of Introduction to Pastoral Counseling, Ministry to the Ill and Dying or Health, and Disease and Spirituality.

National Faith-Based Organizations The following are samples of national faith-based organizations that support faith community nurses formation through professional and religious organizations or denominations:

- Association of Clinical Pastoral Education is considered the recognized organization that provides high quality Clinical Pastoral Education (CPE) programs for professionals of any faith and in any setting (acpe.edu)

- Nurse Christian Fellowship (NCF)—provides information on local NCF groups and contacts, conferences, and NCF resources, including information for the *Journal of Christian Nursing* and other educational resources that may be helpful to faith community nurses.
- Catholic Health Association of the United States (CHA)—holds networking calls for faith community nurses and CE programs that support faith community nursing practice. A directory to Catholic health care organizations and news resources are provided through the organization.
- The Center for Faith-Based and Community Initiatives—supplies information and training, such as toolkits for practice and webinars.
- United Methodist Association of Health and Welfare Ministries (UMA)—provides links to information on the programs and services offered by UMA, including the Resource Center, which offers audio, video, and printed educational resources for staff and governance boards.
- Council of Health and Human Services Ministries, United Church of Christ—provides access to the group's newsletter, ecumenical links, a searchable database of member ministries, publications listings, and information on leadership development programs.
- Lutheran Church Missouri Synod (LCMS) Health Ministries—provides information on standards of care, a listing of suggested readings, organizations, and links to additional information in addition to a regular newsletter for Missouri Synod faith community nurses.

   Some other nursing organizations that offer continuing education for nurses are:
- National League of Nursing (NLN)—provides the latest news in nursing education, conference information, information on NLN continuing education programs, online nursing assessment tests, and overviews of trends in nursing education.
- The American Holistic Nurses Association (AHNA)—provides information on educational opportunities, publications, upcoming events, and links to other related websites.

6.3   Continuing Education and Development Though Faith Community Nursing Organizations

The *Westberg Institute* offers a variety of education and formation support services that are available nationally and internationally. The *Foundations of Faith Community Nursing* curriculum was developed and revised numerous times by this organization and is considered the "gold standard" of basic faith community nurse education. This basic education course has been reviewed and modified for use in several different countries and is available for international use. Beyond this course, the *Westberg Institute* offers preparation courses designed specifically for the faith community educator and coordinator. These courses have been modified for use in other countries as well. The annual *Westberg Symposium* is considered an international educational program for faith community nurse and parish nurse around the world.

This annual symposium addresses a variety of topics pertinent to the specialty practice of faith community nursing including self-care, spiritual formation, evidence-based practice, and research. *Perspectives* is a quarterly newsletter that provides the faith community nurse with the most current information on the practice. The *Westberg Institute* also developed a virtual knowledge platform for the sharing of knowledge and expertise, which will be discussed later in this chapter. The *Church Health Center* also publishes resources for faith community nurses on topics such as the integration of health and faith, advanced spiritual care, and transitional care (Westberg Institute, 2018d).

The *Health Ministries Association (HMA)* provides continuing education and formation resources for faith community nurses, pastors, and health ministry workers. The HMA is a partner with the American Nurses Association in the development of the Scope and Standards of Practice of faith community nursing. The HMA organization offers workshops on the updated scope and standards of practice as new editions are published. The organization's *Faith Community Nurse Mentor Program* links the novice faith community nurse with an experienced faith community nurse to provide mentoring for the new faith community nurse (Health Ministries Association, n.d.).

Faith Community Nurses International (FCNI) has an *Education Committee* that promotes and supports the professional development of the faith community nurse through identifying needs and providing educational resources for their members and the greater faith community nurse community. The Research Committee of the organization promotes and supports faith community nursing research by providing resources related to the development, implementation, and evaluation of research projects; establishing a network of faith community nurse researchers that can provide guidance and expertise to its members; and focusing on the importance of documentation of faith community nursing interventions, outcomes, and activities providing a rich data source for faith community nursing research projects (Faith Community Nurses International, 2018a, 2018b). FCNI research committee coordinated the research Faith Community Research Forum as part of the Westberg Symposium.

Opportunities may arise for individuals or groups to provide a CE activity who are not an approved sponsor for CE. In such cases, the following best practices should be followed to facilitate excellence in programming:

1. Identify an approved sponsor for CE to provide contact hours. Most State Nurse Practice Acts will address this in the Education Section of the Act. State and National Nursing Associations are providers of continuing education and can be a resource for inquiry and support. Connecting with an approved sponsor for CE from the beginning is a criterion for success. The sponsor will guide the planning steps to ensure quality of the program.
2. Identify the learning gap or need of the audience. The learning gap will determine the topic for the CE activity and serve as a context for the goal/outcomes of the program.

3. Find a speaker who is expert in the topic and skilled in presenting. Speakers should be vetted to ensure quality presentation and expertise.
4. Plan the program content to achieve the specified goal/outcomes. It is helpful to have a planning committee which includes a content expert which can be helpful in selecting excellent speakers on the selected topic.
5. Determine how the program goal/outcomes will be evaluated.
6. Determine the contact hours from the program content, anticipated delivery time, and strategies for delivering the identified content.
7. The date, time, and venue of the CE activity should be based on the audience preference/availability which should coincide with the speaker availability and skill set.
8. Market to the target audience at least 4–6 weeks in advance.
9. It is imperative that the CE activity be presented without bias. This can be met by having the speaker and planners complete "conflict of interest" forms. These forms verify that no conflict of interest exists for program developers, sponsors, or presenters. Conflict of interest forms are available from approved CE providers or approvers.

The logistics of conducting the CE activity should be thought out to maximize the desired learning objectives and outcomes. The venue should be selected based on audience ability to access the facility, ease of attending, comfort, and aesthetic environment conducive to learning. Logistical planning may require technology coordination or practice checks for webinars or venues requiring use of technology equipment. Obtaining speaker presentations files for preview and set-up prior to the CE event provides time to deal with any unexpected technical difficulties. Registration needs to be coordinated with marketing to allow for sign-up and payment if necessary and to check-in attendees the day of the event. Determinations regarding refunds should be made prior to marketing the event. Lastly, evaluation of the CE activity is important to determine attainment of goals/objectives/outcomes. Often times, evaluation is required by attendees as part of successful completion to obtain the CE certificate for contact hours.

6.4 Continuing Education and Development Through Virtual Knowledge Platforms

Technology and virtual knowledge platforms support and expand CE opportunities for faith community nurses. *ZOOM* is a free, user-friendly, online program that allows for synchronous and asynchronous meetings. The *ZOOM* connection can be on a computer or mobile device. This electronic platform enhances CE opportunities nationally and internationally. *Free conference call.com* provides a means for audio CE opportunities nationally and internationally. Webinars and Adobe Connect are other available programs used for CE with an associated cost, which may be prohibitive for some faith community nurse users. A virtual knowledge platform is an efficient and effective way to share knowledge, best practices, and research among faith community nurses. This technology can be a means of strengthening web-based knowledge and networking among faith community nurses as an advanced tool for knowledge repositories providing broad social networking (Ziebarth & Hunter, 2016).

6.5   Continuing Education and Development Through a Knowledge Platform for Faith Community Nurses

The *Westberg Institute* was innovative and undertook the development of a virtual knowledge platform for faith community nurses. The purpose of this platform is intended to facilitate the sharing of knowledge, resources, and best practices. This platform benefits faith community nurses nationally and internationally who often practice in isolation and do not have resources for CE or mentoring. The Knowledge Sharing Platform was launched in *Yammer* in 2016. This platform can be accessed by an invitation from the *Westberg Institute*. This innovative electronic platform acknowledges that faith community nursing is the first nursing specialty to develop such a virtual knowledge platform. This platform was created "to (1) collect, store, and manage resources in a repository that is accessible to practicing faith community nurses, (2) maintain a broad stream of faith community nursing communication exchange directed to leaders in nursing, nurse education, healthcare, denominational, and governmental agencies, (3) manage intentional messaging regarding evidence-based and best faith community nursing practices as well as serve as a resource on faith community research, and (4) have an easy-to-use social media component that allows individuals and group "real-time" discussions that incorporate text and attachments" (Ziebarth & Hunter, 2016, p. 3).

There are seven Westberg Institute led groups on *Yammer.* They are (1) *Coordinators and Managers*, (2) *Educators*, (3) *World Forum*, (4) *Research*, (5) *Church Health Center Resources*, (6) *The faith community nursing newsletter, Perspectives Digital Archive*, and (7). *All Network* groups combined number over 1200 faith community nurse participants. The *Perspectives* group provides past newsletters that are uploaded in the shared files for this group. The platform also allows for members of Yammer to create their own groups such as local, regional, state, national, and international faith community nursing organizations. At present, there are over 80 identified groups related to faith community nursing using this platform to communicate and connect. The *All Network* group on the platform is used by many faith community nurses to ask others a variety of questions.

6.6   The Westberg Institute's Position Statements Contribution to Professional Development

The *Westberg Institute* offers resources to faith community nurses directly on best practice through six position statements. Five were published in *Perspectives* starting in the summer of 2015 and continued through the summer 2016. The sixth position paper explores the faith community nurse's role in transitional care. It was shared on

Yammer in the summer of 2018. The seventh position paper addresses "Research and Scholarship" and is included as an appendix to Chapter 25 in this text (Dyess and Solari-Twadell, 2018). The position statements were developed as a result of extensive review of current literature and internal review of leadership within the *Westberg Institute*. The position statements were also presented at the *Annual Westberg Symposium*. The topics for these position statements were chosen based on the frequency of questions the *Westberg Institute* received from practicing faith community nurses. These position statements are housed on the virtual platform, *Yammer*, in the Research Group under files. They are also available and free to the general public by contacting the *Westberg Institute* (https://westberginstitute.org/).

The first position statement published is titled *Faith Community Nursing Compared to Other Nursing Specialties* (Ziebarth, 2015a). This position statement responded to the following questions:

- How is faith community nursing similar to other nursing specialties?
- How is faith community nursing practice different?
- How can faith community nursing be summarized?

The position statement clarified that all of nursing practice is under the legal authority of each state's Nurse Practice Acts and policies. In addition, all are guided by the Nursing: Scope and Standards of Practice. They are also guided by individualized specialty scope and standards of practice (Ziebarth, 2015a).

It also identified the three most noted definitions of Faith Community Nursing, which are:

> … specialized practice of professional nursing that focuses on the intentional care of the spirit as part of the process of promoting wholistic health and preventing or minimizing illness in a faith community.

> … care that supports and facilitates: physical functioning; psychological functioning and lifestyle change, with particular emphasis on coping assistance and spiritual care; protection against harm; the family unit; effective use of the health system; and health of the congregation and community.

> … a method of health care delivery that is centered in a relationship between the nurse and client (client as person, family, group, or community). The relationship occurs in an iterative motion over time when the client seeks or is targeted for wholistic health care with the goal of optimal wholistic health functioning. Faith integrating is a continuous occurring attribute. Health promoting, disease managing, coordinating, empowering and accessing health care are other essential attributes. All essential attributes occur with intentionality in a faith community, home, health institution and other community settings with fluidity as part of a community, national, or global health initiative.

The second position statement published is titled *Faith Community Nursing: Direct Care of "Hands-On" Practice and Glucose Testing* (Ziebarth, 2015b). This position statement responded to the following questions:

1. Should faith community nursing be a "hands-on" versus "hands-off" nursing practice?

2. Can faith community nurses (FCNs) do glucose testing?

The position statement stated that:

Even though there are several faith community nursing interventions that are considered "hands-off," a skill set that all nurses should have is the ability to do a physical assessment. A thorough physical assessment requires "hands-on" the patient's body to auscultate breath sounds, assess lymph nodes, palpate pulses, and assess skin turgor, and so on, especially if the patient was recently discharged from a hospital or has a chronic disease.... (Ziebarth, 2015b)

The position statement reminded us that our goal in demonstrating glucose testing should always be patient self-management and self-efficacy. It stated that, "it is preferred to have the patient demonstrate a finger-stick to the [faith community nurse] than the other way around" (p. 2).

The third position statement is entitled, *Faith Community Nursing and Home Health Nursing* (Ziebarth, 2015c) and clarified the similarities and differences between these two specialty nursing practices. A faith community nurse can practice with the knowledge and skills of a professional registered nurse, but does not replace a home health nurse, if there is a home health nurse visiting a client. The faith community nurse complements, not duplicates nursing care in this situation (Ziebarth, 2015c).

The fourth position statement published is *Wholistic Health* which clarifies the similarities and differences between *Wholistic* and *Holistic* Nursing. The wholistic care that a faith community nurse provides focuses on the intentional care of the spirit as part of the process of promoting health and preventing or minimizing illness (Ziebarth, 2016a). For an in-depth discussion of the use of the terms *wholistic* and *holistic,* please refer to Chapter 3 in this book.

The fifth position statement published by the *Westberg Institute* is titled *Documentation* (Ziebarth, 2016b), which reiterates the professional practice requirement to document the nursing process as stated in the scope and standards of practice and in each state's nurse practice acts. Documentation can protect the nurse against the risk of legal action such as a malpractice law suit. Documentation also is critical for tracking client outcomes (Ziebarth, 2016b).

The sixth position statement addresses faith community nursing and transitional care (Ziebarth, 2018). An in-depth discussion of this topic is offered in Chapter 21. The seventh position paper discusses Research and Scholarship along with reporting on the research agenda for faith community nursing. Further information on this position paper can be found in Chapter 25 (Dyess & Solari-Twadell, 2018).

6.7   Continuing Education and Development Through Nursing Literature

The hallmark of a professional organization is having an associated professional journal. The peer-reviewed *International Journal of Faith Community Nursing* is the official journal of this professional nursing organization, *Faith Community Nurses International.* More information on this organization is provided in

Chapter 17 of this text. The *Journal of Christian Nursing* is a peer-reviewed journal of *Nursing Christian Fellowship*, a religious-based nursing organization which has assisted nurses to integrate issues of faith and nursing since 1984. *Perspectives* the faith community nursing newsletter produced by the *Westberg Institute* includes research news and educational articles, along with faith community nursing practice reflections.

Along with literature specific to faith community nursing, different religious denominations may make information available through printed journals or newsletters. An example is the *Catholic Health Association of the United States* which has several publications that are applicable to faith community nurses. *Health Progress* is the official journal of the *Catholic Health Association* and features articles important to the Catholic health ministry including community benefit, continuum of care, ethics advocacy, and public policy to name a few topics. *Health Care Ethics U.S.A.* is a newsletter jointly published by *Catholic Health Association* and the *Center for Health Care Ethics at Saint Louis University* which provides ideas, ethical analyses, and reflections, leading practices, policies, tools, case studies, and literature reviews from ethicists. Two other publications available only to *Catholic Health Association* members are the *Catholic Health World* newspaper featuring current news and information.

Journals available through general nursing organizations that are not faith based can offer practice support to faith community nurses dependent on the learning or professional development needs of the individual nurse. Databases that help to identify evidence-based practices are the *Cochrane Library* and the *Joanna Briggs Institute*. In addition, The Agency for Healthcare Research and Quality (AHRQ) under the Department of Health and Human Services invests in research and evidence to make health care safer (https://www.ahrq.gov/). AHRQ is a beneficial reference for evidence and research related to specific topics of interest such as strategies to better addiction prevention. Another helpful nursing database is the *Cumulative Index of Nursing and Allied Health Literature (CINAHL)*. This database is the largest and most in-depth nursing research database (https://health.ebsco.com/products/cinahl-plus-with-full-text). EBSCOhost is an online reference system which offers a variety of full text databases including CINAHL (https://www.ebsco.com/about). Nursing databases and literature are valuable resources in identifying topics of interest and CE for the faith community nurse that could provide information on best practices, new disease-specific information, and/or professional development that can enhance the knowledge, skills, and attitudes of the faith community nurse.

6.8   Additional International Educational Opportunities

The first *European Conference on Parish Nursing* was held from November 21 to 24, 2016 at the Deaconess Guesthouse, in Lachen Speyer-dorf, near Neustadt, Germany. Angela Glasser was the coordinator of the conference. Participants at this conference included 16 attendees from Germany, three from Finland, six from the Ukraine, two from the Netherlands, three from the U.S.A., and three from the

UK. The focus of this international conference was "learning from other countries." The keynote speaker was P. Ann Solari-Twadell, who spoke to the role of the congregation in whole person health.

More recently in June 2018, a second *European Conference on Parish Nursing* was held in Finland. Through the work of Reverend Helen Wordsworth, Parish Nursing Ministries, UK in collaboration with parish nursing leadership from other countries, it is anticipated that every 2 years that there will be an international parish nurse conference sponsored by a different country in Europe. This cross fertilization from the participation of different countries enriches the understanding of parish nursing while providing for the development of a wide network of parish nurses to get to know who each other are and enable connection for support, mentoring, ongoing education, and spiritual formation.

6.9 Conclusion

Whether this professional health ministry, which is coordinated through the "call" and work of a registered professional nurse is in the U.S.A., Germany, United Kingdom, Australia, Swaziland, Finland, Croatia or Asia, the nurse that responds to participation in this health ministry is required to ensure that there is regular involvement in ongoing continuing education. Today with the availability of electronic resources the availability of ongoing continuing education for faith community and parish nurses is more available and accessible. Undergirding all continuing education is the foundation of helping people to change their thinking and understanding of the meaning of health. Only through this foundational work will individuals be able to understand the value of personal responsibility for health resources personally and communally.

References

Agency for Healthcare Research and Quality. (n.d.). *Advancing excellence in health care*. Retrieved from https://www.ahrq.gov/
American Nurses Association. (2015). *Nursing: Scope and standards of practice* (3rd ed.). Washington, DC: Author.
American Nurses Association. (2017). *Faith community nursing: Scope and standards of practice* (3rd ed.). Washington, DC: Author.
Catholic Health Association of the United States. (n.d.). *CHA Publications*. Retrieved from https://www.chausa.org/publications/cha-publications
Dyess S, and Solari-Twadell PA. (2018). Scholarship and Research. In Solari-Twadell, P.A. and Ziebarth, D. (2019) Faith community nursing: Changing the understanding of health. Springer, Switzerland.
EBSCO. (n.d.). *About EBSCO*. Retrieved from https://www.ebsco.com/about
EBSCO Health. (n.d.). *CINAHL plus with full text*. Retrieved from https://health.ebsco.com/products/cinahl-plus-with-full-text
Faith Community Nurses International. (2018a). *Faith Community Nurses International*. https://www.fcninternational.org/

Faith Community Nurses International. (2018b). *International Journal of Faith Community Nursing*. Retrieved from https://digitalcommons.wku.edu/ijfcn/

Health Ministries Association. (n.d.). *Health Ministries Association*. Retrieved from https://hmassoc.org/

Ignatian Spirituality. (2018). *The spiritual exercises*. Retrieved from https://www.ignatianspirituality.com/

Lentz, J. (2018). An innovative role for faith community nursing palliative care. *Journal of Christian Nursing, 35*(2), 113–119.

Westberg Institute for Faith Community Nursing. (2018a). *The mission*. Retrieved from https://westberginstitute.org/history-mission/

Westberg Institute for Faith Community Nursing. (2018b). *Philosophy of faith community nursing*. Retrieved from https://westberginstitute.org/philosophy-of-parish-nursing/

Westberg Institute for Faith Community Nursing. (2018c). *Foundations of faith community nursing*. Retrieved from https://westberginstitute.org/foundations-of-faith-community-nursing/

Westberg Institute for Faith Community Nursing. (2018d). *Westberg Institute*. Retrieved from https://westberginstitute.org/

Ziebarth, D. (2015a). Faith community nursing compared to other nursing specialties. *Perspectives, 14*(2), 8–9.

Ziebarth, D. (2015b). Faith community nursing: Direct care or "hands-on" practice and glucose testing. *Perspectives, 14*(3), 8–9.

Ziebarth, D. (2015c). Faith community nursing and home health nursing. *Perspectives, 14*(4), 6–7.

Ziebarth, D. (2016a). Faith community nursing and wholistic health. *Perspectives, 15*(1), 8–11.

Ziebarth, D. (2016b). Faith community nursing and documentation. *Perspectives, 15*(2), 10–11.

Ziebarth, D. (2018). *Faith community nursing and transitional care*. Westberg Institute E Notes. Retrieved from https://westberginstitute.org/

Ziebarth, D., & Hunter, C. (2016). Moving toward a virtual knowledge platform for faith community nurses. *Computers, Informatics, Nursing, 34*, 503–512.

Documenting Models of Faith Community Nursing: Educational Perspectives

P. Ann Solari-Twadell and Ameldia R. Brown

7.1 Faith Community Nursing Organizational Models

Exploration, discussion, and education regarding the different organizational models engaged in supporting faith community nursing programs have been taking place since early in the evolution of this specialty practice. Solari-Twadell presented four organizational models and how these models were positioned to provide essential structure and ongoing education for faith community nursing practice in 1990 (p. 75) (Table 7.1). A workshop at the Annual Westberg Symposium in 1994 also revealed research findings as a result of surveys that were completed by faith community nurses regarding organizational models that were employed to support their practice (Lloyd & Solari-Twadell, 1994). This led to a Matrix Planning Tool rather than a prescribed table of organizational models (Table 7.2). Findings from ongoing studies of the organizational models yielded identification for more direction on what was important in developing a parish nurse program and providing ongoing education than prescribing what should be included in each model. The study of the organizational models which were employed in supporting faith community nursing practice and the programs they function within continued to be studied in 2002. There are pros and cons to each model of faith community nursing. However, education is at the foundation of the development of any model that is being established to support faith community nursing.

The interest in understanding the organizational models was an attempt to learn how the faith community nursing movement was developing across the U.S.A. Faith

P. A. Solari-Twadell (✉)
Marcella Niehoff School of Nursing, Loyola University Chicago, Chicago, IL, USA
e-mail: psolari@luc.edu

A. R. Brown
Department of Faith and Community Health, Henry Ford Macomb Hospitals, Henry Ford Health System, Clinton Township, MI, USA
e-mail: abrown1@hfhs.org

© Springer Nature Switzerland AG 2020
P. A. Solari-Twadell, D. J. Ziebarth (eds.), *Faith Community Nursing*,
https://doi.org/10.1007/978-3-030-16126-2_7

Table 7.1 Models

Models support	Hospital sponsored salaried	Congregation sponsored salaried	Hospital sponsored volunteer	Congregation sponsored volunteer
Orientation	X		X	
Supervision	X	X	X	X
– Pastoral	X	X	X	X
– Nursing	X		X	
Liability insurance	X	?		
Continuing education	X		X	
Physician availability	X	?	X	?
Benefits	X	?		
Peer support	X		X	
Identification of resources	X		X	
Networking	X		X	
Reimbursement	X			

Solari-Twadell (1990), p. 75

Table 7.2 Matrix planning tool to use in developing parish nurse programs

	Institutional paid	Institutional unpaid	Congregational paid	Congregational unpaid
Education and consultation				
Paid or unpaid				
Advertising interview selection				
Basic preparation and orientation				
Continuing education				
Networking				
Liability insurance				
Supervision of nursing and pastoral counseling				
Benefits				
Documentation system				
Position description				
Physician consultation				
Grants				

Solari-Twadell (1999), p. 21

community nursing is very flexible in meeting client's needs as a practice. This ministry and practice usually takes shape around the needs and resources of the faith community and the skills of the nurse. This professional model of health ministry through the faith community nurse responds to the presenting need. The organizational model and practice usually precedes the ministry and the nurse's role and function within the faith community. Today, however, the faith community nursing movement is in a different time, political climate, and developmental period. Rather than letting the development, education, and sustainability depend on the resources and intention of the developers, there needs to be more thought and consideration in developing this ministry and practice to ensure sustainability through documenting fully the contribution this role is making to health care improvement and ultimately quality patient care. Rather than saying a "paid" faith community nursing practice is better than "unpaid," "or "institutional" model is better than a "congregation model" and haggling over form and function, perhaps it is more prudent to study a model that has both paid and unpaid faith community nurses, has sustained over time and is able to document outcomes. How can these models be replicated? The following is a case study exemplifying such a model.

7.2   Community-Based Institutionally Supported Network Model of Faith Community Nursing

This is a model in which a health care system or hospital acts as the convener and host agent for faith community partners that are interested in the ministry of faith community nursing. Paid staff from the health care institution facilitates the relationships with key stakeholders in the faith community and community at large. The institution is the "glue" of the Network in that it acts as a well-organized, funded, and established partner with like values. Through this relationship, accountability is built in through contracts with the faith community and faith community nurse. The Network requires a contract with the faith community and the health care institution. There is also the requirement that the faith community has a separate contract with the faith community nurse. A basic contract is provided by the health care institution and allows for modification by the faith community that is agreed upon by all parties. The health care institution is the primary convener for the faith community nurse through monthly meetings. Faith community nurses are required to attend at least 50% of the Network meetings sponsored by the health care system.

The institution or health care system becomes the lead "Network Administrator" through employment of dedicated paid staff. The Network uses participation and consensus of partners to design projects. Examples of projects that have been implemented with input from faith community partners are a diabetes prevention program, an intergenerational senior safety program and advanced care planning projects. The partners include the faith communities who meet defined criteria. The criteria include that the faith community needs to (1) be located within a specific geographically area, (2) agree to have a contract with the faith community nurse, (3) participate in one network chosen project per year, (4) the *Foundations of Faith Community Nursing* course must be completed, (5) agree to participate in an annual faith community nurse 360 performance appraisal, and (6) support the faith community nurse to use the electronic documentation system developed by the health care institution. As the identified projects are implemented, education is provided by the institution or health care institution to ensure competency of the faith community nurse in the designated project.

Each faith community partner maintains its independence and separate "owner-ship" of their faith community while agreeing to a mission, vision, key objectives, goals, and strategies for the Network. These particular ingredients of the Network are established by a design team made up of institutional employees, different denominations, faith communities, and clergy. The health care institution provides needed resources requested by the faith communities for all Network project designs or as requested by individual partners for projects. The health care institution also serves as a catalyst to direct resources to address health issues, disease patterns, and social needs as identified through an evidence-based community assessment. The institution also provides for and promotes professional development of its partners' faith community nurses and health team members.

The Network often chooses a nursing theory to direct and develop its projects and activities. For example, for this Network, Patricia E. Benner's theory described in her book *From Novice to Expert: Excellence and Power in Clinical Nursing Practice* (Benner, 1984) provided a framework to assist in the formation and devel-opment of faith community nurses. This work engaged these nurses in their own professional development. This was a multi-year project of purchasing the Benner (1984) authored book, using Network meetings to discuss the levels of nursing prac-tice noted in the book and applying this knowledge to advance the faith community nurse. The performance appraisal instrument of the health care institution was also modified as part of this theory application to reflect the levels of nursing practice noted in Benner's (1984) text (Appendix). Data that was collected over the 3-year time frame of this project reflected that the use of this theoretical framework encour-aged the faith community nurses to understand their role as one of professional practice for which they were accountable.

For faith communities that intend to pay their faith community nurses, the salary or payment method is determined solely by the faith community. Different payment methods for paid faith community nurses include: use of a stipend, include only benefits, and/or hourly/salaried payment for services. The money to pay the faith community nurse is generated by the faith community.

Essential to the success of this organizational model is the mindset on the part of each of the members, including the health care system, that each partner has value and brings an important ingredient to the table in assuring the health of the faith community and the community at large. Establishment of a solid working relation-ship requires each party to value the other. The mindset of the health care institution is that "if we go away, the faith community will be able to carry on its' health min-istry with self-sufficiency." The faith community is not seen as being dependent upon the health care institution, but enhanced through a relationship with the health care institution. The health care institution's perception of the Network relationship with faith communities is very positive providing better care of the patient in a cost-effective manner. There is a mutual recognition by the health institution, faith com-munities, faith community nurse, and targeted community populations of the value in maintaining the collaboration and partnership through this Network.

The US government has imposed a regulatory requirement that health care agen-cies with a 501 C(3) tax exempt status tangibly demonstrate and report dollars spent on community benefit based on a systematic assessment of the health needs of the community served (nlm.nih.gov/hrsainfo/community_benefit.html). Increasingly, the community health needs assessment has become a base for which this model of faith community nursing Network can build commonality by acting as a strategic collaborative partner in addressing identified needs.

7.3 Benefits to Partnering or Establishing a Faith Community Network

There are many advantages to a health care institution investing in a faith community network (see Table 7.3). The mission of a faith community is health and salvation, no matter what the denomination (Solari-Twadell, 1999, p. 9). The health care institution in relationship with a faith community can assist that faith community in retrieving and actualizing its health ministry to benefit not only its members, but the

Table 7.3 Institutional health care system benefits for engaging in and supporting a faith community nursing network

1. Social accountability	Faith community nursing is a concrete manner of documenting services to the community at large
2. Market share	Through collaborating with faith communities with like values a health care system is creating and increasing market share which can result in referrals
3. Early access	Faith community nursing supports the health care system to be in relationship with people in the community in their episodes of wellness as well as their episodes of illness creating early access to identification and referral
4. Increase of volunteers	With a collaborative relationship in place with a faith community which encourages service, the health care system or institution could benefit by a ready source of faith-based volunteers
5. Cost-effective care	With the ability to diagnose people earlier in their disease pattern, the cost of an episode of illness would be decreased by earlier intervention and treatment
6. Built in continuum of care	Faith community nurses develop relationships with members at all levels of health. The faith community nurse can refer and follow a client throughout their course of treatment from referral to admission to discharge and ongoing
7. Decreased readmission	Faith community nurses connect and meet regularly with individuals that have recently been hospitalized. The faith community nurse can identify early problems and intervene before the problem necessitates readmission. This results in health care savings for the client, health care system, and insurance company
8. Better health outcomes	The faith community knows the lifestyle and health decisions that clients make over time. Due to that knowledge, the faith community nurse can provide information providers may need regarding the patient, their family, and resources available through the faith community or community at large

(continued)

Table 7.3 (continued)

9. Provision of patient-centered care	By the nature of the faith community nurse role, the nurse tailors the care provided based on who the client is, their culture, personal requests, and faith beliefs and values always taking into consideration the unique needs of the person
10. Stewardship of health resources	Health care today requires that people be better stewards of their personal and communal health resources. Through the work of the faith community nurse, undergirded by the beliefs and values inherent in the faith community, the nurse can educate the individual, faith community, and community at large on a whole person understanding of health, how to make better choices to support health on a daily basis and live those choices counter culture to what may be professed by society at large
11. Community assessment	Health care systems and institutions are often interested in assessing the needs of the community. Through relationships with local faith communities that process may be facilitated
12. Population-based health care	Having the ability to identify populations at risk and deliver programming that can intervene in chronic illness patterns for specific populations is important today. Health care institutions and organizations that network with multiple faith communities may find that in working through a network of faith community nurses that outcomes of health promotion programming can have a more significant impact
13. Advocacy/ health advocate	Today it is more and more important for a patient to have a health advocate that is knowledgeable and understands the changing delivery of health care as well as health care reimbursement. The faith community nurse given the relationship developed with clients over time is in an ideal position to provide that service to clients. Presence of a health advocate can facilitate improved patient care and support to client and patient at end of life
14. Community-based health promotion partner	Many health care organizations struggle with providing health promotion in a cost-effective, organized manner in the community. Through networking with faith communities over time a natural conduit for dissemination of health promotion information, education, and resources can be made available through faith communities
15. Partner in health care reform	True health care reform requires the inclusion of the community as well as innovative strategies that maintain person-centered care, are cost effective, emphasize personal responsibility and include support in addition to ongoing engagement with a continuum of care. A faith community network in partnership with a health care system is a contemporary viable response to this need

community at large. Another benefit is that the health care system is aligning itself with agencies or faith communities that have a similar mission of supporting the best health outcomes and function for its members. For many people they are baptized and buried from the same faith community. In other words, they live their lives in a same geographic area for the length of their life through participation in their faith community. An institution, in partnership with a faith community, can support that individual and their family over a life span creating a consistent market share for the health care system in partnership with multiple faith communities. At the same time, a partnership between a faith community and health care system facilitates the health care system intentionally focusing their resources on addressing identified needs in collaboration with like-minded partners. Faith communities are instrumental in the formation of personal beliefs and values (National Information Center on Health Services Research and Health Care Technology, 2018). When a health ministry is active through a faith community nurse the gospel message of the individual responsibility or being a steward of their personal health resources can be reiterated through ritual, readings, and education provided in the faith community. The ongoing formation of health values through participation in the life of a faith community, that includes a faith community nurse ministry, can assist people over time to make better decisions regarding their health. The consistency of participation in a faith community and the repetitive message that is projected through a health ministry may prevent the development of debilitating and costly chronic disease pattern. The faith community can also foster the idea that "health is not an end in itself, but a means to serve life's purposes" (Foege, 1990). In other words, it is much easier to have the energy and ability to be in service to another, if one is feeling well and is of good health physically, spiritually, and emotionally. The faith community also has a built-in support system for its members. Small groups can easily form over common interests including disease patterns. Also, many individuals establish life-long friends through ongoing participation in a faith community which provides ongoing support. These friends are there to support, bring food, and be present during illness and recovery providing needed support. Faith communities regularly provide educational programs and support groups for its membership (Solari-Twadell, 1997).

A health care institution in partnership with a faith community can provide speakers and small group facilitators. These speakers and facilitators can bring needed expertise to faith community members, faith community leaders, and people from the community at large in a site where most are comfortable in learning new ways to make decisions. For most faith communities, the mindset of "health care as a business" is not present. Resources provided by a health care system to provide education can effectively be disseminated in a knowledgeable manner by a faith community nurse. The institutional Network model of faith community nursing can fill in gaps that most faith communities would otherwise experience as a community seeks to responsibly implement faith community nursing as a part of its ministry. In this model, the institution contributes to its Network members' "amenities" through the signed contract. These amenities include leadership, administrative and professional expertise, knowledge, and development related to the professional practice of nursing, instructional technology, and communication services at levels that most faith communities are unable to provide. Library and research access, a systematic approach to health promotion and care, clinical analysts, pharmacists, physicians, finance specialist, legal support, and a myriad of other professionals essential to health care operations. Resource allocation and access are dependent on the assets and resources of the faith community. For every area of health care that may touch the faith community and its members, the institutional Network model provides the faith community nurse with a contact and "inside" referral to the health care system. Resources such as ambulatory services, urgent and emergency care centers, hospice and home care services, testing areas, affiliated long-term care, public health partners, government agencies, educational resources, and other community partners may be made available.

Faith communities contribute human resources to the Network through the faith community nurse and health ministry team. A partnering faith community serves as a desirable community to focus population health care interventions. Faith communities gain by having health care needs addressed by a person of faith in collaboration with and sometimes guided by an expert, the health care institution. Quality of care services, health education, mutuality of purpose, and accountability to health care regulations can all be enhanced for the faith community through the relationship with a Network and health care institution The faith community, faith community nurse, and health ministry team are able to collaborate with a team from the health care institution through the Network that understands and respects its language, culture, and strengths while addressing its needs and frailties from an approach that integrates science and culture.

7.4   Education for the Faith Community Nurse

Education of partners representing the faith community, institution, and community at large is essential to the development, implementation, promulgation, and sustainability of an institutional Network supporting a faith community nursing program. Most essential is the education of the nurse who is to deliver the service. The *Faith Community Nursing Scope and Standards* states in Standard Twelve "The faith community nurse seeks knowledge and competencies that reflects current nursing practice and promotes futuristic thinking" (ANA and HMA, 2017, p. 73). In addition, the Scope and Standards note that the "faith community nurse bridges two domains and therefore must be prepared in and responsible for both professional nursing practice and spiritual care" (p. 25). Culturally congruent care is also an important content area for faith community nurses to be able to demonstrate competency. Culturally competent care "requires that the nurse has self-awareness of personal cultural identity, heritage and values as well as engagement in life-long learning to understand the culture of others" (ANA, 2015, p. 32). Education includes information not only on the foundation of faith community nursing, health ministry, and spiritual care, but also on the specifics of relationship development. Organizational Structures and information unique to the denomination and community the nurse will be collaborating with is important to include in assisting the faith community nurse to be better prepared.

One creative strategy employed by the health care institution for the purpose of engaging faith community nurses in ongoing education is a *Journal Club*. The faith community nurses can suggest up to three articles that will be distributed and read by all Network faith community nurses. When the nurses convene, they discuss the designated articles drawing out those elements important to their development as faith community nurses. *Case Studies* are another modality that can enrich the development and education of faith community nurses. Faith community nurses in the Network volunteer to present a case from their practice in a "verbatim" format in which the case is described. Faith community nurses can then discuss various strategies for addressing the main problems presented through the case study. *Webinars* are another format for delivery of faith community nursing education through the Network. The use of a webinar does not require the nurse to travel and provides easy access.

Faith community nursing education can also be provided with a focus over time. For example, a series on spiritual care providing continuing education units (CEUs) was presented over a 6-month period through the Network in this case study. The CEUs provided upon completion of this series were a benefit for the faith community nurses who needed designated numbers of CEUs to renew their professional nursing license. Also, through a relationship with a health care system Network, the faith community nurse is invited to attend any continuing education offerings available through the health care system. Educational offerings can provide the latest treatment information and outcomes on specific chronic diseases and ongoing continuing learning opportunities for the faith community nurse.

7.5 Hospital Leadership and Administrators

From the health care institution, designated leaders, administrators, physicians, in patient nurses, and other staff working in and with departments, such as community outreach, population health, ambulatory services, palliative, home, and hospice care, need to be updated regularly about faith community partnerships. Education on the faith community Network needs to extend from the President and Chief Executive Officer to the front desk, including clerical staff responsible for registering patients. Education is strategically designed and delivered in a format to capture the attention of each position providing the essence of the content in a concise, practical, and cohesive manner. Presentations to the Chief Executive Officer and members of the Health Care System Board need to be carefully designed to ensure that the most important information is clearly communicated in an impactful and concise manner. The frequency of the education is another important judgment call. "Just in time" learning may be the most effective, but regular and consistent information flow is the goal to maintain informed decision making.

7.6 Faith Community Leadership and Staff Education

Likewise from the faith community point of view, clergy and the ministerial staff will need regular opportunities to be educated on aspects of faith community nursing, its impact, and the outcomes generated from this Network facilitated health ministry. The faith community nurse may be a primary daily educator. However, purposeful educational offerings for this group of key stakeholders need to be considered in the overall plan of the faith community Network. As the faith community nurse reaches out to the community, potential opportunities for collaboration will occur with leaders and implementers from the executive boards to the delivery drivers. Education is an essential tool for all key stakeholders involved in a faith community Network no matter what their level of involvement. Because faith community nurses interact with and care for clients so close to the clients true life expressions and often accompany clients throughout their health care experience, it is imperative that faith community nurses recognize the uniqueness of their relationship with the clients served. The faith community nurse will use this knowledge and awareness to cross the barriers that exist in health care silos by educating, communicating, and role modeling new ways of addressing gaps in health care.

7.7   Education of the Lay Person

Most important is the education of the "person in the pew" and community members.

Education for this population needs to be determined through an assessment of the congregation as a subset of the community at large. However, ongoing for the lay person are continuous opportunities for them to reframe the understanding of health as "more than being sick" and unable to function at home or at work. The faith community is an excellent location for the "person in the pew" to come to understand health as encompassing the whole person, not only physically, but spiritually, financially, socially, and emotionally. This change in how health is perceived is important not only to individuals caring for their own health, but why the church should be investing in a person's health, health care, and a faith community nurse ministry. Education for the "person in the pew" is where a relationship with a health care system or hospital can be invaluable. A faith community nurse can tap into the educational resources of the health care system, and consult with experts. Experts may also make themselves available to speak to groups in the faith community relieving the faith community nurse of providing all the educational programming.

Creative strategies need to be employed in educating the lay person. The church Bulletin is an important vehicle for ongoing health education. A regular column by the faith community nurse addressing different health topics can be what members think is the most valuable content in the bulletin. Use of bulletin boards, support groups meetings, educational programming pamphlets, retreats, and church meetings as venues for ongoing education is important. Also collaborating with other health-related groups or faith communities that have faith community nurses in joint programming can be fun and take the burden off one person for coordinating such events.

7.8   One Example of Successful Education and Integration of Faith Community Nursing

One Health Care System/Institution realigned its community-related activities through faith community nursing so that it reports to Ambulatory Services and has the status of a clinic service. This formal change in structure occurred after the department to which faith community nursing were aligned, *Faith & Community Health*, led the institution to full recognition status with the Center for Disease Control for Diabetes Prevention Recognized Program (DPRP). The institutional model allowed the faith community Network to collaborate, integrating the highest levels of its organization, for the betterment of patients. Partnering with the American

Medical Association (AMA), its electronic health record (EHR) host, and its Ambulatory services quality management nurse and physician director, a patient registry was developed that gave providers best practice alerts (BPAs) to stimulate a review of patients with elevated A1Cs, BMI, and risk test scores. Based on analysis of the patient, the provider then conferred with their patient and made a decision whether or not to directly refer that patient diabetes prevention program (DPP) classes designed by the CDC and taught by coaches educated through the faith community nurse Network's DPRP. DPP classes have been found to be more effective than Metformin in preventing the decline of Type 2 Diabetes in 58% of those participating in yearlong lifestyle change classes (Knowler et al., 2002). Fifty-one percent of the coaches were Network affiliated faith community nurses or health ministers. Forty percent of the classes were hosted in faith communities, 40% in ambulatory facilities of the institution, and 20% in county-owned recreational/community centers. From a 1-year dataset after implementing the registry, 77 patients were reviewed. The average weight loss was 7.05% (CDC's quality measure 5–7%). Fifty-seven of the 77 reviewed (74%) met all criteria for review by CDC; 43 (75%) of CDC eligible were 65 years or older and met full requirements for benefit reimbursement. If this ongoing care were billed, it would result in $19,135.00 ($445.00 per eligible participant) (Mdpp-cy2018fr-fact sheet 1 17, 2018) departmental revenue for the first year of DPP class participation. The CDC calculates that a $2670.00 cost avoidance is effected in the first year post DPP class per participant (Office of the Actuary, 2016). The American Diabetes Association sites an average cost of $7,900.00 per year per person for diabetes care (American Diabetes Association, 2013).

This potential for growth in revenue, quality, and provider compliance with best practice for the treatment of patients with prediabetes is value added for the faith community Network and only one of its many community and population health interventions. This 3-year project has significantly elevated the sustained operations budget funding for the faith community nurse Network and is now being expanded across the health system. This project would not have been as successful without intense teamwork afforded by the integration of the faith community Network and strategically executed efforts to educate all parties consistently at all levels.

7.9   Conclusion

This case study reviewed the elements, integration, and outcomes of the value of a faith community Network. This collaboration requires investment of health care system resources in dedicated staff, regular communication with all stakeholders and partners, specific allocation of program resources, and sustaining relationships over time with partnering faith communities. The dollars expended were dedicated to health promoting program interventions which resulted in people with preventable, chronic illness having health restored with ability to be productive community citizens. This is the positive outcome of the relationship between "uncanny partners" such as large health care systems and small faith communities, who form a model of community-based care through a strong Network with faith communities and faith community nurses.

Appendix

Faith Community Nurse (FCN)
Core Competencies
Self-Assessment

Name:_____ Date:_____

Network Name:_____ State:_____

Length of FCN Practice: ☐ 0 – 2 years ☐ 3 – 4 years ☐ ≥ 5 years

Years of Nursing Experience: ☐ 0 – 2 years ☐ 3 – 5 years ☐ 6 - 10 years ☐ 11-15 years ☐ ≥ 16 years

I am: ☐ AND ☐ Diploma ☐ BSN ☐ MSN ☐ APRN ☐ MA ☐ PhD ☐ M Div ☐ BSW ☐ MSW ☐ Other:___

FCN Competency	Novice	Advance Beginner	Competent	Proficient	Expert	N/A
Integrator of Faith and Health Role						
1. Understands relationships between faith and health.						
2. Assesses congregation's need and understanding of the relationship between faith and health and identifies opportunities to enhance the relationship.						
3. Integrates spiritual care into all dimensions of the FCN role.						
4. Fosters, promotes and provides opportunities for spiritual care to be discussed.						
5. Provides and documents spiritual care to individuals and groups.						
6. Participates in worship services and life of a congregation.						
7. Attends staff meetings on a regular basis, congregational committees and programs as required.						
Health Counselor Role						
8. Provides health counseling related to health maintenance, wellness promotion, disease prevention and/or illness patterns in individuals/families.						
9. Encourages the client through presence and spiritual support to express and use their faith beliefs.						
10. Maintains confidential client records in accordance with scope and standards of FCN practice and Network policies.						
11. Makes home, hospital and nursing home visits to provide spiritual support and presence.						
12. Promotes stewardship of whole person care.						
13. Collaborates with congregational staff to plan and meet health needs of the congregation.						
14. Participates in Alegent Health/Henry Ford Macomb Hospital initiatives /activities to improve the health of the congregation and surrounding community.						
15. Collaborates with health care professionals and other resources.						
Health Education Role						

(continued)

FCN Competency	Novice	Advance Beginner	Competent	Proficient	Expert	N/A
16. Prepares, develops and/or coordinates educational programs based on identified needs for healthier lifestyles, early illness detection and health resources.						
17. Maintains records of educational programs.						
FCN Competency – Health Education Role continued						
18. Provides congregational leadership, health committee members and FCN Network with information regarding educational programs.						
19. Networks and collaborates with Alegent Health or Henry Ford Macomb Hospital and other resources to promote healthier communities.						
20. Acts as a health resource to other staff of the congregation.						
Coordinator and Educator of Volunteers Role						
21. Identifies and recruits professional and lay volunteers.						
22. Facilitates, and educates volunteers to meet the identified needs of the congregation / community.						
23. Works with others in coordinating and empowering volunteers to integrate whole person health into the life of the congregation / community.						
Developer of Support Groups Role						
24. Promotes, facilitates and/or develops support groups based on identified needs.						
25. Identifies community support groups as sources for the congregation.						
26. Connects individuals with support groups.						
Referral Source / Liaison to Community Resources Role						
27. Provides and documents referrals to services and resources within the congregation and community.						
28. Collaborates with community leaders and agencies to facilitate effective working relationships and to identify new resources.						
29. Develops community contacts to identify and obtain resources and services.						
30. Networks with other FCN's and professionals.						
Health Advocate Role						
31. Encourages clients to use services that enhance their overall well being, and assists them to identify values and choices which foster self care and responsibility for their health.						

(continued)

	Novice	Advance Beginner	Competent	Proficient	Expert	N/A
32. Assists individuals and families in making decisions regarding health, medical services, treatments, and care facilities.						
33. Identifies, communicates and works cooperatively with leaders and agencies to meet health/social justice needs of congregational members and surrounding community, and/or the world.						

Other Competencies continued	Novice	Advance Beginner	Competent	Proficient	Expert	N/A
Website Documentation						
34. Accesses and understands the Network's documentation website.						
35. Documents individual interactions that capture demographics, state of being, health and wellness, disease conditions, interventions, monitoring, referrals, underinsured help, and outcomes.						
36. Recognizes and incorporates cost savings/avoidance projects into individual documentation.						
37. Documents group interactions with ease, capturing differences that are occurring because of these interactions.						
38. Inputs data with ease, including making charts and graphs for reporting purposes.						
39. Uses cumulative documentation reports to evaluate, improve, and adjust ministry goals and Faith Community Nurse practices.						
Management Role						
40. Coordinates all FCN functions in the congregation.						
41. Develops and completes reports regarding faith community ministry activities.						
42. Prepares a budget for development and enhancement of the FCN ministry in the congregation.						
43. Collaborates with funders in planning for and utilizing grants and other donations.						
Professional Development, Education and Research Role						
44. Participates in continuing education to meet identified learning needs.						
45. Participates in FCN Network meetings sponsored by Alegent Health or Henry Ford Macomb Hospital.						
46. Acts as a preceptor to students from Schools of Nursing, seminaries and other health care disciplines.						
47. Seeks to enhance personal spirituality through Faith Community nurse meetings, prayers, and other spiritual development activities.						
48. Participates in a regular ministry appraisal process setting goals and objectives (personal and ministry).						

(continued)

49. Participates in research related to Faith Community nursing when necessary consent and approval have been obtained.						
50. Represents FCN Network and / or congregation in community and educational programs / activities.						
51. Serves on committees or boards to represent faith community nursing locally, statewide and/or nationally.						

Signature:_____   Date:_____

Other Self-Appraisal Questions

1. Identify one major accomplishment during the past year. What was the key element success?

2. Identify any major difficulties you have encountered during the year, and the possible causes of those difficulties.

3. Were your parish/faith community nursing ministry goals for the past year accomplished? If not, why?

4. What are the goals for your parish/faith community nursing ministry for the coming year? What support do you need to achieve them?

5. On a scale of 1-5, with 1 = poor, 2 = fair, 3 = good, 4 = very good and 5 = excellent, how successful is your faith community nursing ministry? Identify factors influencing this score.

Additional comments?

Please sign once completed.   **Signature:**_____   **Date:**_____

References

American Diabetes Association. (2013) Economic costs of diabetes in the U.S. in 2012. *Diabetes Care*, *36*(4), 1033–1046. pp-cy2018fr-fact sheet 1 17 2018; Fact Sheet: Final Policies for Medicare Diabetes Prevention Program Expanded Model in the Calendar Year 2018 Physician Fee Schedule Final Rule.

American Nurses Association. (2015). *Nursing: Scope and standards of practice* (3rd ed.). Silver Spring, MD: Nursebooks.org.

American Nurses Association and Health Ministry Association. (2017). *Faith community nursing: Scope and standards of practice* (3rd ed.). Silver Springs, MD: Nursebooks.org.

Benner, P. E. (1984). *From novice to expert: Excellence and power in clinical nursing practice.* Menlo Park, CA: Addison-Wesley. Nursing Division.

Foege, W. (1990). The vision of the possible: What churches can do. *Second Opinion, 13*, 36–42.

Knowler, W. C., Barrett-Connor, E., Fowler, S. E., Hamman, R. F., Larkin, J. M., Walker, E. A., et al. (2002). Reduction in the incidence of type 2 diabetes with lifestyle intervention or metformin. *New England Journal of Medicine, 346*, 393–403.

Lloyd, R. C., & Solari-Twadell, P. A. (1994). Organizational framework, functions and educational preparation of parish nurses: A comparison of survey results. In *Proceedings of the Eighth Annual Westberg Symposium, Ethics and Values: A Framework for Parish Nursing Practice,* September 21–23, Northbrook IL, pp. 107–114.

National Information Center on Health Services Research and Health Care Technology. (2018, December). *Community benefit/community health needs assessment.* United States Library of Medicine. Retrieved from: www.nlm.nih.gov/hsrinfo/community_benefit.html

Office of the Actuary. (2016, March 23). Centers for Medicare & Medicaid Services Certification of Medicare Diabetes Prevention Program.

Solari-Twadell, P. A. (1990). Models of parish nursing: A challenge in design. In P. A. Solari-Twadell, A. M. Djupe, & M. A. McDermott (Eds.), *Parish nursing the developing practice* (pp. 57–76). Park Ridge, IL: Lutheran General Health Care System.

Solari-Twadell, P. A. (1997). The caring congregation: A healing place. *Journal of Christian Nursing, 14*(1), 4–9.

Solari-Twadell, P. A. (1999). The emerging practice of parish nursing. In P. A. Solari-Twadell & M. A. McDermott (Eds.), *Parish nursing: Promoting whole person health within faith communities* (pp. 3–24). Thousand Oaks, CA: Sage.

Advanced Education: Advanced Practice Nurse as a Faith Community Nurse

8

Kathryn A. Dykes and Felicia Dawn Stewart

8.1 The Faith Community Nurse with Advanced Graduate Level Preparation

The *Institute of Medicine* (IOM) is affiliated with the *National Academies of Science*. By intention it strives to provide leadership on health care. In October 2010 through a collaboration with Robert Wood Johnson Foundation a consensus report titled "The Future of Nursing: Leading Change, Advancing Health" was published. The purpose of this work was to make action oriented recommendations to direct the future of nursing. The four recommendations from this report are:

- Nurses should practice to the full extent of their education and training.
- Nurses should achieve higher levels of education and training through an improved education system that promotes seamless academic progression.
- Nurses should be full partners, with physicians and other health care professionals, in redesigning health care in the U.S.A.
- Effective workforce planning and policy making require better data collection and information infrastructure (IOM, 2010).

Given the recommendation from this report, it is important that faith community nursing reflect on the different preparation, skill levels, and expertise of those nurses engaged in this specialty nursing practice. Table 8.1 includes an overview of educational preparation and corresponding skills that different nurses may bring to faith community nursing. The idea of nurses prepared at the graduate level contributing to the growth and development of faith community nursing is not new. McDermott and Mullins reported early research findings on the demographics, employment,

K. A. Dykes (✉)
Department of Geriatrics and Long Term Care, Prevea Health, Green Bay, WI, USA

F. Dawn Stewart
Department of Nursing, Saint Mary-of-the-Woods College, Saint Mary of the Woods, IN, USA

© Springer Nature Switzerland AG 2020
P. A. Solari-Twadell, D. J. Ziebarth (eds.), *Faith Community Nursing*,
https://doi.org/10.1007/978-3-030-16126-2_8

Table 8.1 Faith community nurse role differentiation by education

Educational preparation	Minimum preparation	Graduate level preparation	Advanced practice registered nurse
Role performance	1. Baccalaureate or higher with preferred preparation in community-focused or population focused care 2. Current experience as an RN using the nursing process 3. Knowledge of assets and resources in the community 4. Specialized knowledge of the spiritual beliefs and practices of the faith community 5. Ability to implement Scope and Standards of Faith Community Nursing (ANA and HMA, 2017, p. 25)	1. Prepared at Masters or Doctoral level 2. Have advanced skills, abilities, knowledge, judgment 3. May serve as faculty or clinical preceptors in schools of nursing in addition to faith community nursing position 4. May have experience in course development, research and clinical oversight 5. May be administrators of healthcare systems 6. May be in leadership positions such as hold Board positions 7. May provide consultation services 8. May be prepared in counseling 9. Integration of theoretical and evidence-based knowledge (ANA and HMA, 2017, p. 26)	1. Completed an accredited level program preparing for practice as a certified nurse practitioner 2. Successfully passed a national certification exam specific to the advanced practice registered nurse specialty preparation 3. Holds advanced clinical knowledge and skills to provide direct care to patients/clients 4. Practice includes greater depth and breadth of knowledge, synthesis of data, increased complexity of skills and interventions 5. Increased role autonomy 6. May include prescriptive authority 7. Holds a license to practice as a nurse practitioner 8. Integration of theoretical and evidence-based knowledge 9. Influence and measure treatment outcomes (ANA and HMA, 2017, p. 27)

recruitment, motivation, satisfaction, and frustration, as well as personal and professional evaluation. At that time, Dr. McDermott was faculty at Loyola University Chicago, School of Nursing and Mullins a graduate student. Magilvy and Brown (1997) were one of the first to highlight the contribution that nurses with advanced nursing education may bring to the development of then, parish nursing. In fact "the authors believed that parish nursing to be an advanced practice role, with the minimum educational preparation being a master's degree" (p. 69). This article noted that "program planning, implementation and evaluation in addition to outcome research" was consistent with faith community nursing (p. 71). Dyess and Chase (2010) noted that "to better address desired health care for adults living with chronic illness in America today, health care dialogues need to acknowledge that health care can be provided not only in acute environments, but also in a variety of community settings that include communities of faith" (p. 42). Through the role of the Advanced Practice Nurse (APN) with additional preparation as a faith community nurse health care can be enhanced through the integration of advocacy, research, evidence-based knowledge, theory, and consultation with the basic roles of educator, referral agent, and health counseling being added not only to the health care dialogue, but the life of the faith community. This independent practice role is particularly fitting for actualizing additional education, professional expertise, life experience, and spiritual maturity of the APN who is "called" to the role of faith community nursing. An APN can serve and advocate for the people of their parish community in ways that no other staff member is prepared to do.

The most recent "Faith Community Nursing: Scope and Standards of Practice," 3rd edition, 2017, included standards of practice for the APN role in faith communities. Another skill that advanced nursing education often is associated with is grant writing. Through identifying funding that is available from different external resources, following the guidelines for the development of a proposal and applying for a grant, new opportunities can be made to members of faith communities through the role of the faith community nurse.

The following describes such an opportunity that was developed through the development and awarding of a grant written by an APN.

8.2   The Setting

The program titled "Si Se Puede" (Yes, You Can) was conducted in an inner city, Roman Catholic faith community in northeast Wisconsin. A large number of the members are elderly, English-speaking "Anglos." The parish has a large number (over 50%) of newly arrived Mexican immigrants from small rural areas of Mexico. The level of education of the Mexican immigrants is less than grade 6. The immigrants English-speaking skills are poor. Their health literacy skills are low. They live in poverty. Those with jobs work in low-paying employment in meat packing plants, often with rotating shift work. The immigrants hope for overtime work on weekends due to the opportunity to earn more for their families. Many of them are "living in the shadows" and make sincere efforts to avoid the mainstream of society. This Roman Catholic faith community has had a non-paid faith community nurse since 1997.

8.3   The Faith Community Nurse

In the past the faith community nurse had written small grants to support some of the faith community health and wellness activities, but the funding went directly to program materials or to materials to improve the health of the members of the faith community. The faith community nurse had been working toward her Master's in Nursing Education/Geriatric NP (dual emphasis) until the degree was earned in 1996. Some of the projects submitted in her advanced nursing education program included "mock" grant submissions for projects that could be carried out in a setting with demographics similar to this faith community. After graduation, this faith community nurse submitted some of the applications developed as part of her advanced nursing education to community agencies. She was very successful with a 100% success rate receiving 4 out of 4 small grants, ranging from $5000–$10,000.

This faith community nurse is bilingual (English/Spanish). In addition, she had many community connections as a result of volunteer work on behalf of many vulnerable and marginalized demographic groups. These volunteer experiences included being a phone counselor for the community Crisis Center, a victim advocate for the Sexual Assault Center, an English as an Additional Language tutor for the Literacy Council, a sponsor for Hmong refugees resettling in the area, a Bible study leader for a group of Catholic inmates at a local maximum security prison, a volunteer Health and Safety Instructor for the Red Cross (CPR, First Aid, Advanced First Aid, Basic Life Support and the Babysitter Course) in both English and Spanish, Board Member for the Alzheimer's Association, and emergency assistant for the local performing arts center. This faith community nurse was also involved regularly with faith community activities, such as Eucharistic minister both within the faith community and at one of the local hospitals weekly, a lector for Roman Catholic masses, religious education instructor for primary grades, faith community social justice committee and faith community council member. Professionally, the faith community nurse who is also an APN is a full time geriatric nurse practitioner at a local clinic. In this capacity, she is instrumental in outpatient service, including a memory clinic for persons with dementia, and nursing home rounds 4 days a week in the community.

8.4   The Grant Application Process

"Si, se Puede" is a culturally congruent diabetes education program for Spanish-speaking participants. It addresses whole person health while including not only the participant, but also their family members and significant others. A community Health Worker (prometoro/a) model is integral to the success of the program which was managed by this APN faith community nurse.

This faith community nurse, due to her collaboration and many community contacts, was approached by NEW-AHEC (North East Wisconsin Area Health Education Center) with an invitation to be a community partner with them in a major grant application. There was a call for proposals for grants up to $500,000 each from the *Wisconsin Partnership Fund*. This grant, if awarded, while offering life changing opportunities to improve the health of the community, would also carry increased responsibilities for the faith community nurse in terms of commitment of time and energy, Also if awarded, this grant challenged how things "have always been done" through the faith community. The faith community nurse presented the grant opportunity and collaboration to the pastor, the council of the faith community and staff. Through this process the decision was made to pursue this grant opportunity.

The AHEC leadership, in partnership with the faith community nurse and faith community leadership, identified community partners to provide letters of support for the grant application. The letters of support were provided by faculty from local health professional preparation programs in nursing and dietetics, the County Health Department, local Hispanic organizations, local primary care clinics, the community free clinic, the University of Wisconsin, School of Medicine and Public Health, and the Aging and Disability Resource Center, among others. These different agencies and institutions who offered support through providing letters for the grant application had previous favorable partnerships with the two lead agencies, AHEC and the Roman Catholic faith community.

The process of applying for the grant was time intensive and required many meetings. Partnering agencies had to determine what their role would be in working with the target population as well as writing up the various portions of the grant for submission. There were not only positive benefits to consider, but also some of the negative aspects of involvement, such as time involvement of agency and institution staff and developing a budget for inclusion of this program. Budget development for the grant was a detailed and difficult process that required speculative input from all parties involved.

Budget development from each participating agency including the faith community was needed to determine the amount to request from the funder in order to successfully implement and evaluate the grant project. For example, if students from the schools of nursing and dietetics were to participate, what financial considerations were needed to be included for faculty, staff, materials, products, and labor costs.

Proposed program development was necessary in order to identify a basic class format, the number and type of staff needed to carry out the program, and the development of additional activities associated with the basic diabetes education course. It was the University of Wisconsin School of Medicine and Public Health and the AHEC leadership that proposed the idea of utilizing Community Health Workers (prometora-os) to facilitate the activities of the program. The Community Health Workers would have significant input into the material included and how it would be presented. However, the faith community APN and University of Wisconsin professors would evaluate the content based on evidence-based practice. The identification of materials needed over the life of the grant and the cost of these materials was very important to the successful implementation of the grant programming

Although the faith community APN had a previous one hundred percent success rate in applying for smaller grants over time, the expertise of the AHEC leadership and their experience in applying for large scale grants was significant. A task which was daunting to the faith community advanced practice nurse was actually a great opportunity to learn the "next step," i.e. applying for larger scale grants. Her previous experience on a small grant allocations committee was also helpful in knowing how to write the grant. In the future, all the grant writing experience, both through her advanced practice education and this grant writing experience would prepare the faith community APN to apply for future larger grants to support the health programming for the faith community.

When the grant and general class outline was submitted, there was a period of waiting to hear from the grant allocations committee. There was initial excitement in learning the grant had made the first "cut" of applicants. Suggestions were made by the grant funder to revise the submitted program and grant to increase the chances of funding. There was a request to add other components following the completion of the class sessions. Follow-up sessions such as support groups, exercise groups, nutrition or cooking classes using dietetic interns, focus groups to add qualitative research in addition to the pre- and post-test questions related to diabetes to report quantitative research were a few of the suggestion made to enhance the success of the grant process. The support of the University of Wisconsin School of Medicine and Public Health in developing research questions and methods, as well as obtaining the Institutional Review Board approval for the research that would be conducted as part of the program was invaluable to the success of the grant process.

Eventually the grant proposal made the final cut and a grant of $411,000 over 3 years for the "Si Se Puede Program" was awarded. As anticipated, the grant came with additional responsibilities and commitments.

8.5   Grant Program Implementation

Identification of staff for the basic education program was significant to the success of the proposed grant programming. There were a number of possible candidates. The criteria for a Community Health Worker or "prometoro/a" were met by a number of the applicants. However, a married couple actually exceeded the standards for the grant-funded position. They were very willing to assume the role of community Health Worker. The couple, a physician, and a registered nurse from Mexico were highly educated, but not licensed here in the U.S.A. Therefore, they could not practice in their professional capacity in this country. The applicant who practiced as a physician in Mexico did not speak English at a proficient level. His wife, who was educated as a nurse was more proficient than her husband. They were highly respected in the Mexican community and in the faith community due to their education and knowledge of health and wellness matters as well as their Spanish language proficiency. They were "naturals" to fill the prometoro-prometora role for "Si Se Puede." Some additional staff were selected for child care and positions to assist the Community Health Workers with class. In addition, these assistant positions did set up and clean up, and screened class participants for blood pressure and blood sugar during the classes. The faith community APN was present for all of the classes acting as a liaison/interpreter for dietetic and nursing students, offering transportation to and from classes for anyone who did not have a ride, and assisting with class presentations, answering questions and supporting the Community Health Workers and participants.

The faith community advanced practice nurse began meeting with the Community Health Workers and community partners to prepare the content for the class sessions. The material to be covered was selected in terms of what goals were to be achieved: "Learning to Live with Diabetes," "Using the Glucometer," "Preventing Complications," "Nutrition," "Nutrition and Exercise," and "Managing Stress" were identified as the titles of the sessions to be offered.

The classes were free and offered in Spanish. There was a process to determine the best days of the week and time to offer the classes in order to promote ease of attendance for all sessions. Most of the diabetes classes in the community were offered during weekday "business hours"—that is, Monday through Friday and between the hours of 8 and 5. Through a process of recruitment and then polling the potential participants in detail, it was determined that the time most participants could come to a diabetes class would be Sunday late mornings. This was also a normal time that many would be attending Spanish Mass with their family. Transportation was offered in case a participant did not have a vehicle or ride to class as the buses did not run on Sundays. It was important to the grant that participants attend all the sessions or they would not count as having completed the program. The participants, however, really wanted to attend the sessions as they developed a supportive relationship with one another. Child care was offered for very young children, but children of school age were encouraged to attend with their parents.

The classes were based on the concept of whole person health and included the families and significant others of the participants. The first session focused on learning to live with diabetes. This was a very emotional class for many of the participants and those family members who were present. After introductions, participants were asked what their reaction was to learning about their diagnosis with diabetes. This particular demographic group came from a third world country environment: rural Mexico. Most of them and their children were very tearful. They stated that they were going to die young, have an amputation or two, go blind, etc. None of them thought that they had any control over the disease or its management.

Mantras were developed based on the concept that each person believes "I am not a "diabetic," I am a person with diabetes." The mantras were posted around the classroom and were reviewed and re-stated at the start of each week's class. This was the basis of each participant taking charge of their life and their disease. Family members learned how to become a support to their loved ones. This was the first time most of the participants had talked about their feelings with their family members and the participants realized how deeply their children cared for them and wished them well. This class session motivated the participants and their families to learn how to manage their diabetes in the remainder of the sessions.

The second session focused on the use of the glucometer and what the readings meant. This was also an opportunity for the participants to share their feelings about pricking their fingers and testing blood glucose levels throughout the day. As part of the session, each family member was asked to prick their own finger to experience what the participants with diabetes were feeling two or more times a day. They were taught how to offer support, when able, such as placing their hand on the person's shoulder when they did their glucose testing.

The nutrition session offered a game which was based on points for carbs and how to make selections from a buffet of artificial food items that are available in the community—both from American fast food culture and from the traditional foods they were eating at home. The children and adults all enjoyed this method of learning through active participation. Posters regarding food choices were made by dietetic students. Post-graduate classes on nutrition focused on traditional recipes which were converted to a healthier version by the dietetic interns. The recipes were actually prepared by one of the families in attendance and all were given an opportunity to taste the revised version of the traditional recipes.

The exercise session was led by the prometoro who was a sports medicine physician in Mexico. He was good natured and fun to work with. He taught how to stretch to "warm up" and how to "cool down" following each light exercise session which was accompanied by uplifting Latin music. All ages enjoyed this activity and it was practiced regularly in an exercise group for "Si Se Puede" graduates. The prometoros held exercise sessions, primarily walks in the park, for families, in order to support them in their need for regular exercise.

The session on managing stress used all the senses. Aromatherapy, dimming the lights, guided meditation, personal meditation, progressive relaxation, deep breathing, listening to music, and other methods were taught to participants and their families to reduce stress. This was another session in which many tears were shed as people discussed what the stressors were in their lives. All participants openly shared with others in the group, as their support of each other grew during the sessions.

8.6   Program Support

Important to the recruitment of participants was the development of marketing materials, a program logo, a website for the program and PowerPoint presentations to share the program and its results with others. As a result of the grant award, an invitation to present the findings of this project was received resulting in participation in the initial State of Wisconsin Community Health Worker Annual Conference.

When each completed session of six classes was accomplished, a special graduation or recognition program was held honoring those that had finished the work entailed in each class. For many of the participants, who had a sixth grade education or less, this recognition was a source of great pride for them. Each individual was presented with a certificate of completion, and some graduation gifts, including a laminated placemat illustrating the "plate method," a medic alert bracelet or necklace, a photo of them holding their certificate, either with or without their family/friend. As more sessions were completed, previous classes were all invited to the recognition sessions. The participation in the recognition sessions grew larger following the completion of each six week series. Each recognition session included games which involved information from the classes they attended to reinforce knowledge beyond the class time. Prizes were awarded for correct responses. Again family members and significant others were invited and participated. In addition, a blessing was offered in church following the Sunday Mass in Spanish for anyone who wanted ongoing support and prayers.

The bilingual staff of the "Si Se Puede" program also provided assistance scheduling appointments with the participant's health care providers. This assistance included interpreting at their health care appointments, applying for low cost medications and test strips as well as reporting their diabetes self-management results to their provider.

It should be noted that the education, skills, and life experience of the faith community APN was applied to many of the activities involved in the implementation and evaluation of this program grant. For example, in setting up the time for the diabetes classes, the faith community advanced practice nurse needed to know when the target audience would be available. For example, knowing that most participants worked first or second shift Monday through Saturday and needed the family or neighborhood car to get there, most of them need a babysitter while they are at work, knowing that overtime is often offered at work and that extra work takes priority over anything else. In addition, knowing that some days and times are in conflict with other popular faith community activities and programs was essential to program scheduling. It was important for the reunions or graduations of participants, to avoid Sundays during baptisms as the faith community staff and members were often invited to attend these celebrations.

8.7   Additional Considerations

Evaluation strategies also had to be carefully considered. Which method of surveying would be the best for the literacy levels of the target audience? These decisions did not necessarily come from the faith community advanced practice nurse's education, but from the knowledge and teamwork of those representing the participating agencies and institutions involved in the grant. Through collaboration, authentic communication, dedication, and respect for each other, professionals and community workers who were integral to the development and implementation of the grant worked closely together to ensure evaluation of the project was comprehensive. Important to this process were the English to Spanish speakers through the Literacy Council, and knowing the daily living patterns of the target audience through years of direct contact and friendship. The Community Health Worker or "promotors input" was also significant to the final programmatic and evaluation decisions.

The input of the Community Health Workers or "prometoros" was also valuable in planning program activities. The promoters were included and invaluable in making administrative decisions to determine the details of class delivery. From the type of logo, colors used, and types of food to discuss during class sessions, the acceptable family meals and alternatives to integrate into the class along with when to include the family in sessions and activities to ensure that an intervention would be successful over time, their input was invaluable.

Grant writing is a skill that is part of the education of the APN. This skill is useful in applying for start-up, continuation, and activities which branch off from a primary grant program such as exercise groups for children or families and food/dietary education for families. For example, enhancing multi-cultural education related to diabetes and the Spanish-speaking patient is an important goal for University Dietetic Interns and RN, BSN, and NP students. Having the Community Health Worker's/prometoros take the students on tours of local Hispanic grocery stores to see what products and food items are available was helpful in understanding their patients' educational needs in their future practice. Adding the education of professional students of various disciplines enhances the impact of the program beyond the target audience and their families. These documented activities increase the likelihood of receiving additional funding.

Knowing the importance of faith and family to the participants of this culture is important. Inclusion of faith-based cultural practices within the class sessions and self-care was key. For example, during the class session on "Managing Stress," using popular Bible passages featuring Jesus in a comforting or healing role were used in practicing "guided imagery" or meditation in a quiet session. This combined with aroma therapy, supportive religious music in the background, and journaling helped incorporate faith into coping and managing stress. The strong religious beliefs of the faith community APN as well as her experience with guided imagery, meditation, types of prayer, music, knowledge of religious hymns and journaling skills were significant to these class sessions. The Community Health Worker's faith was equally important, or more so, than that of the faith community nurse. The ability for them to be open, authentic, and plan together was instrumental to each successful class session.

Experience with research was important for this faith community APN in collaborating on the development of the pre-and post-test questions used for quantitative research, and the focus group questions employed for the qualitative research in evaluating each participant's experience. Again, the contributions of doctoral prepared staff from the partnering organization were extremely valuable for this aspect of the program and provided credibility to the evaluation material developed and resulting outcomes of the program. Good data is always useful and increases the potential for future funding. The involvement of doctoral students in writing questions for the focus groups, conducting the focus groups in Spanish and interpreting the results of the focus groups provided for excellent learning experiences and are always appreciated by funders.

Information Technology (IT) staff were needed and assigned from the University partner. Specific data entry programs were developed for the grant-funded program, as well as programs to tabulate results of research questions, and capturing the responses from the focus groups in an accurate manner. The development of these programs involved many long meeting, which included the faith community APN, Community Health Workers or prometoros, and community partners who were committed to and invested in reporting the results in a comprehensive manner.

It should be noted that the faith community APN who served as the Grant Program Coordinator needs to attend copious meetings. It is essential that this faith community nurse has the interpersonal skills, patience, and knowledge needed to communicate with partners from many different disciplines as well as many different educational and skill levels. In other words, the faith community advanced practice nurse will be required to know at least a little bit about many different things and resourceful enough to be prepared and present for each meeting. Sound knowledge of the current medical gold standards for diabetes treatment, prevention, and management through lifestyle changes was necessary to provide a solid basis for expected outcomes for the "Si Se Puede" program.

The human resource aspect of the program development was also a vital role for the faith community advanced practice nurse. Hiring for all grant-funded positions was fundamental to the success of the grant project. From the screening of the child care providers, checking whether they were certified or not while meeting the faith community criteria for background checks was one category. Screening drivers for those who needed assistance with transportation, considering their personality, communication style, knowledge of Mexican culture, level of respect for the participant was another consideration. Facilitating the contributions of the nursing students, dietetic interns, IT staff, data entry staff, university faculty and researchers, marketing, payroll tested the ability of the faith community APN to keep multiple agendas in the forefront. Each of these contributors needed job descriptions which included qualifications and criteria for performance evaluations. As Grant Coordinator, the faith community APN was responsible for completing all of these documents.

Inclusion of family members was a very important ingredient to the success of the program. Beginning with the first class session titled "I am a Person with Diabetes, Not a Diabetic," when the participants were asked to talk about how they felt when they first got the diagnosis of diabetes many of the children who participated tearfully expressed how they feared that their parents would not survive for very long and would not be able to work or support their family. The Community Health Workers needed to be skillful in order to facilitate this first class session with the high level of emotion evoked by the session's activities. This was an empowering session if managed in a skillful manner.

Family members were included throughout, such as each being offered the opportunity to prick their own finger in order to understand what their family member was going through, and by offering support at home. Family members were encouraged to reduce their own risk of diabetes by following the same diabetes healthy diet as their loved ones were following and by keeping unhealthy snacks out of the home environment so as not to tempt their loved one.

Each class session and graduation/reunion session involved adult learning principles in reviewing key points from past sessions. Use of all the senses, active participation, repetition, building on past knowledge, and rewards were all significant to the review portion at each session. Use of adult learning principles was a part of the advanced practice nursing preparation for this role and essential to class sessions as well as the graduation/review sessions.

Rewards for correct responses during review sessions were all meaningful to the health and well-being of the participants and their family members. Rewards were as simple as dental floss, toothbrushes, foot creams, or more significant such as gift cards for farmer's market or grocery stores, diabetic socks, gasoline gift cards for transportation to appointments, appointment calendars, notebooks for record keeping of blood glucose levels and blood pressures Graduation awards were also considered important by participants. Graduations were celebrated with a healthy meal, and gifts which was a source of great pride for the population, as many of them had not even graduated from grade school.

The extension of activities beyond the basic diabetes course was important and required the same knowledge of the culture, adult learning principles, daily living activities, and health literacy level of the participants. The exercise group needed a strong leader, and the basic Community Health Workers were all busy working with the basic course, which was ongoing in terms of marketing, promotion, soliciting new participants as well as conducting the courses, graduations, and review sessions. Looking for new Community Health Workers to take the lead on exercise classes, cooking classes, and support groups was a constant activity that needed to be regularly tended to be the Grant Coordinator.

The dietetic interns were very helpful in developing converted recipes for those submitted by the participants so that they were diabetes friendly. Many conversions were highly successful and the participants agreed they did not taste much different than the original high carb or high fat version. A cookbook was developed from the course and was a very popular item for sale by the faith community at Christmas and throughout the year. Each recipe contained a story from the contributor of the recipe about the family traditions they associated with the foods.

Again, staff skilled at editing, layout, and printing were needed for this "off-shoot" project to be successful.

8.8   Conclusion

The faith community APN can work to the full extent of her licensure through leading grant-funded projects which have the ability to impact individuals, families, and populations over time. In addition, a faith community APN can work as a full partner with physicians, educators, funders, and other key stakeholders in changing not only the systems for the delivery of care, but the lives of the individuals that interface with these systems.

Through reflecting deeply on faith beliefs, personal values, culture, skills, and talents while at the same time being open to expanding personal and professional skills, knowledge and attitudes, the faith community nurse with advanced nursing education is in a key position to be an instrument of change.

References

American Nurses Association (ANA) and the Health Ministry Association (HMA). (2017). *Faith community nursing: scope and standards* (3rd ed.). Washington, DC: American Nurses Association.

Dyess, S., & Chase, S. K. (2010). Caring for adults living with chronic illness through communities of faith. *International Journal for Human Caring, 14*(4), 38–44.

Institute of Medicine. (2010). *The future of nursing: Leading change, advancing health.* Washington, DC: National Academies of Science.

Magilvy, J. K., & Brown, N. J. (1997). Parish nursing: Advanced practice nursing model for healthier communities. *Advanced Practice Nursing Quarterly, 2*(4), 67–72.

Part III

Changing the Understanding of Health: Faith Community Nursing Development

Perspective from the Pastor and the Faith Community

9

Helen Anne Wordsworth

9.1 Faith and Health: A Concern of the Faith Community Internationally

9.1.1 Historical Overview of Faith and Health in the Life of the Faith Community

Prayers for healing and healing services have been a feature of the life of various denominations since the beginning of the early church. Monasteries and convents were involved in the establishment of hospitals and the care of the sick. For example, a history of the Cathedral at Peterborough, England, reveals that the monks offered care and prayer for healing with the local community as far back as 1100 AD (Mellows, 1980). In the sixteenth century priests sometimes cultivated herb gardens from which they would take medicinal remedies for common ailments. An example of an herb garden can be seen near Shakespeare's burial site in Stratford, England, UK.

It was not very long ago that churches were key organizations in the provision of health services across the world. The modern missionary movement began with the founding in 1792 of the Baptist Missionary Society by William Carey, quickly followed by the Church Missionary Society and the London Missionary Society. But it was a little later, during the nineteenth century that churches began to include medical professionals among those they sent to various countries. The first medical missionaries were sent from the Edinburgh Medical Missionary Society, formed in 1842 (Stanley, 1992). In some countries the churches remain the largest providers of health care, but the responsibility for this may have been delegated to large institutions that have little to do with the local church. In other places the influence of the church is waning due to increased state and private provision (Flessa, 2016).

H. A. Wordsworth (✉)
Parish Nursing Ministries UK, Peterborough, UK

Westberg Institute for Faith Community Nursing, Memphis, TN, USA
e-mail: Helen.w@parishnursing.org.uk; wordsworthh@churchhealth.org

© Springer Nature Switzerland AG 2020
P. A. Solari-Twadell, D. J. Ziebarth (eds.), *Faith Community Nursing*,
https://doi.org/10.1007/978-3-030-16126-2_9

9.2   The Role of a Nurse in Health Ministry

In the nineteenth century, the health care offered by the German Lutheran church under Pastor Fliedner inspired both Florence Nightingale in her quest to understand nursing care, and the formation of the nursing community of St John the Divine in London (McDonald, 2010; Community of St John the Divine, 2018). Deaconesses in Lutheran, Episcopal, Methodist, and Baptist traditions were required to do nurse training before or at the same time as theological preparation. These were mirrored in the Catholic and Orthodox traditions by the nursing orders in convent communities. A 1902 photograph of a parish nurse outside her cottage opposite Christchurch in Beckenham, Kent, was discovered at a visit to that church when they were exploring the possibility of a contemporary parish nursing service. Many of these early Christian nursing services across the world have become integrated into more comprehensive health programs, administered by state, non-profit, or private organizations. In the process, some of the Christian influence has been lost. In response to this trend, the World Council of Churches set up a "Christian Medical Commission" in the 1960s to explore what the future role of the church should be in relation to health. They reported in 1981 and stated that:

> Medicine must not only abandon the separation of body, soul and spirit but must also understand the human person as a being in relationship to other persons, to the environment, and to God (World Council of Churches, 1981).

However, partly due to the influence of Greek philosophy and "Enlightenment" thinking, Western congregations moved away from the wholistic integration of body mind and soul in the latter part of the twentieth century and towards a more compartmentalized approach to theology: doctrine, worship, evangelism, charismatic renewal, and church growth became prioritized. Social action, where seen as part of the gospel imperative, was delivered in a way that did not include faith discussion or prayer with those served. This is demonstrated by the statements produced by the Lausanne conferences on world evangelism. Progression was seen from a view of evangelism and social action as two separate, but necessary activities in 1974 (Lausanne Movement, 1974) to a more integrated perspective in 1989 (Lausanne Movement, 1989). In 2010, the Lausanne Conference concluded that churches should work with the disabled and sick, empowering them in self-care and service delivery, rather than simply offering care to them (Lausanne Movement, 2010).

9.3   The Importance of Faith Community Nursing in Advancing the Mission for Health in a Faith Community

In the majority of European countries parish nurse/parish nursing remains as the predominant language to describe what is called faith community nursing in the U.S.A. Additionally, nurses are involved in providing services through faith communities in Europe, they may refer to, but are not required to acknowledge the scope and standards of nursing developed in the U.S.A. Although there is a shared history, the terminology differs. Thus, in this chapter you will observe the use of both terms parish nursing and faith community nursing interchangeably.

In 2008, a study was commenced in England, UK to discover the effect that the appointment of a parish nurse had on the mission of the local faith community (Wordsworth, 2015). The findings demonstrated: (a) a significant increase in volunteering; (b) an increase in the church's contact time with people outside of the faith community; (c) an increased profile of the faith community in the community at large; and, (d) an increase in the breadth of interventions that the faith communities were able to provide in response to need. All 15 participant ministers said they would recommend a parish nurse ministry to another faith community. Twelve of them suggested a strong commendation. This study has helped more faith communities to see the value of parish nursing ministry and the number of active parish nursing services has grown in the UK from 28 in 2008 to 87 at the time of writing.

9.4 Purpose of a Health Ministry

Where a significant proportion of the population attend a faith community, and where health care is only accessible to those who can afford it, there is a very pragmatic reason for developing a health ministry within the faith community; it enables a greater percentage of the people in a given area to have access to educative, preventive, and supportive care. However, if the theological foundation for health ministry is examined, it can be seen that notwithstanding the size of the congregation, there is a Biblical rationale for whole person health. It is built upon the Hebrew and Christian concept of body, mind, and soul being a unified whole. That means that a person's faith-life affects all of their existence, their physical and mental health as well as their devotional life. God wants people to experience life "in all its fullness" (John 10:10), even if people have to live with certain health or environmental restrictions. Christ commissions His disciples to

...heal those who are ill and tell them "the Kingdom of God has come near to you" (Luke 10:9).

Furthermore, the missional purpose of God that occurs throughout Jewish and Christian writings commissions the faith community to reach out to those who are not believers and offer them the same kind of care as given to those who are faith community members. The mission of Christ is for the world, not just for His church, and He works to extend His kingdom even if His followers choose not to get involved. So any health ministry commenced by a faith community has a missional purpose, both within the faith community and with the faith community to others. Faith Community nursing then should be a missional activity, not just a health service for those who attend a faith community. But faith communities cannot serve God and others to the best of their ability unless they take care of their own health, so where a faith community nurse only has time to see members of the faith community, she/he is engaged in equipping them for service in the community. One way of demonstrating this is for a nurse to give faith community members resources that they can use to help improve the health of their neighbors.

Health is a gift from God that the church and individuals have a responsibility to look after and share. Faith community nursing seeks to turn upside down any false dichotomy between faith and health, for we do not find such a division in the scriptures or in the ministry of Jesus Christ.

9.5 Significance of a Faith Community Nurse as a Member of the Pastoral Team

So what does a faith community nurse do that contributes towards this understanding of health and faith?

9.5.1 Health Promotion/Disease Prevention

A faith community nurse is educated in health education and knows the significance of living a healthy lifestyle on the prevention of disease. Evidence-based advice may be given in group sessions, individual conversations or via noticeboards/magazines/social media on such subjects as nutrition, exercise, smoking cessation, drug and alcohol awareness, mental health, ageing, men's health, dealing with grief and loss, child development, immunization, sexual health, and antenatal classes. Simple screening can be undertaken, for example, to detect hypertension, diabetes, and cancer, so that early treatment can be accessed and complications prevented. Those leaving a hospital or recovering from acute disease can be monitored and supported back to work. Health assessments can be offered to people with chronic conditions and care plans discussed. Care givers can be helped to live as full a life as possible, while caring for their friend or relative. Those near the end of life can be supported to receive interventions which will alleviate suffering.

A study of 15 churches that had a parish nurse compared to a control group of 77 churches that did not showed that the parish nurse churches offered four times more physical health interventions than the control group and twice as many mental health interventions (Wordsworth, 2015).

9.5.2 Spiritual Care

Spiritual care involves fostering good relationships with family friends and others; a sense of meaning and purpose in life; the search for peace and resolution of conflict; and transcendence, the connection with God (or a higher being), which includes living with His values, prayer, care for creation and concern for His world (Büssing, Balzat, & Heusser, 2010). Faith community nurses offer intentional care of the spirit which means that they may address all of these issues in an integrated way with physical and mental health care. For some people, this helps them to reawaken or strengthen an earlier experience of faith. The study referred to above showed that spiritual and community interventions by the faith communities that had a parish nurse were also significantly increased (Wordsworth, 2015). People of all faiths and those that profess no faith are served by faith community nurses. This specialty nursing practice does not promote proselytization: faith community nurses are aware that they are working with vulnerable people and must respect each person's faith position. But an encounter with a faith community nurse may enable a person to pray or to explore faith and they may find this helpful to their sense of health and wellness. As with other interventions, referrals may be made to other appropriate chaplains or groups, if the patient, or client requests such information.

9.5.3   Multiplication of Ministers

Having a faith community nurse on the ministry team increases the number of staff available to help meet the health and pastoral care needs of the faith community. She/he may work closely with an existing pastoral care team, enhancing and supporting their work by being available to them for advice when a visit reveals health concerns. But this is not the only advantage. Part of the faith community nurse's role is to recruit, train, and coordinate volunteers to help families with everyday shopping or transport to appointments. They may, for example, help to organize a health fair or clinic, or assist with a walking club. This responds to the Biblical theme of every member's vocation, where all may experience a sense of call to a role that makes the best use of their gifts, passion, and personality.

9.5.4   Promoting the Health of the Ministerial Staff as Well as the Faith Community

There is an inspiring example of the way in which the faith community nurse may care for the health of the ministerial staff in the state of Oklahoma in the U.S.A., where the Catholic archdiocese has employed a faith community nurse just to care for their priests (Archdiocese of Oklahoma News, 2018). Ministerial staff may feel reluctant to share their health problems with members of the faith community, and may have little inclination to attend health appointments which result in them sharing the same waiting room as the members of their faith community. Equally, they may feel unable to share concerns with their overseers, for fear of influencing future career moves. Furthermore, ministers of faith communities are among those with an increased risk of mental illness or burn out, and the presence of the faith community nurse in the team may help to promote better lifestyle balance, encourage healthy nutrition and exercise, or identify early stress-related symptoms.

9.6   Role of the Congregation in Advocacy

9.6.1   The Faith Community's Role in Assisting People to Think: Applying Values and Beliefs

A faith community nurse will be writing articles in the faith community magazine or newsletter that help the members to think through their understanding of health-related values and beliefs. The aim of this article is to stimulate discussion among their families and friends that will result in health-enhancing action, be that at an individual or community level. An example of this is in Stockport, England, where the nurse only has a few hours each week to serve a large faith community. So, in order to increase the impact of her work she gives everyone two or three copies of her hand-outs with the instruction that they are to share them with the people who live near them, but do not attend church. In this way, the local community is empowered to think more pro-actively on health issues.

9.6.2   Promoting People in the Congregation to Become More Politically Active in Relation to Health

Whatever the local context, the faith community can be encouraged to become more aware of the issues surrounding health provision and more active in supporting health providers. A parish nurse in a faith community in Cambridgeshire, England has provided the city hospital with three of its governors in the last few years, and six of its chaplaincy volunteers. It also has a city councillor who works hard to ensure that poorer people do not face discrimination when it comes to health and social care. The faith community provides a night shelter for homeless people and advocates on their behalf. And it hosts a food recycling day each week when those who need it are provided with food. This kind of activity is common in many faith communities across the world, but a faith community nurse can be the catalyst in both suggesting ideas for action to relieve assessed local need, and inspiring faith community members to personal involvement.

9.6.3   Communal Advocacy for Changes in Local Community Related to Health

The environmental context for health and wellness has been shown to be influential to many diseases. It is well known that poor hygiene and lack of sanitation lead to outbreaks of gastrointestinal infection; air pollution in cities increases the incidence of childhood asthma, and smoking to lung cancer. A faith community with a faith community nurse can address some of these environmental issues by campaigning for more public health inspectors, less use of cars with high emissions, more cycle paths, and more smoking cessation programs. They can also add weight to local campaigns for better access to healthcare facilities, more play areas for children, more breastfeeding facilities in the local mall, or more places where people can exercise safely. They can model these improvements by encouraging people to share cars to the faith community or use bicycles, to join walking clubs or get involved in sporting activities. In the global scene, they can promote the purchase of fair trade goods, which will help to provide health care for people in developing countries.

9.7   Relationship of the Pastor and Faith Community Nurse

9.7.1   Collaboration

For some pastors, this may be the first time that they have worked closely with a health professional colleague. It is important to recognize that there will be learning requirements around how collaboration and communication take place. The faith community nurse will be working under confidentiality guidelines pertaining to professional regulatory bodies, and so will only be able to share information with the consent of the client or patient. This can be a problem for the minister and the pastoral care team who share a caring responsibility for the same people that approach the nurse. In anticipation of this potential conflict, a communication policy should be developed around the sharing of sensitive information. Where the nurse feels that the involvement of the minister or pastoral care team is desirable, she/he commits to asking the client's permission for this and vice versa. Documentation is kept confidential to the nurse, and a suitable secure storage facility is required.

9.7.2   Respect

It is both important and a Biblical injunction that the team is seen to respect one another, so the faith community nurse and minister will need to ensure they do not speak negatively about another member of the team or each other. A culture of respect seen at the leadership level will filter through the congregation and help to prevent conflict.

Some of the faith community may feel more inclined to talk to the faith community nurse rather than the minister of the church, and this can lead to lack of confidence in position or feelings of inferiority on the part of the minister. Where finances are tight and the faith community or the minister make decisions about staff termination of employment, this could escalate into a major threat to both the faith community nurse and minister. A recent questionnaire was circulated among ministers that had worked with a parish nurse for more than 2 years and these were some of the comments received:

Parish Nursing has been the most significant ministry in mission that I have encountered in 25 years of leadership.

Having a Parish Nurse as part of our ministry and outreach has so demonstrated God's love for the whole person to many within & outside the Church.

Having a Parish Nurse helps us to provide more holistic pastoral care and offer sound health and well-being advice to our parishioners.

A Parish Nurse has opportunity to pray and read scripture with patients, if so desire, in a way that is denied to other health professionals. This is much appreciated, especially by clients who have visual limitations.

It shows the community we care strongly about them. Advice is freely given to people who may feel uncomfortable talking to their GP.

Parish nursing has been a great opportunity to be an integral part of our local community and show just how relevant our Christian faith can be.

By swift referrals, our Parish Nurse has most definitely saved/prolonged the life of individuals over the years (Parish Nursing Ministries UK, 2018; Wordsworth, 2018).

9.7.3 Partnership

Regular meetings should be arranged between minister and faith community nurse so that good communication can be facilitated. These should be held in a place where other people are present or nearby, so that there can be no suspicion or accusation of untoward behavior. The development of a position description that takes account of the strengths of both the faith community nurse and minister will help towards collegial working. An understanding of each other's gifts, personality, and passion will enable a stronger partnership. Where appropriate, the minister may invite the faith community nurse to take part in prayers for healing, or give an account of his/her work in the annual business meeting or reporting structure. And where the patient's consent is obtained, referrals may be made from one to the other.

9.7.4 Leadership

The faith community nurse is responsible for the efficient and effective leadership of the faith community nursing service and must therefore develop good leadership skills. She/he must be able to think strategically, plan for succession, inspire volunteers, and ensure that the service is well managed. To this end, she/he will have selected a team of supportive members of the faith community, sometimes called a health cabinet, who can help to develop vision, raise funds, offer practical help with various health initiatives and pray for the work. The nurse will also identify people in the congregation who can act as visitors where loneliness or practical household support is required. If there are other health professionals in the faith community, the faith community nurse will ensure that they are invited to offer their skills where appropriate, given that the faith community nurse remains the leader of the health team.

9.8 Congregations as Agents of Change in the Understanding of Health

9.8.1 Application of Scripture to Understanding of Health

9.8.1.1 Whole Person Health
Robinson (1952) points out that the Greek concept of body and soul being separate is not found in the Old Testament and goes on to argue that it is not present in the New Testament either. This is acknowledged by Wilkinson (1998) in his work on healing. In the first words of Genesis, we find that Spirit and water combine to form the earth (Genesis 1:2). In the laws for living given to Moses (Exodus 31:18), we find the integration of both spiritual and physical elements. In the books of wisdom and the prophets spiritual life is connected with social justice, community cohesion, and compassionate action. In the incarnation God (Spirit) comes to be with His people as Jesus is conceived in the Virgin Mary's womb (Luke 1:35). And in Jesus' life and ministry spirit and body combine as Jesus brings physical healing along with forgiveness of sins, or growth of faith. Supremely, body and Spirit combine in the passion, death and resurrection of Jesus. And at Pentecost, God sends His Spirit upon his disciples (Acts 2:1-4), enabling them to do things that their physical and mental capacities would not otherwise be able to do. The promise of Jesus's return (John 14:1-3) has both physical and spiritual elements. These concepts give faith community nursing a fundamental understanding of health as whole person health.

9.8.1.2 Stewardship of Health
The belief that health is a gift from God brings us to the question of how we look after it. In his letter to the Corinthians, the apostle Paul writes that a believer's body is the temple of the Holy Spirit and instructs the readers to honor God with their bodies (First Corinthians 6:19-20). He is warning them against immorality, greed and drunkenness. And writing to Timothy, Paul urges steadfastness in suffering like a soldier, perseverance and obedience like an athlete, and hard work like a farmer (Second Timothy 2:1-13). All three need to be careful of their health in order to continue their work. Paul himself talks about having a "thorn in the flesh" and having suffered much for the sake of the gospel yet God gives him strength to continue his work without being crushed, or destroyed (Second Corinthians 12:7-10). We have to guard against burn-out or preventable disease because each of us has a God-given task to accomplish.

9.8.1.3 Caring for One's Neighbor
For faith communities, not only encouraging care of self, but emphasizing care for our neighbors is important. The faith community nurse will help them to do that more effectively, whether they are people of faith, people of other faith or no faith. The key learning example to this is the parable told by Jesus of the Good Samaritan, where someone who was a hated and mis-understood stranger, risks his life, his reputation and his money to minister to the needs of a traveler from a different culture who had been attacked and wounded (Luke 10:25-17). Just as the Samaritan delegated the task of care to an innkeeper, so faith community nurses may delegate

the everyday help that a suffering neighbor might need to members of the congregation. But he/she will ensure that those who are asked to volunteer will be recruited, educated, coordinated, and valued so that they are not overwhelmed or taken for granted. In one faith community in rural Lincolnshire, the faith community nurse was commissioned along with fourteen volunteers that she had already recruited. They have stayed with her, forming a deeply significant team of helpers in the village where the church is based.

9.8.2 Stewardship of Health Resources

Whether or not the country has a state funded or privately funded health service, health resources may be thinly spread and not able to cover all that is needed. Home health nurses or district nurses have target times to work with and may not be able to spend as much listening time as is needed by patients with complex conditions. Faith community nurses can manage their own time and may therefore be able to offer more active listening. They may be able to connect the patient or client with the most appropriate source of help, navigate them through the health services, and advocate for them where needed. They can prevent unnecessary visits to the doctor's office by holding an advice clinic at the church and where someone needs an urgent hospital or doctor appointment they can expedite that through the professional relationship that they will have built with other health providers. The preventive work they do can relieve pressure on the health service and save money in the longer term. All of this leads to better stewardship of the health provision that a country, state, or commercial provider can offer.

9.8.3 Preparation of the Faith Community

The issues surrounding the commencement of a faith community nursing service needs to be well understood by the faith community in order for the service to become well established and sustainable. To achieve this, it is important to connect with a national, regional, or denominational infrastructure association for faith community nursing. An example of where this has been helpful is provided by Parish Nursing Ministries, UK (Parish Nursing Ministries UK, 2018). They have developed a step by step process to help faith communities of all denominations prepare the way. It begins with an enquiry sent from the nurse and/or the faith community from the website, in return for which a free enquiry pack is sent, giving basic information about the nature, structure, and accountability of a parish nursing service. It includes an option to request a visit to the faith community by a trained advocate, so that as many of the members of the faith community as possible have access to a presentation about parish nursing. The next option is to have a regional coordinator allocated to the church. This is a registered nurse who is able to help the leadership develop a vision, mission, and risk analysis for their service. Help with recruitment is the next step, followed by training for the selected nurse and ongoing support as the service develops. A review is offered at the beginning of the fourth year along with the opportunity to attend a refresher course. This process has enabled faith communities to be more informed at the beginning of a faith community nursing initiative and is beginning to demonstrate greater sustainability and professional support. It does however require funding, and so the church pays start-up fees and an annual contribution to the non-profit national infrastructure organization.

9.9 Conclusion

Faith communities and pastors need to appreciate the theological rationale for appointing a faith community nurse in order for the initiative to be sustainable in the long term. This involves helping the clergy, faith community leaders and members to understand the essential inclusion of health as a major element of the Christian gospel. This chapter has defined health as a gift from God to be experienced by all members of a faith community and shared with the local community. It has included insights from a research project that looked at the effect of parish nursing on the mission of a faith community. It has described the ways in which the clergy and faith community can participate in the ministry of health. It also has shown how valuable the faith community nursing can be as part of the missional activities of a faith community and has suggested a way in which countries can provide the infrastructure and support to enable the growth and sustainability of the practice.

References

Archdiocese of Oklahoma News. (2018). Retrieved April 20, 2018, from http://www.archokc.org/news-2/1685-priests-nurse-to-remind-clergy-members-of-the-importance-of-health-1685

Büssing, A., Balzat, H. J., & Heusser, P. (2010). Spiritual needs of patients with chronic pain diseases and cancer – validation of the spiritual needs questionnaire. *European Journal of Medical Research, 15*, 266–273.

Community of St John the Divine. (2018). Retrieved June 28, 2018, from http://csjd.org.uk/history.html

Flessa, S. (2016). Christian milestones in global health: The declarations of Tübingen. *Christian Journal for Global Health, 3*(1), 11–24. Retrieved April 13, 2018, from https://doi.org/10.15566/cjgh.v3i1.96

Lausanne Movement. (1974). Retrieved April 20, 2018, from https://www.lausanne.org/content/covenant/lausanne-covenant

Lausanne Movement. (1989). Retrieved April 20, 2018, from https://www.lausanne.org/gatherings/congress/manila-1989

Lausanne Movement. (2010). Retrieved April 20, 2018, from https://www.lausanne.org/gatherings/congress/cape-town-2010-3

McDonald, L. (2010). *Florence Nightingale at first hand; vision, power, legacy*. London: Continuum.

Mellows, W. T. (1980). *The Peterborough Chronicle of Hugh Candidus*. Peterborough Museum Society.

Parish Nursing Ministries UK. (2018). Retrieved April 20, 2018, from www.parishnursing.org.uk

Robinson, J. A. T. (1952). *The body*. London: SCM Press.

Stanley, B. (1992). *The history of the Baptist Missionary Society* (p. 233). Edinburgh: T&T Clark.

Wilkinson, J. (1998). *The Bible and Healing: A medical and theological commentary*. Edinburgh: Handsel.

Wordsworth, H. (2018). Unpublished work commissioned by Parish Nursing Ministries UK, Peterborough.

Wordsworth, H. A. (2015). *Rediscovering a Ministry of Health: Parish nursing as a mission of the local church*. Eugene, OR: Wipf and Stock.

World Council of Churches. (1981). *Conference proceedings*. Christian Medical Commission.

From the Perspective of the Faith Community Nurse

Faith Roberts and Kathie Blanchfield

10.1 In the Beginning: Reverend Granger Westberg's Vision for Whole Person Health

Responding to the "call" to be a faith community nurse offers a professional nurse the opportunity to practice in a faith community as a minister of health. Thanks to the vision of Reverend Granger Westberg (Westberg & McNamara, 1987), faith community nursing delivers whole person health in the real place of healing, a faith community. In his vocation as a pastor, chaplain, and medical school faculty, Reverend Westberg understood that healthcare needed to change to be inclusive of spiritual care He understood how vital nurses are to providing care to the whole person including the body, mind, and spirit (Westberg, personal communication, December 1977). Lane (1987) in a classic article titled *Care of the Human Spirit* challenged nurses to understand the unique opportunity they have to deliver whole person care at the bedside. Reverend Westberg led the movement for faith community nurses to deliver whole person care in the faith community setting (Westberg & McNamara, 1990).

10.2 Faith Community Nurses Respond to Their "Calling" into Ministry

Sulmasy (1997), a priest, physician, and well-respected author, notes many healthcare professionals understand the spiritual aspect of their calling and want to attend to the spiritual aspects of healing. He also notes that because a healthcare

F. Roberts (✉)
Carle Foundation Hospital and Carle Physigan Group, Urbana, IL, USA
e-mail: Faith.roberts@carle.com

K. Blanchfield
Lewis University, Romeoville, IL, USA
e-mail: Blanchka@lewis.edu

© Springer Nature Switzerland AG 2020   145
P. A. Solari-Twadell, D. J. Ziebarth (eds.), *Faith Community Nursing*,
https://doi.org/10.1007/978-3-030-16126-2_10

professionals practice is in a secular setting, they can be hesitant to address the spiritual aspects of care with patients. Yeaworth and Sailors Yeaworth & Sailors (2014) assert that faith community nurses not only minister to the whole person, but that this is the hallmark of this specialty practice.

Initially, faith community nurses may be uncomfortable in providing spiritual support to members of the congregation. This discomfort can happen when surrounded by faith leaders and staff who seem to do this effortlessly. Marty (1990) discusses the advantage faith community nurses have when practicing in a faith community. He shares that in society there seems to be two languages related to faith. In a religious setting, matters of faith can be discussed directly without hesitation. In other areas of a secular society, this language may not be discussed for fear of offending others. When faith community nurses follow their "calling" into in a faith community, they can focus on matters of faith, as well as caring for the physical and mental aspects of health (Solari-Twadell, Djupe, & McDermott, 1990).

10.3 Preparation for the Practice of Faith Community Nursing

It is imperative that the nurse understands the beliefs of the faith community in which they practice. Many times, families attend the same faith community throughout their life. Other times, teens may leave and no longer follow the beliefs of the faith, but still consider the faith community, their home as they grow older. One cannot assume that each person will have and practice the same faith traditions. With this understanding in place, the faith community nurse learns many ways to support spiritual needs of those cared for by this role. A few of these ways may include: (a) listening, (b) praying with and for individuals, (c) leading prayer at meetings, (d) discussing what supports spiritual health, (e) being present to offer intentional spiritual support in a calm supportive way, (f) asking others who have gone through the same difficult time in their lives to provide support to others when needed, (g) leading days of reflection, (h) developing grief support groups, and (i) sharing reflections about their own spiritual growth.

10.4 Where to Start: Collaboration with the Faith Community's Leader and Staff

The first step for the novice faith community nurse after attending the *Foundations for Faith Community Nursing Course* is meeting with the faith leader and staff. Some nurses educate, some focus on program development, and others choose a home visit ministry that fulfills a need in the faith family. For a novice faith community nurse, the initial work is on relationship building with staff and members of the faith community. Collaboration is a key aspect of the practice. Without the ability to collaborate with the membership, community agencies, and healthcare systems, faith community nurses find themselves isolated in their ministry (Blanchfield & McLaughlin, 2006; Dyess, Opalinski, Saiswick, & Fox, 2016; Schroepfer, 2016).

It is imperative that both the faith leader and the nurse understand their individual roles and how the roles are enhanced by collaboration. A discussion of what skills and knowledge they each bring is a solid starting point. The nurse should be aware that the faith leader may not have worked with a faith community nursing program before and might feel threatened. The best way to educate is to point out what was learned in their faith community nursing course and what the nurse sees as their way to contribute to the faith leader's team (Catholic Health Association of the United States, 2016). A faith community preparation course and formal nursing education is different than the education received at a seminary, rabbinical school, or religious studies. Faith community nurses can excel when they share their expertise in health education and in care of the whole person. Once the decision is made about how they can collaborate together, both the nurse and the leader will be better equipped to meet the needs of the faith community together.

An example of collaboration between the faith community nurse and faith leader is addressing documentation of the care of the client and the need to maintain private health information confidential. Faith leaders and staff members may be aware of the Health Insurance Portability and Accountability Act (HIPAA), but may not understand the responsibilities that the faith community nurse has regarding the confidentiality of patient information and documentation if connected to a health care organization. Confidentiality is a part of the legal and ethical responsibilities of every registered nurse. This ethical perspective of nursing practice goes way back to Florence Nightingale (Gretter and Committee for the Farrand Training School for Nurses, Detroit, 1893). Whether or not HIPAA is involved, keeping information private, unless permission is given, is a professional obligation and a legal responsibility.

When discussing concerns with a member of the faith community, an easy way to gain permission to share this information would be this statement, "I have enjoyed our time together. I want to inform the pastor of your struggles. Is that alright with you?" Once permission is granted the nurse is free to share *only need to know* information with the faith community leader. Note this permission was given for the leader, not for all of the staff. Another statement that may be useful would be "I am honored that you trusted me enough to share your concerns about the bullying your daughter is facing. I think our youth leader would be an excellent source of support for you and your family. He knows so much about difficult relationships. Is it alright with you if I share this information with him?"

Faith community nurses need to take the lead in educating others about their professional responsibilities as outlined in their state's practice act and guided by their scope and standards of practice (ANA and HMA, 2017). A faith community nurse should carry professional liability insurance. The paid or unpaid status of a faith community nurse does not remove this requirement. The paid or unpaid status of a faith community nurse does not remove the need to document the care provided. There are electronic as well as paper options for documentation. While faith community nurses are not a high liability risk, they may give advice, which could be misinterpreted. It is vital that all care given be recorded (Harris & Longcoy, 2016). Chapter 19 details of documentation expectations and resources available.

Faith community nurses need to explain to their patients that they will be keeping confidential records on pertinent information and this information will be kept secured. It is not unusual for the faith leader, staff, or others to ask the nurse for information about members that they are concerned about. This is how people show their concern and willingness to help each other. Faith community nurses cannot respond unless directed by the patient to do so. Members will frequently give this permission and ask the faith community nurse to tell others so they can receive support and prayers. This permission must be documented in writing.

There are important exceptions to confidentiality. Nurses are mandated reporters of child and elder abuse. The leader and staff need to understand the professional responsibility that a nurse has to notify the state authorities of any suspected abuse. Faith community nurses also need to report any information they have about an individual they suspect is intending to do harm to themselves or to others. Reviewing the faith community nurse's professional responsibilities surrounding issues of confidentiality will help others to see the nurse as a trusted resource.

Nurses should also be alert to any conversation that begins with "I want to tell you something, but you cannot tell anyone else." Before agreeing, the first response should be "I am not able to do that if you or someone else is being hurt or are thinking of harming yourself. I can help you with either of those two areas, but I cannot keep it to myself."

10.5 Exemplar: Collaborating with Others

A frequent need for confidential collaboration between the faith community nurse and the faith leader is in meeting the needs of isolated elder members. In one instance, the faith leader received a call by "Sarah's" frustrated daughter. She explained that her mother refused all help and had an infected leg ulcer and that her landlord was threatening to evict her because of the foul odor. The daughter mentioned that the only person her mother trusted was her volunteer communion visitor from church. The faith leader called the faith community nurse and together they developed a plan to collaborate with the communion visitor to make a home visit. The plan was to provide spiritual support and nursing interventions to problem solve.

The home visit started with prayer and was followed by a discussion based on the medical needs of Sarah. Sarah made her own dressings for her leg ulcer and used a plastic bread bag, which was tightly wrapped around her leg with rubber bands. The faith community nurse reflected that she could not embarrass Sarah by directly referring to her home-made wrappings, but with the communion visitor's help, encouraged her to unwrap her dressings. The faith community nurse recalls that she kept praying for guidance. "As I knelt down in front of her, I knew I was on holy ground." She remembered thinking that what she said next could either help her to trust me or turn her away. The faith community nurse focused upon how grateful she was to fully understand what the client was going through. When the assessment was finished, the faith community nurse explained to Sarah that she needed immediate medical care. She reluctantly agreed to a home visit by a doctor. She was firm about the fact that she had no physician and that she would not leave her home unless a doctor made a home visit to her. She also gave us permission to share this information with the faith leader.

The faith leader, communion visitor, and faith community nurse collaborated about how to arrange for a doctor to make a home visit who spoke Sarah's native language and engaged others in community referrals. Additionally, a community ambulance was asked to be on call and a hospital was alerted to a potential admission. The community paramedics were notified of when this home visit would take place and Sarah's daughter was also asked to be present.

Before the intervention at her home, some whom were consulted suggested that Sarah wanted to be left alone to die at home. It was explained by the faith community nurse that Sarah had isolated herself because of a sense of fear and shame. Fear because she could not figure out how to control this raging leg ulcer and shame over the foul odor that this ulcer emitted. It was stressed that Sarah also needed spiritual support and decision-making support to help her make the right decision.

The faith community nurse recalls feeling that advocating for Sarah was a privilege that came with her faith community nurse role. "I knew how isolated she was and how much she needed urgent medical care. The home visit was a success with Sarah reluctantly agreeing to go to the hospital for care. When the paramedics arrived, the first paramedic through the door was from our faith community. I sensed that this was the work of the Lord and that all would be well."

When the faith community nurse visited Sarah at the hospital, the foul odor was gone and she was sitting up in bed talking to everyone who entered her room about what a difference this care made for her and that her leg and life had been saved! "This intervention happened early in my ministry as a faith community nurse. I believe it helped us to understand the power of prayer and collaboration to deliver whole person care to members of our faith community" (Blanchfield, 2002).

10.6   Introducing Yourself and Your Ministry

Introducing yourself and your role to the faith community is a critical first step. If you belong to a faith community that has more than one gathering, a photo of yourself in the newsletter, or as part of a display will help acquaint others to this new role. Some nurses say "I have been going here for years everyone knows me." However, if the faith community nurse always attends the 11:00 worship service others who attend the 9:00 service may not recognize them. The introduction should be brief and positive. "My name is …… and I have been a nurse for … years. I look forward to hearing what health education needs you have. I am more than willing to set up programs that will meet those needs. My initial ministry will be New Baby visits. The members of the *Health Cabinet* supporting this work are _____".

Along with a photo, this introduction lets people know who you are without deluging them with too much information.

There are different boundaries issues for the faith community nurse. Often, the nurse is also a member of the faith community, where the practice is located. The faith leadership and staff can aid in setting boundaries by intercepting calls and not giving personal home phone numbers. Having posted office hours will also help. An individual who does not set boundaries may wind up spending more time with their faith family than with their own family. Review the faith community nurse role with loved ones and have them assist in setting reasonable expectations. In the acute and ambulatory settings, nurses spend too much time doing things others could do. The same can happen in the worship setting. Before accepting a request, stop to ask yourself, is this my responsibility? Or, could someone else respond to this request? Delegation is key to a successful program.

10.7 Multiplier of Ministers: The Health Cabinet

Reverend Westberg knew that faith community nurses need an enormous amount of help with this ministry. As a former pastor, he knew there were many people who could be called upon to help meet the needs of the faith community. He believed that a *Health Cabinet* would be an asset. Reverend Westberg compared this to the fact that most homes have a medicine cabinet that everyone in the house uses to take care of health needs. He felt the *Health Cabinet* would serve the same need. This health cabinet is a resource for the faith community nurse to help meet the congregation's whole person health needs (Westberg, personal communication October, 1997).

The faith leader might have suggestions for whom to invite to be a member of the *Health Cabinet*. Members who are healthcare professionals can be invited to share their knowledge. Other leaders of the church can be invited to participate, such as a youth group leader, leaders of the women's or men's groups, a leader of volunteers, or a support group leader. There may also be members from outside of the faith community invited such as members of the fire department, paramedics, and police. Faith community nurses must carefully discern how to draw people from outside healthcare who are interested in assisting. For instance, elementary educators have taken courses on how to design bulletin boards. If the entire cabinet is made up of providers, therapists, and nurses, there is a danger of creating a mini-hospital or operate from a medical model. The cabinet is there to promote whole person health and wellness.

Cabinet members can also help bring resources to the faith community and to the surrounding community. Programs around identified health and safety needs can be put together using the contacts of the members of the health cabinet. Police can come to the congregation to present programs such as gun safety, active shooter drills, informed use of the internet, along with identifying building hazards and safety issues in the physical surroundings of the worship space. Paramedics can do programs on when to call 911 and what information to give over the phone about entrances and barriers to getting to the person in need. Educators can come to do programs about how to support children being healthy, how to enhance learning, what to limit with use of electronics and games online, as well as social media security and parental guidance with posting on social media. Additionally, programs about preventing and stopping bulling can be addressed to children and parents. A reward for faith community nurses and volunteers happens when members testify to how these programs made a difference.

The health cabinet can help plan various large health events such as a health fair, which allows for partnering with the health department to deliver vaccines, partnering with schools of nursing to do vital sign screenings, or with a medical center to do well children's physicals and back to school physicals. These events can be opened to the whole community as outreach.

10.8   Exemplar: No Time—A Positive Outcome from Health Fairs

"Mark" was a young father with a high-pressure job and a growing family. He entered the gym that had been transformed into an *Adult Health Fair*. In greeting, Mark told the faith community nurse he was here to pick up his daughter who was helping. He was encouraged to take advantage of the fair by having his blood pressure (B/P) taken. He said: "Thanks but I have no time." Fortunately, it took a few minutes to find his daughter. In the meantime, Mark agreed to have his B/P taken. His B/P was 190/110 with a pulse of 88. Symptoms of hypertension were discussed and Mark was counseled to call his doctor to get immediate help or go to the ER because of his elevated blood pressure and pulse. He indicated that he had no time for this. As he left, the faith community nurse asked permission to call him in a few hours to see how he was doing. He agreed. When the follow-up call was later made, Mark reported that he went to the hospital because his wife insisted he call his doctor. He was advised to go to the ER with his B/P reading. Mark called the faith community nurse 2 days later and his wife sent a thank you note addressed to all of the members in the *health cabinet*. Mark was found to have a heart condition that he most likely was born with and now needed treatment. His doctor told him his life was saved that day in the church gym. The faith community nurse remarked, "God's healing presence is everywhere" (Blanchfield, 2014a).

Novice faith community nurses are looking for programming ideas. Table 10.1 describes multiple ministry offerings from the faith community nurses of a large Midwestern program, which serves over 200 congregations and mosques.

Table 10.1 Faith community health ministry programs

General	Nutrition/Scripture/Exercise
• "3 Attitudes to Change—Grief, Guilt and Gloom"	• Cooking for One
• Bike Rodeo	• Heart Healthy Potluck
• Blood Drive	• Men in the Kitchen
• Donor Sabbath	• Soy Snacks
• Elizabeth Ministry	• Keeping your mind fit
• Flu Shots	• Thin Within
• Grief Share/Divorce Care	• Exercise Class/Yoga/Pilate
• Health Fairs: Senior, Adult, Teen, Young family	• Walk to Bethlehem
• "Humor–Laughter of the Heart"	• Walk to Jerusalem
• "Living with Chronic Disease"	• Walking with the Lord
• New driver blessing	
• Stress Management	
• "Stroke Series"–3 weeks	
• "The Bones, The Body and The Bible"	
• Vial of Life	
• Wellness Website	
• "Who Wants Mom's Lemon Pie Plate"	

10.9   Population Health

A concept that helps guide faith community nurses is to think of the congregation as a setting that by its nature is an excellent place to practice population healthcare. Faith communities are a group of people that are drawn together around a shared faith belief (Gotwals, 2018). Here is an explanation about population health from a respected textbook:

> Population Health embraces a comprehensive agenda-the healthy and unhealthy, and the clinical and nonclinical as well as the public sector and private sector. While there are many determinants that affect the health of populations, the ultimate goal is the same: healthy people comprising healthy populations that create productive workforces and thriving communities (Nash, Fabius, Skoufalos, Clarke, & Horowitz, 2016).

Notice this definition of *Population Health* does not mention the spiritual aspect of health. Faith community nurses provide spiritual interventions along with population health interventions. Being embedded in this faith community allows the nurse to be actively involved with members throughout their lives. Nurses participate in the gatherings of the faith community. They are privileged to know members and their families, and to be at the right place and time for members to reach out in times of need for health information and referrals. One example is a study by Shackelford, Weyhenmeyer, and Mabus (2014), which found faith community nurses are successful at connecting "hard to access" populations with preventative health information. The goal of this study was to reach at risk populations with early breast cancer detection information. The results were that nine faith community nurses reached more than 500 study participants.

Healthcare systems are focusing upon delivering *Population Health* and are looking for opportunities to collaborate with groups such as faith communities to support delivering health and wellness services in the community. Faith community nurses can take advantage of this opportunity to collaborate with healthcare systems by offering to host health education programs and wellness activities. The host faith community has an excellent opportunity to be welcoming and receptive to members of the community while providing both members and community members with health information (Blanchfield, 2014b).

Population health and the role of a nurse navigator has grown in importance for many healthcare organizations. Orientation to this role includes how to build a trusting relationship with patients. Faith community nurses are the original nurse navigators and do not need to build trust with their faith family as they already have established relationships. Church Health in Memphis, Tennessee has an excellent navigator program that emphasizes the bond already present between the faith community nurse and congregation (Church Health, 2016).

10.10   Exemplar: Preventing Readmissions—Scale Buddies

As the number of congregants with congestive heart failure (CHF) continues to increase, basic care of this chronic condition is important to prevent hospital readmissions. CHF requires strict monitoring of daily weight. A cardinal fear of older adults is falling and the idea of stepping up 2–4 inches on a scale causes anxiety. Cardiac nurse navigators note that morning phone calls for weights are often misleading because they can tell the person is not being truthful. Many health care professionals are unaware that expecting an older adult to look down at a scale to read the number can increase anxiety due to a fear of losing their balance. One faith community nurse came up with the idea of "scale buddies." Scale buddies" are adults who go to each other's homes and stand next to the person while they get on the scale and look down for them to read the scale. What several have done is "buddy up" and get both weights done and recorded. While some "scale buddies" get the weight and go, others stay and visit. As usual a creative ministry was developed by someone who understood not just the diagnosis, but how a simple request for a weight could create anxiety for a person (Roberts, 2018).

10.11   Reaching Out to the Community

Faith community nurses can offer many types of health programs both to the faith community and to members of the surrounding community. Health fairs, immunization mornings for children and adults, self-care education programs, along with chronic care and wellness screenings can be offered by the faith community nurse and the health cabinet. These offerings can also be staffed with volunteers and professionals from community healthcare systems. Everyone benefits from this arrangement. A health care system has visibility in the community and can use this opportunity for providing health services to the community as part of their community benefit report. The faith community nurse and members of the Health Cabinet can reinforce the need for follow-up and can plan additional whole person health initiatives as a result of interacting with participants in these programs (Blanchfield & Reifsteck, 1998; Dyess et al., 2016; Schroepfer, 2016; Shackelford et al., 2014; Yeaworth & Sailors, 2014).

A bonus of faith community health programs and health fairs can happen when the staff and leader participate by taking advantage of these health services. When a faith leader and staff stand in line to receive their influenza injection along with other members of the congregation, they are role modeling self-care and the importance of taking time to get an immunization.

10.12 Exemplar: Growing in Ministry of Health

After two years of offering onsite health fairs it was determined that it was time to expand the health and wellness programs and reach out to the community by opening these programs up to members of the surrounding community. The faith community was blessed to have many healthcare professionals that were affiliated with several healthcare systems.

With the help of the members of the Health Cabinet, a plan for two health fairs, one for children and one for adults was developed. This expanded into offering back to school physicals and immunizations for children and college students. This was a partnership with the township to offer immunizations at reduced cost. The medical center was approached for help with the school physicals. The head of the Pediatric Residency Program brought ten residents to do the school physicals. Also, there to help were instructors and students from two colleges of nursing. The gym and classrooms were transformed into a clinic. The parking lot was transformed into a Health and Safety Fair. More than 250 immunizations were given, and more than 140 school physicals were completed. A written grant supported 30 car safety seats for infants and children. The police did safety car seat checks and gave out car seats to those who needed these for their children (Blanchfield, 2014b).

10.13 Intentional Integration of the Spiritual Dimension

The best medicine in the world will not bring down a blood pressure of someone who cannot afford to pay for the medication. Many people have insurance, but co-pays can add up to a point where care is delayed in lieu of other bills. Faith community attendees are struggling with debt and student loan commitments. The anxiety that comes with poor financial health may also impact physical illness. Denominations have responded to this with an increase in faith driven money management courses.

Faith community nurses often experience the effects of family dynamics on whole person health. When a person or a relative is seeing the end of a marriage or a job, grief is present and can affect their health. If a person has not heard from or has a contentious relationship with a family member, this too can affect their health. This adverse effect is evident when all treatment plans are being followed, but symptoms persist. The seminal studies by Dossey (1998), demonstrated that underlying grief, anger, or anxiety may affect an individual's physical response to disease. Practicing faith community nurses see this through increased blood pressure, digestive issues, and increased stress on a daily basis. Someone who is emotionally wrought over a loss of job, marriage, or life situation may not be interested in taking their medications as scheduled. Someone who aches for a connection with others may not pay attention to physical changes they are experiencing. The studies on family caregivers highlight the signs of self-neglect the caregiver might be experiencing in order to make sure the ill family member receives needed care (Miller, 2008). Support groups for family caregivers often focus on the caregiver's health and emotions instead of all the conversation focusing on the ill relative. The faith community nurse has the advantage of being able to add relational and financial health in supporting whole person health.

10.14   Exemplar: Financial Health

A coordinator of a large faith community nurse program in the Midwest, the program includes an Islamic Mosque among the faith organizations. The faith community nurse coordinator received a phone call from one of the Muslim nurses inquiring whether or not setting up education on mandatory car insurance would be acceptable. Before answering, an inquiry for more background was requested. This was not a topic that had ever been pursued in a health ministry class. The community setting is a university town with a large graduate student population of more than 22,000. Forty percent of graduate students originate from the Middle East and a significant number of these students are Muslims. What the nurse discovered was that while the university sent information about many aspects of living in the U.S.A., the state mandate for car insurance had not been covered.

Unfortunately, one of the graduate students was in an accident and it took all of the money the family had brought for his education that school year to pay the associated costs. The faith community nurse pointed out that because of this lack of knowledge the financial health of this family had been severely affected. This was post 9/11 and returning home was not an option. The ability at that time for this family to re-enter the states would be tenuous at best. The impact to this family was the loss of a year of study, a delayed degree, and increased pressure on their budget. The nurse at the Mosque was sensitive to the fact that in this case, poor financial health could also affect relational health. Together with the two faith community nurses serving at the Mosque, a program was developed on mandatory car insurance including three quotes from insurance brokers in the community. This program on mandatory car insurance was met with interest and appreciation. It is now offered every August to new graduate students and their families (Roberts, 2018).

10.15 Blood Pressure: Truly a Vital Sign

Another factor faith community nurses need to keep in mind is how blood pressure (B/P) can be an indicator of other health issues that are present for an individual. For many faith community nurses, a blood pressure ministry is used as a way to be visible on the day of worship. Any attendee can get their blood pressure checked at a local clinic or store that has an automatic machine. The difference when coming to a faith community nurse screening is the presence of a caring professional nurse that has been educated to listen carefully and to integrate health and faith.

10.16 Exemplar: Blood Pressure and Spiritual Care

An 82 year-old female presented for B/P following the 10 AM service. Her B/P was 170/94. The first response from the nurse was "Did you remember to take your pill today?" The response was "yes," which cued the nurse to look at this person and seize the moment. "Wow…that is a rather high blood pressure for you. I can see here that your last three were all much lower. Is something going on? Anything you want to talk about?"

It is not uncommon when a B/P is elevated and medication has been taken to see the actual mind-body-spirit response. The reply to the faith community nurse could be "I have been worried about my son, his marriage is in trouble" or "this Tuesday will be one year since my husband died." By being present in the moment and listening carefully, the nurse sees hypertension as a physical response to an emotional concern.

Grief can re-trigger throughout the life span and present with a physical response such as an elevated blood pressure. An elevated blood pressure might also be the physical sign of someone struggling with family separations, broken relationships, or addiction in the family. Assessing physical responses should include questions about relational health.

During a home visit, the faith community nurse is on holy ground (O'Brien, 2018). The sacred space might be at a table with a candle or statuary, a rolled prayer rug in the corner, for others it is the table next to the recliner with church bulletins, scripture, prayer beads, and devotionals. For many though, it is in the kitchen, on the refrigerator door. On this appliance there might be magnetic letters from children or grandchildren, a favorite scripture, church bulletin, family photos or a yellowed Erma Bombeck column. When viewing these remembrances the faith community nurse can get a sense of what is sacred or most valued in the home and to the individual (Roberts, 2018).

10.17 The Spiritual Gift of Presence

There are many benefits for both the faith community nurse and for the patients they see. The art of presence is something that takes the precious commodity of time and offers the precious gift of self. To truly listen to another and absorb their words, rather than focus on what to say in response, is to be present. To be open to the spirit and to know that in silence much can be learned that will help the interaction reach a deeper level. In order to minister to the whole person, faith community nurses must draw on their and skills and knowledge. Instead of focusing on physical interventions, the focus may be on hearing and empathically responding to the spiritual or emotional challenges facing the person.

Presence is a nursing intervention that is a core competence to all faith community nurses. In today's world, the mantra has become "I'm busy." In reality, who isn't? It is in the small moments of life that spirits bond. The initial question in the U.S.A. culture has been "Hi, how *are* you?" It has now changed to "Hi, what do you *do*?" Many nurses have experienced caring for a patient and focusing on titrating the IV pump, vitals, or treatments and just as the nurse is preparing to exit the room, the patient grabs their hand, squeezes it and says "Thanks hon." Moments like that stop the clock and bring the nurse to the present. Presence is a gift because many do not expect the full attention of another person.

Todays' health care world is one filled with technology and a pervasive false sense of urgency. It truly is a skill to simply "be" with another person. Isolation and loneliness do not fall to one generation. A new mother on an 8-week maternity leave can feel alone. A young widower in his forties might feel out of place at a church grief group. A person no longer able to drive, may be lonely and longing to have fellowship.

Faith community nurses many times have the gift of time to practice presence. When engaged with a faith community attendee, consider taking a breath to bring about a sense of calmness. Focus on the other person's words, body movements, and vocal pitch. By focusing solely on listening the faith community nurse will increase awareness of not just what is said, but how it is said. It is said that every person just wants someone to hear their story. For faith community nurses that practice presence, the ability to be present and just listen is an acquired skill.

10.18 Exemplar: Practice of Presence

One of the first things a faith community nurse may observe is that working in a faith community is very different than an acute care setting. Another key learning is that being a faith community nurse can be isolating. Some faith community nurses may be the only nurse working locally in their denomination. Collaboration includes sharing experiences with others walking the same road. Meeting with a more seasoned faith community nurse at a local diner for a Pepsi or talking over the phone helps a new faith community nurse to be more comfortable in providing spiritual care. Praying with each other helps to be more familiar with differing styles of prayer. Often nurses may have a "Find it, Fix it" mentality. It is important to recognize that not everyone can be, or even wants to be "fixed." Confidence can grow as the nurse becomes more comfortable with the art of presence. The more the nurse practices presence, the better the ability to focus on what the client is saying or needs.

All faith community nurses come to this specialty with different experiences and expertise. One evening, a faith community nurse received a call from a pastor asking for the nurse to go to a church member's home immediately as they were actively dying and the pastor was unable to get there. The faith community nurse hung up the phone and the anxiety and negative self-talk began; "I don't do this" "I have never done this" "What am I supposed to do?" When the faith community nurse arrived at the home of the client, a cousin greeted the nurse. The cousin told the nurse that the woman who was dying was surrounded by her adult children in the front room. She also shared that all three of the adult children had left the faith they had been reared in when young. One was an agnostic, one a Buddhist, and one a Scientologist. The faith community nurse took a deep breath and entered the room. Two adult sons and one daughter hovered over their beloved mother. The woman who was dying was a life member of the congregation with a reputation as a strong witness to her beliefs. The faith community nurse prayed "Please Lord let me say something that shows kindness, please Lord help me do this right." At that moment all three adult children joined hands and beckoned the faith community nurse to join in as they sang a traditional hymn from their denomination. This evening ended up not about who believed what, it was about how you help a family say good-bye. That evening had nothing to do with their own spiritual journeys as much as helping their mom join her Creator (Roberts, 2017).

10.19 Spiritual Strength Programs

A faith community nurse can offer *Spiritual Strength Programs* that are uniquely suited to the faith community setting. Certain problems can cause spiritual distress because of shame and isolation surrounding the problem. These problems can be difficult to discuss and can cause individuals and families to keep secrets. Examples of these problems are addiction, mental illness, and suicide, infidelity in marriage, domestic violence, hoarding, depression, anxiety, and compulsive shopping. Shame around these problems can cause individuals to not address the issues or to not seek help. All of these problems are human afflictions that can be dealt with by being sensitive to the spiritual drain that these conditions can have on individuals, families, and communities.

Faith community nurses, in collaboration with the *Health Cabinet*, can bring in resources from the community. In addition, members of the community who have been successful in overcoming one of these problems could be invited to present a *Spiritual Strength Program*. Inviting Alcoholics Anonymous into the faith community sends a powerful message. Survivors of domestic violence can educate the faith community and provide resources. Loved ones of someone who died by suicide can facilitate a sensitive discussion about such a tragedy. Out of these *Spiritual Strength Programs* informal or formal support groups can develop. This is the advantage the faith community nurses partnering with and practicing in a faith community.

10.20   Exemplar: Spiritual Strength Programs

In providing Spiritual *Strength Programs*, it has been reported that most attendees do not look up or greet anyone. Beginning the program with a prayer is helpful in decreasing anxieties. No one is asked to introduce themselves, but the following question is asked, "what do you hope to receive after attending this program?" Then presenters share what they hope to accomplish.

An example of one program is *Loving Outreach to Survivors of Suicide* (LOSS). This program addresses family members of someone who died by suicide. A *Health Cabinet* member who was an ER Physician started this program by sharing that he was also a survivor of losing a loved one by suicide. After he shared what helped and what did not help him, everyone seemed to want to talk about their lived experience. When the program was over, the conversations continued in the parking lot. Many small groups of attendees gathered sharing stories and phone numbers. As a result of this program, the faith community was known as a site that hosted a support group for the LOSS Program.

Spiritual Strength Programs are usually received well. Here is a list of program titles:

1. Spiritual Strength for Addiction to Alcohol
2. Spiritual Strength for Addiction to Drugs
3. Spiritual Strength for Facing a Long-Term Health Condition
4. Spiritual Strength for Supporting Those with Depression
5. Spiritual Strength for Survivors of Suicide
6. Spiritual Strength for Facing Memory Challenges
7. Spiritual Strength and Resources for Caregivers of Loved Ones (Blanchfield, 2013)

10.21   End of Life Care Planning

Nurses who have experience working in acute care understand that the hospital setting is not the ideal setting to initiate end of life planning. When nurses practice as a faith community nurse, one of the benefits is the impact that place has. There is a difference in helping people to create their own *End of Life Planning* in the faith community setting versus in an acute care organization. Nurses know that ideally this planning needs to be done when individuals are not in a crisis or severely ill. The *Gunderson Lutheran Medical Foundation* (Gundersen Lutheran Medical Foundation, 2014) understood this when they created the *Respecting Choices* program to educate people about the need for *End of Life Planning*. This program comes complete with papers that address the person's wishes and identifies who should speak for the individual if they cannot speak for themselves. This program is clear and practical as it moves the reader through the necessary steps of end of life planning. The *Respecting Choices* program also complements the *Five Wishes Form for End of Life Planning* (Aging with Dignity, 2011).

The faith community setting is an ideal place to educate members about what is involved with creating an Advanced Directive for care at the end of life. End of life planning programs are opportunities for collaboration with faith leader. By offering programs on this topic, faith community nurses can share Godly wisdom in planning individual end of life arrangements before the need arises. The faith leader can validate the need for this end of life planning and explain how this does align with teachings of the faith. These programs can be set up to have attendees come with loved ones so everyone is educated at the same time. Then, at the program, documents are available to be filled out. Note that most states differ on what is required, and the nurse must be aware and use the correct documents. Any adult may witness these documents, including a faith community nurse.

10.22 Exemplar: Family Struggles with End of Life Care Planning

After collaborating with the faith leader to present several well-attended programs about *End of Life Care Planning*, the faith community nurse was called by a couple who attended one of the programs. They asked the nurse to make a home visit to discuss their family's response to their plans. When the nurse arrived, it became apparent that their discussion did not go well with their four adult children. The parents told the nurse that they felt that this was an act in accordance with their faith and that by filling out these forms they would not only be expressing their wishes, but also be stating their belief in God and in an afterlife. The problem arose when their adult children could not agree upon whom would take responsibility for the legal aspects. So, they refused to be named as a healthcare power of attorney if one of their parents could not speak for themselves.

This caused the parents a great deal of emotional and spiritual distress. During the home visit, time was taken to consider the spiritual needs that were not being met. Both felt that they were faithfully planning for their end of life care according to how they felt God wanted them to do this. They realized that once these plans were in place, they would feel a sense of peace. This sense of peace would reinforce their beliefs as they prepared for the care they believed was best. In their initial discussion with their children, they did not share this spiritual dimension. Instead, they focused upon the legal and medical aspects of these plans.

After time was dedicated to reflecting about the spiritual aspects of *End of Life Planning*, the couple decided to make this the focus of their discussion with their children. Fortunately, this meeting went very well. The parents felt supported and affirmed in their faith beliefs. After the father died, the mother stated that she had great comfort in her husband's end of life care and in her children's support during this sad time. She stated she did not fear what would happen when her time came because of her faith and of her children's participation and understanding with carrying out her husband's wishes. This is another example of the sense of peace and satisfaction a faith community nurse can facilitate by providing support for *end of life planning* (Blanchfield, 2011).

10.23   The Size and Demographics of a Faith Community

The size and demographics of a faith community can impact the practice of a faith community nurse. This knowledge can guide the nurse in how to approach program planning to address health needs. If the size is 200 members, and demographics are older, program planning will look different than if the faith community has mostly young families. Depending upon the size and demographics, faith community nurses need to determine what is the best use of their skills and time. In smaller faith communities, where everyone knows each other, it may be expected that the faith community nurse makes frequent home and hospital visits. In larger ones, the use of volunteers may be necessary (Butler & Diaz, 2017).

In large faith communities of 2000 or more, nurses have to make difficult choices about how to best use their time and resources. It is imperative for faith community nurses to take the time to recruit and to support volunteers to make it possible to multiply their services. The nurse needs to communicate the needs and put frequent notices in the bulletin.

In rural areas, there is often a shared responsibility towards health care. In one small town, a bi-monthly blood drive is staffed by three faith communities. One hosts the mobile van, while another registers and completes paperwork, and a third prepares a meal. This small community has done this for years and boasts of a donor group averaging 100 donors every 2 months. In a town with a population of 125,000, two faith communities on the same main thoroughfare decided to share a health fair. One faith community hosted young family and teen health education. At the other faith community, adult and senior education was offered. This collaboration resulted in strong attendance, while focusing on specific audiences.

10.24   Exemplar: Small Congregation Learns from an Elder

A small Lutheran faith community in the Midwest averaged a Sunday attendance of 175–200. This faith community was predominately farm families and very close. An energetic and thoroughly organized faith community nurse sprang into action upon hearing that a member was home on bed rest for 7 weeks. A problem with a pregnancy necessitated complete bed rest for this young mother of two. She and her husband were shell-shocked trying to figure out how the house would function and how their two sons age seven and five would get to their activities. The nurse met them at their home and reviewed what was needed and went to work organizing volunteers. She made an excel sheet. She had an online *meal train* setup with likes and dislikes. She designed it so it would kick out someone who entered a meal that had already been taken, to avoid three lasagnas in 1 week. Her absolute favorite was the baseball schedule for the 7-year-old child. She had the dates and location of each game with a square for drop off and pick up. Announcements were made the previous Sunday that volunteers were needed to help this family.

Sunday morning found the faith community nurse behind a table with a box of pens and signup sheets. To her dismay, an older gentleman came up and signed up for every drop off and pick up for every game. She stated "You can't do that" "Why not?" he replied. "Because you are taking all the spots." He smiled, sighed and looked at her… "Honey, did you ever play ball? Whoever takes the boy, has to pick him up, because they have to stay for the game. On the ride back, you tell him what he did well and what he could do better. You offer to throw a couple balls with him later in the week. And you tell him that the other kid is a jerk and don't worry about him." The faith community nurse eyes filled with tears as she realized that while she had focused on an extremely large *to do* list, this gentleman was focused on helping a little boy feel safe and cared for during a time of incredible upheaval in his home (Roberts, 2018).

10.25 Exemplar: Faith Community Nurse Lived Experience in a Large Metropolitan Congregation

The pastor agreed to have a faith community nurse join the 15-person parish staff as the first faith community nurse. A faith community had 5000 families. During the meeting with the pastor, it was emphasized how faith community nursing would enhance several existing ministries. The faith community already had a ministry to the homebound, a grammar school of 800 children, a youth group, a group for seniors, and a grief support group, along with many others. The faith community nurse stressed that working alone would not be beneficial. Instead the faith community nurse worked to multiply the ministers by recruiting volunteers. The pastor encouraged the faith community nurse "call" forth others to share their gifts within the congregation. With this wisdom, the faith community nurse soon realized how God works. As volunteers came forth a *Health Cabinet* and *a Nursing Cabinet* were developed. Fortunately, it was easy to recruit volunteers when the faith community nurse "met" parishioners in the grocery store, in the gym at children's games or sporting events, and at the faith community. Once, the concept of faith community nursing was explained, there were many willing volunteers. Volunteers stated that this *health ministry* would allow them time to engage with people, while sharing their knowledge and skills. The volunteers celebrated being part of responding to God's "call" to care for others.

The *Health Cabinet* had 20 members. Most were healthcare professionals with different backgrounds ranging from nurses and doctors to nutritionists, psychologists, and teachers. A few were elected community officials or part of the fire department and paramedics. The *Nursing Cabinet* had 15 nurses from more than ten different healthcare agencies. Each nurse brought unique experiences and resources to help plan healthcare programming aimed at promoting health and wellness in the faith community and in the community at large. The difference between the *Health Cabinets and Nursing Cabinets* was a matter of focus. The *Health Cabinet* focused on promoting health by reaching out to the greater community, as well as their faith community. The *Nursing Cabinet* focused upon collaborating with other parish ministries and providing needed help to external individuals and groups. A regular meeting time facilitated evaluation of the programs offered, the need to develop new health programs, and to help those who were dealing with chronic illness. Inherent in this work was the regular celebration of the hundreds of volunteer hours that were devoted to the health ministry.

The *Health Cabinet* collaborated with other parish ministries. The *Health Cabinet* worked with the youth minister to develop programs on spirituality for teens and recruited teens to help with other large health programs. In addition, the cabinet worked with the grammar school teachers to develop health awareness programs for various grade levels. The senior citizen group welcomed health information, as long as there was no interference with bingo. A brown bag pharmacy program broke the ice with the seniors. These various collaborations resulted in being able to reach more people. Soon, there was regular scheduling of joint programs on the parish's annual calendar.

Through joining two different groups of faith community nurses, support and additional ideas for developing this *health ministry* presented themselves. Meeting monthly to pray together, to share stories, to share lessons learned, and to advocate for more health resources in the community was foundational to these networking sessions. The faith community nurse groups provided an excellent source of support. In addition, through collaboration, interdenominational health programs were facilitated.

An example of collaboration occurred when an urgent call for help was received from the grammar school principal. A mother of one of the school children needed a bone marrow transplant and was anxious to find a donor. Through working together, within 2 weeks a bone marrow donor drive was held. With God's significant help, more than 200 donors participated and more than $12,000 was donated to this cause. This health initiative helped this large faith community to come together to support one member in need. This was a reminder that God would take care of delivering what was needed as long as others joined together and responded to His call (Blanchfield, 2014b).

10.26 Conclusion

Faith community nurses are able to readily transfer both their knowledge and skills to a faith community setting. The satisfaction from being a faith community nurse comes from the ability to apply professional nursing while integrating faith into everything that the faith community nurse does. Being a faith community nurse fills a part of the heart of the faith community nurse that has been asking more from nursing.

Faith community nurses have the privilege of becoming a part of a faith community, being with faith community members in their most intimate moments is a privilege. Through this work the faith community nurse is a known, respected, and trusted source of health information. Faith community nurses do not shy away from grief, illness, death, shame, anger, or guilt and know that every day they are privileged to share sacred times. The focus is not on productivity, but in caring and sharing the power of prayer and faith. A favorite quote from a small town parish nurse is "I would much rather give my gifts and talents as a registered professional nurse to this church then make one more covered dish for this congregation. While this comment resonates with many, I understand that God has gifted me with skills and knowledge that may help others".

References

Aging with Dignity. (2011). *Five wishes*. Tallahassee, FL: Author.

American Nurses Association and Health Ministries Association, Inc. Scope and Standards. (2017). *Faith community nursing: Scope and standards of practice* (3rd ed.). Silver Spring, MD: Nursesbooks.org.

Blanchfield, K. C. (2002). Homebound with shame: Caring for the spiritual, emotional and physical needs of an isolated elderly person. *Journal of Advocate Health Care, 4*(2), 37–40.

Blanchfield, K. C. (2011). The spiritual dimension of facilitating advance directives planning: The congregational setting as a vital resource. *Hektoen International, 4*(2).

Blanchfield, K. C. (2013). *Spiritual strength programs*. Presentation at faith community nursing preparation course, Lewis University, Oak Brook, IL.

Blanchfield, K. C. (2014a). *The outcomes of health fairs*. Presentation at faith community nursing preparation course, Lewis University, Oak Brook, IL.

Blanchfield, K. C. (2014b). *Ethical and legal aspects of community collaborative partnerships*. Presentation at the 2014 Westberg Symposium Church Health Center, Memphis, TN.

Blanchfield, K. C., & McLaughlin, E. M. (2006). Parish nursing a collaborative ministry. In P. A. Solari-Twadell & M. A. McDermott (Eds.), *Parish nursing development, education and administration* (pp. 65–81). St. Louis, MO: Elsevier.

Blanchfield, K. C., & Reifsteck, S. M. (1998). Parish nursing: Holistic care within a congregation. *Viewpoint, 20*(2), 11–12.

Butler, S., & Diaz, C. (2017). *Nurses as intermediaries in the promotion of community health: Exploring their roles and challenges*. Retrieved from https://www.brookings.edu/wp-content/uploads/2017/09/es_20170921_nurses_as_intermediaries.pdf

Catholic Health Association of the United States. (2016). *Improving the lives of older adults through community partnerships: Healing body, mind and spirit*. Retrieved from https://www.chausa.org/docs/default-source/eldercare/improving-the-lives-of-older-adults-through-faith-community-partnerships_final-oct-192016.pdf?sfvrsn=0

Church Health. (2016). *Congregational health promoter training leader guide*. Memphis, TN: Author.

Dossey, L. (1998). *Healing words: The power of prayer and the practice of medicine*. New York: Harper.

Dyess, S. M., Opalinski, A., Saiswick, K., & Fox, V. (2016). Caring across the continuum: A call to nurse leaders to manifest values through action with community outreach. *Nursing Administration Quarterly, 40*(2), 137–145. https://doi.org/10.1097/NAQ.000000000000157

Gotwals, B. (2018). Self-efficacy and nutrition education: A study of the effect of an intervention with faith community nurses. *Journal of Religion and Health, 57*(1), 333–348.

Gretter, L., & Committee for the Farrand Training School for Nurses, Detroit. (1893). *Nightingale pledge*. Retrieved from https://www.vanderbilt.edu/vanderbiltnurse/2010/11/florence-nightingale-pledge/

Gundersen Lutheran Medical Foundation. (2014). *Respecting choices advanced care planning*. Retrieved from www.respectingchoices.org

Harris, M. D., & Longcoy, R. (2016). Collaborative efforts in the community: Faith community nurses as partners in healing. *Home Healthcare Now, 34*(3), 146–150.

Lane, J. A. (1987). Care of the human spirit. *Journal of Professional Nursing, 3*(6), 332–337.

Martin, M. (1990). Forward. In P. A. Solari, A. M. Djupe, & M. A. McDermott (Eds.), *Parish nursing the developing practice* (pp. 1–8). Park Ridge, IL: National Parish Nurse Resource Center.

Miller, J. E. (2008). *The caregiver's book: Caring for another, caring for yourself* (2nd ed.). Fort Wayne, IN: Willowgreen.

Nash, D. B., Fabius, R. J., Skoufalos, A., Clarke, J. L., & Horowitz, M. R. (2016). *Population health: Creating a culture of wellness* (2nd ed.). Burlington, MA: Jones & Bartlett Learning.

O'Brien, M. E. (2018). *Spirituality in nursing: Standing on holy ground* (6th ed.). Burlington, MA: Jones & Bartlett Learning.

Roberts, F. B. (2017). Presentation at Bay Care System Faith Community Nurse Retreat, Tampa, FL.

Roberts, F. B. (2018). Presentation at Faculty Preparation Training Westberg Institute, Memphis, TN.

Schroepfer, E. (2016). Professional issues: A renewed look at faith community nursing. *MEDSURG Nursing, 2*(1), 62–66.

Shackelford, J. A., Weyhenmeyer, D. P., & Mabus, L. K. (2014). Fostering early breast cancer detection: Faith community nurses reaching at-risk populations. *Clinical Journal of Oncology Nursing, 18*(6), E113–E117. https://doi.org/10.1188/14.CJON.E113-E117

Solari-Twadell, P. A., Djupe, A. M., & McDermott, M. A. (Eds.). (1990). *Parish nursing: The developing practice*. Park Ridge, IL: National Parish Nurse Resource Center.

Sulmasy, D. P. (1997). *A healer's calling: A spirituality for physicians and other health care professionals*. Mahwah, NJ: Paulist Press.

Westberg, G. E., & McNamara, J. (1987). *The parish nurse: How to start a parish nurse program in your church*. Park Ridge, IL: Parish Nurse Resource Center.

Westberg, G. E., & McNamara, J. W. (1990). *The parish nurse: Providing a minister of health for your congregation*. Minneapolis, MN: Augsburg.

Yeaworth, R. C., & Sailors, R. (2014). Faith community nursing: Real care, real cost savings. *Journal of Christian Nursing, 31*(3), 178–183. https://doi.org/10.1097/CNJ.0000000000000075

From the Perspective of the Physician

Glenn Scott Morris

11.1 A Physician's Role in Faith and Health

11.1.1 The Early Years

During my first year at Yale Divinity School, I got to know David Duncum, who taught at the divinity school, but whose full-time job was the chaplain of Yale Medical School. He invited me to meet with him at his medical school office to talk about my desire for ministry and what form it would take. I had always known my professional path would link faith and health, but as a first year seminarian, I didn't have a clear picture of how.

The medical school at Yale is literally on the other side of New Haven from the divinity school, and it is hard to get from one school to the other. I was waiting to meet with David in his small office, and after sitting there for a few minutes I looked at his desk. It was cluttered and disorganized, but on the corner I saw an 8 × 10 thirty-page pamphlet titled, "How to Start a Church-based Health Center." Its author was Granger Westberg. I picked it up and began reading through it. The idea was simple. The plan called for using the basement of a church and integrating people's health care with a physician, a social worker, a nurse, and a pastoral counselor. Along with a few pictures, the pages described how the integrated care worked.

That was it—a church-based health clinic.

From that point on it felt like a "calling." It seemed that God said to me, "This is what you will do." It wasn't emotional. If anything, it was intellectual, but it felt true and pointed. This is what I was going to do with my life. I blocked out of my head other options. Nothing would stop me. I was "called." Or was I just stubborn? Ever since I was young and began reading the Bible for myself, particularly the Gospels,

G. S. Morris (✉)
Church Health, Memphis, TN, USA
e-mail: Morriss@churchhealth.org

© Springer Nature Switzerland AG 2020
P. A. Solari-Twadell, D. J. Ziebarth (eds.), *Faith Community Nursing*,
https://doi.org/10.1007/978-3-030-16126-2_11

I was convinced the church didn't do enough to live out the healing dimension of the gospel.

So I arranged to go to Hinsdale, Illinois, a suburb outside Chicago, where Rev. Granger Westberg was operating a church-based health clinic out of a church and see how it was done. I spent a month of my summer break absorbing everything Granger had to teach me about whole-person health care. By then, Granger's interests were already widening to the possibilities of what could be done for whole-person care by expanding the role of nurses. Since I hadn't even been to medical school yet, my head didn't keep up with that new frontier. It would be years before I realized I had been wrong not to pay more attention.

After finishing seminary and becoming credentialed in the United Methodist Church, I did go to medical school and complete a residency in family medicine. During residency, I even had the chance to be part of a sort of trial run at opening a church-based clinic to provide care for an underserved population. Then I moved to Memphis in 1986. A major pull was that it was one of the poorest cities in America. I took a job with the local health department, introduced myself to the pastor of a downtown United Methodist Church, and bravely pursued whatever far-fetched connections began to emerge in a city where I was determined to open a faith-based clinic to care for the working uninsured. The next year, we opened the doors of *Church Health* in a rehabbed house with one doctor—me—and one nurse with a small support staff. We saw 12 patients the first day. Now, more than 30 years later, *Church Health* sees patients in another renovated home, a repurposed former Sears distribution center known as "Crosstown Concourse." We have been the doctor of record for seventy thousand patients. In more than three decades, our mission hasn't changed: to reclaim the church's biblical commitment to care for our bodies and spirits.

Present day.

In many ways Memphis is still Memphis after all this time. It's still on the list of poorest cities of America. It's still a place rife with issues that compromise the health of individuals and entire segments of our population. We are almost exactly 50% white and 50% black, with small percentages of other ethnicities and multiple nationalities. We have low-wage earners and people with high wealth. We have large employers and small businesses barely scraping by. Zip codes divide economics and access to health care. Multiple large medical systems work with nonprofits like *Church Health* in county-wide initiatives to try to close the gaps, but the challenge is ever-present. We have plenty of health care obstacles to go around, requiring every strategy we can collectively come up with.

Locally, *Church Health's* clinical services are the organization's flagship, providing a true primary care family practice medical home as well as walk-in urgent care services. *Church Health* partners with most hospitals, labs, and diagnostic centers in the area to provide services to an underserved population base. From its beginning, *Church Health* has operated a full-time medical clinic open from 7:00 a.m. to 9:00 p.m. It is staffed with 12 full-time practitioners, but also supported by 1000 physicians throughout the city who volunteer their services both at *Church Health's* site and by seeing patients in their own offices. The volunteer physicians, who represent a range of specialties, make it possible for patients to receive diagnostic testing, laboratory services, and hospital admissions, all without charge. Any medical problem can be cared for without an uninsured or underinsured patient in a low-wage job receiving a large medical bill—or going without care for fear of such a bill. Medical subspecialists generally treat patients in their own offices, but over the last few years retired doctors have been holding regular clinics at *Church Health's* location and then referring patients to former partners for surgery when needed. Other medical services include a 24-chair dental clinic, a large eye clinic, physical therapy, and a behavioral health center that emphasizes care around substance abuse. A low-cost pharmacy also is available.

Because the mission of *Church Health* is to reclaim the church's biblical commitment to care for our bodies and spirits, from our inception we have integrated wellness and medical care while addressing the spiritual needs of those we serve. This is central to our whole-person model of care. A wellness mentality includes thinking not just about the illnesses presenting in the exam rooms, but also about other parts of physical, spiritual and emotional that affect an individual's quality of life. While offering the best medical care we can, we also help people experience greater whole-person wellness, a philosophy that aligns our physicians and staff with the essence of faith community nursing. I should have been paying more attention to Granger Westberg during my seminary summer break.

From our beginnings, *Church Health* has worked to find new ways to engage the faith community in the creation of health ministries for the whole person, leading us to work in areas beyond the clinic and in the public health arena. For instance, education is fundamental to changing health outcomes over a lifetime. We can wait in the clinic for people with lower levels of education to turn up with higher levels of preventable diseases, or we can begin to change those outcomes decades before they happen. *Church Health* has run a preschool named *Perea* for 20 years. The name comes from Jesus' location when he said, "Let the little children come to me." When they enter as 3-year-olds, most of the children are behind national standards of development. By the time they leave two years later, most meet or exceed those standards, giving them a solid foundation for future years of schooling. Education changes prospects for a range of socioeconomic factors, and all of them influence health outcomes.

One of *Church Health's* most successful programs in faith communities has been training congregational health promoters. Virtually every faith community has someone—usually a woman, sometimes a nurse—who has the trust of the faith community on multiple levels. People are already going to her for advice. *Church Health* offers an eight-week training program on basic topics. Through *Church Health* community resources people may not be aware of, such as nutrition, mental and emotional health, common health issues such as hypertension, diabetes, and understanding medications are covered. *Church Health* addresses prenatal, well baby, and women's issues. *Church Health* even stares sexually transmitted disease in the face—yes, in the faith community.

Over the decades, the influence of *Church Health's* model has widened. Engaging communities of faith with the mission of reclaiming the biblical commitment to care for our bodies and spirits has meant moving beyond Memphis and into formats that travel the miles to other cities. A thriving resource development arm targets faith communities with books, curricula, and devotional materials exploring themes of faith and health. The flagship product is *Church Health Reader*, a quarterly magazine, along with other publications aimed at faith community nurses.

But more hands are always better. As a Chief Executive Officer, I know faith community nurses are an important arm of our ministry. As a physician, I'm confident they are a leading force in the way forward in patient care. I have come to see the severe limits to what traditional Western medicine has to offer people we care for. All too often, our only resource is giving patients pills that have limited effectiveness or that might actually do harm. Doctor's offices are often thought of as a place to get a pill even when the prescribing physician knows that the pill will have little impact on the person's problem. And then we collect a fee. In the American health system, it's too easy for the fee, or at least keeping up with the daily appointment schedule, to become the focus of the visit rather than an improved health outcome of the person in front of us. Faith community nurses, with their core value of whole-person care that never separates spiritual care into a separate category, help keep us grounded. The more exposure physicians have to faith community nurses, the more they will see that the specialty practice offers a missing link in traditional American medicine.

11.1.2 New Tools for Health Care

At *Church Health*, all begin with an understanding of health where, along with the World Health Organization, health is recognized not about the absence of disease. Instead, it is about a life well lived. Our purpose must go beyond just living where we only breathe in and breathe out. Instead, we should be helping people achieve what we have come to see as the goals for living. I define them as having more joy in your life, having more love in your life, and being driven closer to God. But more joy, more love, and being driven closer to God have little to do with the doctor.

In the years that *Church Health* has cared for people in Memphis, it is noted that two-thirds of our patients seek treatment for illness that healthier lifestyles can prevent or control. We realized that if we want to make lasting difference in our patients' lives, the most effective strategy is encouraging overall wellness in body and spirit. We can put salve on what hurts at the moment, but what does that change? At a fundamental level, we must transform what the words *well* and *health* mean in the minds and hearts of most people. We've developed a *Model for Healthy Living* (Morris, 2017) that communicates our heart for healing and wholeness in body and spirit.

Many people seen in our clinic, and in our large wellness facility, are isolated both from sustaining relationships and from understanding themselves in a way that lets them make healthy choices. In many instances, common diseases, such as obesity, diabetes, alcoholism, substance abuse, high blood pressure, high cholesterol, and related heart disease, can be prevented or well managed. They do not have to become crises. But this depends on identifying what's wrong in the first place, and these answers are not likely to show up in lab work discussed in a medical appointment.

How can we help our patients treat not only others but themselves with the kindness and patience and love that would lead to better health? This question led to developing our *Model for Healthy Living*.

Life is a complex web, interconnected in every dimension. When a relationship is out of sorts, we feel out of sorts spiritually as well, or we can't concentrate at work. If we're eating fast food in the car between meetings, exercise is the last thing on our minds. Sitting all day at work and all evening in front of the television can lead to lying awake in bed staring at the ceiling.

Change is a process that brings results in the long term. In that context, the Model for Healthy Living is a tool for individuals to use to take charge of their own health, and it reflects that true wellness is not just about our bodies but about the interconnectedness of body and spirit in the ways that we live. Here are the seven key dimensions of the *Model for Healthy Living*.

Faith life—Faith traditions vary widely, but at the core, a faith life helps us build a relationship with God, our neighbors, and ourselves. This affirms that we are body-and-spirit beings created and loved by God. We can explore a richer faith life and enjoy the benefits this experience will bring to overall wellness.

Medical care—Doctors have education and experience, but we know ourselves better as individuals than any doctor ever will. Even doctors sometimes are the patient. When it comes to medical care, we bring something important to the conversation. We can build a partnership with a health care provider that lets us participate in managing our health care.

Movement—When we consider the way the parts of the body are hinged and rotate and reach in every direction, it's easy to see that God means for us to move. It's part of how we celebrate our body-and-spirit connection to God. No matter what our physical activity level is now, we can discover ways to enjoy movement.

Work—We were made to work, and the value of work is intrinsic. We can appreciate the skills, talents, and gifts we bring to our work situation, whatever it is, and find meaning for our life through our jobs or volunteer commitments.

Emotional life—It's easy to turn to unhealthy habits in response to stress, whether it's food, mindless television, excessive spending, alcohol, or something else. In the moment, we feel better, even though we know it's bad in the long term. Through understanding our feelings, it's possible to make changes to manage stress in healthier ways.

Nutrition—Good nutrition builds strong bodies that can lead us to being whole people better connected to God. What we eat matters. Whatever our eating habits are now, we can increase our understanding of how food affects our overall well-being and make food choices with more intention.

Friends and family—God, Jesus, and the Holy Spirit were the very first relationship. Even God exists in community. Coping with life is sometimes hard, but friends and family make it easier. Giving and receiving support through relationships contributes to our health.

In the fall of 2011, I received a call from Deborah Patterson, then Executive Director of the *International Parish Nurse Resource Center*, asking whether *Church Health* would be interested in having the *International Parish Nurse Resource Center* move from under the umbrella of the *Deaconess Foundation* in St. Louis, to become part of our work in Memphis. It was an intriguing proposition. I was only given a few days to consider the offer. There were very few physical assets to transfer—a closetful of pins and papers. None of the resource center's four employees would be moving to Memphis. The primary resource was the rights to the curriculum used to educate parish or faith community nurses and the *Annual Westberg Symposium*. That was it.

After considering the offer for a day, I made my pitch to our senior leaders. With some trepidation they saw what was possible. I then arranged to see the Chair of the Board, who was a keen business person and also loved the work we did to care for the poor in the name of the church. He heard me out and then asked point blank, "Now why exactly are we interested in the nurses in Paris?" It was apparent I had not done a very good job explaining to him what parish nursing was all about. I went at it again, and he agreed it made sense, and so the *International Parish Nurse Resource Center* came to Memphis and became the *Westberg Institute*.

The *Model for Healthy Living* meets faith community nursing. In my mind as a physician, the Model is a practical tool in the hands of faith community nurses to care for the whole person. The *Model for Healthy Living* is more than just a chart on the wall. It's a communication method, a planning tool, a health care strategy in which both providers and patients can actively participate. More and more, the *Model for Healthy Living* has come to the center of everything that happens at *Church Health*. It's not that we have changed what we believe about the importance of any of the areas of the *Model for Healthy Living*—we've always offered exercise opportunities and counseling, and health coaching—but over the years we have increasingly grabbed hold of new opportunities to put our convictions into action.

Faith community nurses, on the front lines in faith communities, can carry the *Model for Healthy Living* into working with the people they serve. It opens up a level of conversation that happens around *Church Health*, but does not happen in the vast majority of doctor's appointments elsewhere. A health care system that revolves around fees and reimbursements simply does not reward time spent talking to patients about understanding how appreciating the gifts they bring to their work can positively improve their health or probing how well they are nurturing relationships with friends and family because of the health benefits of supportive relationships. It takes time to get people to open up about the topics in the *Model for Healthy Living*, and it requires a degree of trust-building that doesn't occur in a fifteen-minute appointment slot. But it can happen in the context of relationships that faith community nurses have with members of faith communities or community groups they support with their professional skills, and we can begin to see improved health outcomes that do not rely simply on pills and procedures. *Church Health* has made a commitment to the *Westberg Institute* and faith community nursing because physicians and hospital systems need faith community nurses as much as faith communities do.

Unfortunately, many have become addicted to the next breakthrough the pharmaceutical companies put before us on TV and have developed an unholy love affair with technology. We believe we can live our lives any way we want to and it won't matter, because when we are broken the doctor will use that technology to fix us; only the technology is not that good and the doctor is not that smart. God gave us our bodies for a reason, and we have an obligation to care for them. This is why health systems need faith community nurses to draw us back into a better understanding of the connections between body and spirit and between faith and health. We won't have better health outcomes without being open to exploring these connections not just theoretically, but in the lives of real patients, which faith community nurses do every day.

Rev. Granger Westberg was right to see nurses as a bridge between medicine and ministry that offers enormous promise. The specialty practice of faith community nursing is still in its infancy and continues to find its legs in the complicated health world. Faith community nursing is a resource in the medical community that should only enlarge over the coming decades. It's a specialty nursing practice with emerging opportunities even beyond the "nurse in the church" vision of Rev. Granger Westberg.

As a physician, I see patients one after another. There is never enough time to go beyond just the simplest ways of helping people achieve their goals in life. I am all too often treating self-limiting viral illness with medicine that has limited benefit. What I long for is a network of faith communities where faith community nurses can go in-depth to help people live healthy lives so they can better engage God's desires for them. When I talk to faith community nurses—or even hospital administrators—I talk about "Mrs. Jones" a lot. Mrs. Jones is in every faith community in the world. She has some medical issues that may be major or they may be minor. She might have a chronic condition that isn't well-managed, but easily could be before it turns into something that puts her in the hospital. Perhaps she doesn't understand her blood sugar fluctuations or hypertension medications. Maybe she lives alone and doesn't think it's worth the bother to cook most of the time. Maybe Mrs. Jones has already been in the hospital, and now the question is how to keep her from ending up there again.

But Mrs. Jones loves her faith community and the people there care about her. She's been singing in the choir for 30 years, and every kid in the youth group was in her arms as a toddler. Until her knees started hurting so much, she wouldn't think of missing Thursday morning Bible study. When the prayer chain needs to be activated, Mrs. Jones gets the first call.

Mr. Smith might not have much in common with Mrs. Jones on the surface. He's newer to the faith community, helps with upkeep of the church grounds, and as a young single dad is figuring out little girl braids and soccer schedules. But when he gets hurt at work and faces an unexpected surgery, a complicated recovery, and related depression, he enters a foreign, vulnerable place.

For every Mrs. Jones or Mr. Smith, a caring faith community nurse is the portal between the medical care people assume they're getting—though this isn't always the case—and the nonmedical support that helps bring about more joy, more love, and more closeness to God by leveraging the strengths of congregations as caring social systems that already exist and already are predisposed to want Mrs. Jones, Mr. Smith, and their families to thrive.

Faith community nurses educate and explain medical information and systems that people receiving health care don't always absorb just because technically it was provided to them. They discern the difference between presenting evidence-based practice and the "try it, it can't hurt you" approach when it actually could hurt you and doctors may not even know what Mrs. Jones is trying. They help collaborate and navigate medical and social services systems that the "person in the pew" would not know how to do, especially during a period of overwhelming illness. They advocate, whether medically or simply by letting people in the congregation know there is a need that could easily be met with a transportation schedule, a meal train, or a few phone calls that lessen social isolation, sustain connection to the faith community, and support transition between hospital and home.

In other words, faith community nurses are not checking off boxes. They're looking people in the eye and assessing how they're doing with life, not just illness. The sooner physicians and hospital systems see faith community nurses as partners in sustaining health, the sooner we'll see greater measurable impact of faith community nursing on health outcomes.

We have our work cut out for us.

11.1.3 The Promise Before Us

The book of Numbers recounts the story of the Hebrew people approaching the border of the land God had promised to them hundreds of years earlier in a promise that Abraham's descendants would inhabit the land. Now the Hebrews were reluctant to trust God's plan. They sent spies into Canaan to survey the land that, God said, "I am giving to the Israelites" (Numbers 13:2). The promise was already there.

Moses gave instructions. Go somewhere you have never been and collect data. That's the heart of what Moses said. And be bold. Why should they not be bold? Going into the promised land was what God planned for them to do all along. But they hesitated. They did send spies into the land and collect accurate data. The land was full of everything the Hebrews would need: flowing milk and honey, grapes, pomegranates, figs—a strong agricultural foundation.

Fortified cities.

Large people.

The objective data itself was accurate. The interpretation was where most of the spies went wrong. Without conducting experiments, they concluded the "giants" could not be conquered. Abort the mission. The fortified cities were greater than God's promise. And fear spread. The people were afraid to do what God called them to do and go into the land God promised to give them. The glory of the Lord appeared to all the people, the manifestation of God's presence (Numbers 14:10). This could have been God's pleasure but was instead judgment. Instead of triumph, a watershed moment gave way to rebellion—and forty years of wilderness wandering. But still God's promise was before the people.

Years later, in another cycle of revolt and despairing season of "Are we all to perish?" the people's doubts were overt. They doubted Moses' leadership. They doubted God's provision. They doubted God's plan. And the Lord sent poisonous serpents that bit the people, and many died (Numbers 21:6). That got their attention. Repentance came quickly, and Moses interceded.

We might think God could have made the snakes disappear just as quickly as God sent them. Why not dry them up in the desert or send them down a warren of holes? Getting past obstacles and back to God's plan is not that simple; it requires something of us—an act of faith. In this case, God told Moses to make a bronze serpent on a pole. Anyone who looked at it would be healed of the consequences of the snake bites.

It's only when the Hebrews could trust God to deliver them that they were able to enter the Promised Land. I am confident that faith community nursing is moving into a wider and deeper future than even Rev. Granger Westberg imagined. It's time for faith community nursing to set aside its doubts, look with faith on the bronze serpent, and trust God that we are ready to enter the promised land God calls us to.

Are there giants? Yes.

- Do some of them have letters like MD after their names? Yes.
- Are some of them hospital systems facing challenges without an understanding of how faith community nurses can help? Yes.
- Are some of them running research programs? Yes.

But Moses told the spies both to collect the data and to be bold. So as faith community nursing moves more deeply into meaningful roles alongside physicians and conquers the Promised Land, let us be bold. My fear is that faith community nursing been bitten by doubt: not taken seriously, underpaid or not paid at all, ignored. I don't doubt that many in my medical profession are unaware of the value of faith community nursing and operate with the conviction that anything with the word faith in the title has little or nothing to do with medical science. Others simply haven't heard of the specialty practice of faith community nursing. Many who may have encountered the term, or the older language of parish nursing, are unaware of the healing potential of creative partnerships between medical institutions and faith community networks.

Going back to Egypt starts to look good. There we can undertake something small and safe and leave the giants be. But when we lift our eyes to the healing bronze snake, with all its perplexity, we prepare to quell our doubts and take on the giants.

As a physician, I don't have to tell nurses that what they bring to the table is not always valued as much as it should be. Bringing along a specialty practice about which most doctors know very little to the table is a giant task. But conquering it will change health outcomes in the Promised Land.

Eyebrows still raise when a faith community nurse turns up with a patient at an appointment or a discharge session or is listed as an individual authorized to receive confidential information. Creating awareness of the existence of networks of faith community nurses in the communities in which physicians practice is a giant task. But conquering it will change health outcomes in the Promised Land.

Increasing organized connections between faith communities and health care systems, with faith community nurses as the connection points of communication and collaboration, is a giant task. But conquering it will change health outcomes in the Promised Land.

Rev. Granger Westberg's first venture into parish nursing started with a pilot program in a handful of churches partially funded by a hospital. From the start the vision was not only "nurse in the church" but also "nurse in the church connected to the medical system." The movement has grown to tens of thousands of nurses in thirty-one countries trained in the core values and practices of faith community nursing, many of whom are well connected to faith community settings. While there is still work to do to help clergy understand the ways faith community nurses can enhance ministry within a congregation and see the links between spiritual health and physical health, far fewer faith community nurses also have connections to hospital systems.

Hospitals want to prevent readmissions, which can be expensive to their bottom line, but most attempt to do it by hiring community health workers to check up on Mrs. Jones because it is less expensive than a faith community nurse, or even part of the salary of a faith community nurse. In addition, the effectiveness of faith community nurses requires working with volunteers—members of faith communities—that hospitals cannot control. However, the community health workers have less training and education, higher turnover, and less personal investment in the health outcome of Mrs. Jones than the faith community nurse and the army of volunteers that sincerely care about keeping Mrs. Jones out of the hospital, because they would rather see her back at Thursday morning Bible study and choir practice.

It is for this reason that we must not be afraid of going into Canaan and boldly collecting data. Our job is not to be intimidated by what we see, and therefore misinterpret the data, but rather keep our eye on God's faithful promise. The data we collect, in the form of research that stands up to scrutiny in the medical community, will demonstrate the effectiveness of the work faith community nurses do.

We know the work of faith community nurses improves lives by addressing the whole person, body, and spirit, and helping people find the abundant life God means for them to live. We know that this work reduces health care costs by preventing disease, preventing advancement of disease, preventing hospital readmissions, and promoting and empowering healthy living choices. Anecdotally, we can tell the stories of every Mrs. Jones or Mr. Smith we have known and the difference faith community nursing has made. What we need is organized data that we can share on a wider level. Sometimes we have seen the need for quantitative research as a giant that is easier to avoid.

Just the opposite is true.

Church Health has supported faith community nurses involved with transitional care and reducing readmissions by undertaking research with two separate health care systems. Comparing similar patients who benefit from faith community nurse intervention with those who do not has shown positive result in reducing the length of hospital stay and reducing readmissions within 30 days and even up to 6 months. This is just one piece of the burgeoning field of research needed to slay the giants.

What do the other giants look like? What do the tools for slaying them look like? This is an occasion for imagination, not intimidation. We need to build on our successes to show both clergy and medical professionals that faith community nurses are critical to both a life of faith and improved health outcomes.

When I first met Rev. Granger Westberg, I never imagined that I, as a physician, would become a true believer—an evangelist, even—for faith community nursing. Now, I do not see how medicine can move into the promised land of better care for the whole person without embracing the role of faith community nursing as the much underused arm of health care.

Reference

Morris, S. (2017). *Model for healthy living* (Vol. 7(4)). Memphis, TN: Church Health Reader.

Further Reading

Model for Healthy Living. (n.d.-a). found at http://chreader.org/model-healthy-living/
Model for Healthy Living. (n.d.-b). found at https://www.youtube.com/watch?v=WXWSm5M6fJU
Morris, S. (2016). *Model for healthy living introduction with reflections*. Memphis, TN: Church Health.

Faith Community Nursing: From the Perspective of the Health Care System

Lois Ustanko and Karla J. Cazer

12.1 Traditional Relationships Between Health System Organizations and Faith Communities

Health systems often reflect on their founding principles when connecting to faith communities. Collaboration between faith communities and health systems is nothing new. Traditionally, most modern hospital systems trace their existence to people of faith who provided financial support and other resources to build hospitals. Rosenberg (1995) commented that the evidence of faith-based hospitals is seen in the legacy of names. Saint Vincent, Mount Sinai Presbyterian, Mercy, and Beth Israel are all charitable hospitals that began to care for abandoned children and the poor. Traditionally, hospitals were designed to respond to acute health conditions, but in this day and age, must also respond to chronic health issues. As length of stay in the hospital decreases and a growing number of aging struggle to live alone at home, it is only natural that the health system and the church re-discover the shared benefit of working together for the good of the people they mutually serve.

To qualify for a tax-exempt status, non-for-profit hospitals are expected to provide community benefit programing. This originally meant charity care for the poor and uninsured. Now the *Internal Revenue Service* requires non-for-profit hospital organizations in the U.S.A. to adopt a more focused, intentional implementation strategy to meet the community health needs identified through a community health needs assessment (Additional Requirements for Charitable Hospitals, 2014). The *population-health management model* that rewards providers for keeping patients healthy has recognized that health and socioeconomic factors are closely intertwined (Casey & Cull, 2018). As

L. Ustanko (✉)
Clinical Services, Edgewood Vista, East Grand Forks, MN, USA
e-mail: lois.ustanko@edgewoodvista.com

K. J. Cazer
Faith Community Nursing Center, Sanford USD Medical Center, Sioux Falls, SD, USA
e-mail: Karla.cazer@sanfordhealth.org

© Springer Nature Switzerland AG 2020
P. A. Solari-Twadell, D. J. Ziebarth (eds.), *Faith Community Nursing*,
https://doi.org/10.1007/978-3-030-16126-2_12

a result, hospitals are investing in community health initiatives, such as nutrition and housing (Hussein & Collins, 2016). Ziebarth (2016), wrote about the benefits of having a faith community nursing initiative as part of a hospital's *community benefit* programming. She used a five-finger response/illustration to address why a hospital may value and support a faith community nurse program and encouraged rehearsing a concise elevator speech. The five reasons are "…the faith community nurse program's connection to the hospital's mission and vision statement, continuity of care in the community, new community partnerships and grant opportunities, organizational and national health goals are met, and the mandate of community benefit." Faith communities and faith community nurses are excellent partners for hospitals to impact community health in multiple ways (Health Research & Educational Trust, 2016).

12.2 Power in Partnerships

12.2.1 Case Study: A Midwestern Experience

Sanford Health located in the Dakotas opened two hospitals: one in Sioux Falls, South Dakota in 1894 and another in Fargo, North Dakota in 1908. In Fargo, the launch of the "Parish Nurse Project" was kicked off on May 5, 1991 (Quigley, personal communication, February 21, 2014). It was suggested that an affiliated faith community model would be used as a method of promoting health where people lived, played, and prayed and emphasized the potential to reach people of all ages (Vitalis, personal communication, March 1, 2014). Meanwhile, parish nursing, now referred to as faith community nurse, emerged in the Sioux Falls area around 1996, using an institutionally paid model. The health system provided education and administrative support to the faith community nurses. The health system recommended that the nurses be paid. Some faith communities chose to engage faith community nurses as unpaid staff members. Regardless, the faith community nurses all have access to hospital-based continuing education, orientation, mentoring, documentation, networking, consultation from the program coordinator, as well as opportunities for grants from the health system.

The faith community nursing coordinators for each region are employees of the hospital and help faith communities envision their potential to be places of whole person health and healing. The majority of faith leaders and nurses, who express an interest in establishing a faith community nursing role in their faith community, may be unaware of the theological foundations of health, healing, and wholeness. The coordinators help educate them about the practice. They also help faith communities understand that preaching, fellowship, worship, service, and advocacy are all directly related to health and well-being. They share that a faith community nurse program can become a concrete expression of their mission of health (Anderson, 1990). This coordinator may help the faith community:

- complete a health needs assessment,
- prioritize needs and develop a program, which best fits the specific faith community,

- develop a role description for the faith community nurse,
- professionally develop the faith community nurse,
- measure outcomes of the faith community nursing ministry, and
- ensure accurate records are kept regarding services provided by the faith community nurse.

A newsletter has also been produced by the faith community nurse coordinators. Through the newsletter, faith community nurses learn about health related resources available not only in the health system, but also across the community. The newsletter is also distributed to inter-professional team members in the health system and community agencies, so they are informed of what is being offered in the faith communities to promote health and well-being.

12.3   Addressing Health from a Whole Person Perspective

Faith community nurses frequently show the health care system how to be mindful in caring for all dimensions of the body, the mind, and the spirit to achieve whole person health and well-being. The faith community nurse understands that the definition of health is so much broader than the mere absence of disease and that healing can occur even when physical or mental health is not fully restored. In fact, some of the healthiest people living in communities may be individuals living with physical disabilities or serious, acute, or chronic illnesses when considering physical activity, engagement within the community, spiritual maturity, and other lifestyle factors (Centers for Disease Control, 2017).

Modern medicine is amazing, but health and healing can also be impacted by social determinants. Social determinants can impact health outcomes sometimes more than access to expert medical providers, high technology, and state-of-the-art facilities (Artiga & Hinton, 2018). Faith community nurses are experts in knowing community resources and can assist community members with financial needs they face as their health status changes. Some examples are: (a) when a patient is discharged from the hospital and does not have the financial resources to purchase medical equipment. The faith community nurse will often look for other funding options or for organizations that offer services or medical equipment at low or no cost. (b) A faith community nurse can ensure that a client has food by accessing the local food pantry or by engaging a faith community-based meal ministry. (c) The faith community nurse can facilitate transportation for patients for follow-up medical appointments.

Faith community nurses often demonstrate to the health systems that health care begins in the community with prevention. Examples of this are when faith community nurses share innovative community-based approaches: (a) responding to food insecurity by sending food home in the backpacks of children who live in poverty (American Hospital Association, 2018), (b) engaging with local developers and housing authority to create safe and affordable housing (Butcher, 2017), and (c) providing primary and secondary screenings in community schools, emergency homeless shelters, and local community centers.

In one case, the hospital saw that the faith community nurses focused on non-traditional factors and care for the whole person. This awareness influenced the health care system as a whole to address social determinants by embedding a whole person assessment within the patient's admission electronic medical record. In addition, this admission assessment includes questions that help identify community members who are experiencing homelessness. Faith community nurses become the community-based bridge for getting health system services to those in need. The faith community nurse can organize a food drive or use faith community volunteers to distribute food to the homeless (Erie United Methodist Alliance, 2017).

12.4 Inter-Professional Education to Integrate Faith and Health

Ongoing professional development ensures that nurses are current practitioners of safe and expert care. A health system can offer a wide array of services to develop clinical excellence in nursing practice, including local faith community nurses. The health system provides:

- continuing education sessions prepared by clinical experts,
- health ministry conferences to promote spiritual development,
- networking opportunities to create awareness about community resources,
- newsletters that reference evidence-based practices, and
- the *Foundations for Faith Community Nursing Course* to prepare registered nurses for this role.

The education sessions provide opportunities for networking between faith community nurses and other inter-professional members from both the health system and community agencies. These opportunities break down barriers between inter-professional members. The faith community nurse is a valuable, contributing member of the inter-professional team to collaborate "with" to empower patients to promote their health across the continuum and over time (Harris & Longcoy, 2016).

Faith community nursing programs associated with health systems typically host regularly scheduled meetings. For example, monthly department meetings can be made open to case managers, registered nurse health coaches, social workers, chaplains, and other staff from community agencies, including faith community nurses. During these meetings, participants learn about evidence-based approaches to dealing with health issues such as chronic disease self-management, family caregiver stress, and current recommendations for hypertension screening. In addition, through this networking opportunity, the attendees build strong relationships, share best practice models, and develop an increased awareness of community resources.

Health systems that offer the *Foundations for Faith Community Nursing* course base content on the curriculum developed through the *Westberg Institute*. The primary reason why health systems offer this course is to promote the preparation of faith community nurses in regions where health systems exist. The health system can also offer scholarships for the course to health system employees and members at affiliated faith communities. This funding ensures that the faith community nurse novice will have the information and skills needed to practice with basic knowledge.

Sometimes nurses from a health system attend the *Foundations for Faith Community Nursing* course not because they want to become a faith community nurse, but because they want to learn how to be responsive to the spiritual needs of the patients they are caring for on a daily basis. They may work in the cancer center, the palliative care unit, the intensive care unit, and other settings where patients and families are trying to cope with transformational life issues. Nurses learn to deliver spiritually responsive care in a manner they have witnessed by faith community nurses who have interacted with their patients (Johnson, personal communication, September 10, 2017). Upon completion of the course, these nurses return to the workplace prepared to offer spiritually relevant whole person care and community health. In addition, some decide to become engaged in an existing faith community nursing program, establish a new program, or participate in health promoting activities (Schanilec, personal communication, April 26, 2018).

12.5   Addressing Health Issues Upstream

When payment is based on fee-for-service, a health system is financially rewarded for clinic visits and hospital stays. This is reactive "illness" care as clinicians try to restore individuals to health after they develop complications from acute or chronic illnesses. Today, payment is shifting to accountable-care-organizations that manage the health of a population. In this approach, insurance plans and health systems are motivated to support methods to prevent illness, better manage chronic health conditions, and transition patients to less expensive locations for end-of-life care. A faith community nurse's approach is consistent with the triple aim of enhancing the patient experience, improving health of populations, and reducing cost of health care (Institute for Healthcare Improvement, 2018).

Faith community nurses provide primary, secondary, and tertiary care in their communities. For example, most faith community nurses offer the primary intervention health education newsletter articles. They offer secondary prevention through health screenings, like monthly blood pressure screening. The health system can make motivational interviewing training accessible to these nurses, so they can use the tertiary intervention of health coaching to help individuals with hypertension in making lifestyle changes. A few of the nurses use the tertiary intervention of offering stroke support sessions to individuals who suffer from complications of uncontrolled hypertension and their caregivers. Some of the interventions offered by faith community nurses include but are not limited to:

- writing health related articles in bulletins or faith community newsletters,
- offering health screenings, and
- teaching self-monitoring of blood pressure or blood glucose.

Faith communities—churches, synagogues, mosques, and temples—can be excellent partners of a health system in disseminating health information and raising awareness about available resources. This information and resources enable individuals to make good decisions about their health and medical care. Faith communities have established communication networks and core values that are consistent with community-based health programs. Religious institutions are also one place where large numbers of community members, particularly older adults, regularly gather. Sussman (2018) reported that 60% of individuals over the age of 65 still attend faith community services weekly. Medical-religious partnerships are particularly effective in reaching rural and minority communities, especially when there is enthusiastic support from faith and lay leaders (Bolwerk, 2016). Faith community nurses remove barriers and make care accessible (Parham, 2018).

12.6 Evidence-Based Approaches to Meeting Community Needs

Faith community nurses have been effective partners in the success of a number of the health system initiatives including advance care planning, caring for those in poverty, hypertension, diabetes management programs, and fall prevention, just to name a few. The priority for initiatives in many health systems is driven by the triennial *Community Health Needs Assessment* (CHNA) and grounded in evidence-based programs. The specific health concerns will vary from one faith community to the next, so it is important for the health system to collaborate with the faith community to complete a health needs survey.

Decisions need to be made based on the health needs, available time, and resources present within both the health system and the faith community. In most cases, the health system identifies the evidence-based approach to the health issue and provides the training or tools while the faith community nurse becomes the trusted health professional to deliver the program to community members. A program can be carried out in a specific faith community, in combination with other faith communities that have similar needs and interests, or in coordination with a community program that is designed to address the identified health issue. All successful plans include: (1) goal(s)/objective(s); (2) a defined target population; (3) action needed and/or steps to meet the goal/objective; (4) identification of resources needed and a means for evaluating outcomes after the plan is implemented.

Many of the needs identified in health system's community assessment have been consistent with findings in national health surveys. Disease-specific programs created included those addressing stroke, heart disease, diabetes, cancer, foot-care, depression, and dementia. In addition, education increasing awareness about community services such as assisted living, skilled nursing facilities, home health, palliative care, hospice, and prescription assistance providers. Sessions for increasing proficiency with self-management have focused on medication management, home safety, and preparing for provider appointments. On-site screenings have provided cholesterol checks and mobile health screenings, which use EKG and ultrasound technology to assess for carotid artery occlusions, peripheral arterial disease, abdominal aortic aneurysms, atrial fibrillation, and osteoporosis. The health system has helped in participating faith communities establish and train care teams to promote independent living of their seniors by assisting with visitation, transportation, shopping, and light chores inside and outside the home. The health system has also armed faith communities with necessary tools to establish effective support groups for a variety of situations such as cancer survivorship, bereavement, exercise, and weight reduction.

Some of the more common evidence-based programs implemented by faith community nurses include:

- *Respecting Choices®* approach to advance care planning (ACP) in which trained facilitators ask if there are faith or cultural considerations that need to be incorporated within the written health care directive.
- *Stepping On* or *A Matter of Balance* a falls prevention program, which includes strategies that encourage lifestyle changes to promote independent living.
- Stanford University's chronic disease self-management program, which requires participants to set goals and create a plan to reach this goal with the assistance of the faith community nurse. There is strong evidence that chronic disease self-management (CDSM) programs like this improve health outcomes for individuals with a wide array of chronic conditions (Brady et al., 2013).
- The *National Diabetes Prevention Program* (DPP), which is a structured lifestyle change program that has been developed specifically for people who have prediabetes or are at risk for type 2 diabetes.

The faith community nurse may also make on-site health screening accessible such as:

- Audiometry testing offered through mobile screening clinics.
- Mobile heart and vascular screening that involves three modalities including ultrasound screening to identify abdominal aortic aneurysm and carotid artery disease, finger-stick blood screening to assess lipid levels and glucose levels as well as C-reactive protein and liver enzymes, and an electrocardiograph to detect atrial fibrillation.

Faith communities in metropolitan communities can have up to 5000 registered members. Gallup polls (Newport, 2015; Pew Research Center, 2014) show up to 32% of adults in the Midwest attend faith community on a weekly basis, thus faith communities are excellent sites to offer health education. The faith community nurses not only offer educational sessions, they also incorporate health education into weekly bulletins, faith community newsletters, and include links on the faith community's website. Some of the healthy living education sessions offered include:

- *Faith Communities Alive!,* which promotes healthy eating at Sunday morning coffee, during *Vacation Bible School,* and at all faith community gatherings by offering healthy food options.

- Physical activity programs including structured walking programs such as the *Walk to Bethlehem,* as well as the use of gym space to offer basketball leagues, pickle ball, or Tai Chi.
- "Doc Talks" sessions in which an expert provider is accessible to offer a brief presentation on identified topics. Even more importantly, providers are available for open dialogue with participants.
- Cooking classes where participants learn to make meals that are not only nutritious, but also delicious. These classes are also social events as participants get to eat all of the dishes that are prepared during the session.

12.7   Role of a Faith Community Nurse in Life Transitions

The faith community nurse supports individuals of all ages and stages of life navigate through life transitions. The faith community nurse provides whole person care during illness, injury, and sometimes frightening life situations. Through listening and assisting individuals during these difficult times, the faith community nurse helps members find meaning in their health experience. Through presence, the individual is reminded, he or she is not alone. During the visit to a homebound member, communion can be shared, and arrangements can be made to receive other sacraments. The nurse can be invaluable to individuals during the following transitions:

- A first-time mother who is overwhelmed by all of the changes taking place in her life.
- Pregnant women who lack resources, ensuring they enroll in programs for which they may be eligible. The nurse may also provide guidance with breastfeeding, educate the new mom on anticipated growth and developmental milestones of the infant, and screen for postpartum depression.
- Patients being discharged from the hospital. When faith community nurses work with patients who have been discharged from the hospital, there is more adherence to the treatment plan including taking medications as prescribed and better communication with providers (Morris & Miller, 2014).
- During clinic visits, some health systems have developed the process for adding the faith community nurse as an identified care team member on the patient's electronic medical record.

12.8   Engaging Faith Community Nurses in Innovative Ways

Faith community nurses are also leading the way in helping the health system address gaps in care and in meeting the needs of those who are poor or vulnerable in communities. A few health systems have designed innovative approaches for placing faith community nurses in emergency shelters, clinics for the homeless, clinics and other locations that fill the gap in rural communities. These innovation practices include:

- Homeless Shelters: Although all people are guaranteed access to emergency care, those who are homeless and lack insurance, go without basic health care services, such as health promotion and chronic disease management. Through partnerships with the shelters, health systems are able to provide care to the medically underserved, high-risk homeless population who often have chronic or complex conditions including hypertension, diabetes, heart disease, and respiratory conditions as well with mental health disorders and addictions.

- Collaborating Faith Communities: Rural faith communities are experiencing a decline in resources as rosters and contributions are decreasing. A lone rural faith community is less likely to have the capacity to engage a faith community nurse. Several faith communities may pool their resources to ensure a nurse is accessible to members, which is vitally important due to the lack of community service providers and the great distances individuals must travel to reach the urban hubs.
- Bridging the Gap: The "Bridging the Gap" pilot project aims to implement three sustainable strategies to assist older adults in rural communities living full, meaningful lives with dignity, independence and vitality. The strategies include: (1) placing an educated faith community nurse in the community to offer whole person health services; (2) implementing chronic disease self-management programs to equip community members to successfully manage their chronic conditions; and (3) providing a nurse-led, mobile clinic that reaches members in the community. The local faith leaders refer members to the clinic and come to the *Bridging Center* to offer spiritual support or counseling if the faith community nurses' assessment indicates spiritual distress.
- Faith Leader Health: Often faith community nurses make themselves accessible to help their faith leaders develop personal improvement goals if they desire to do so. Some denominations employ a faith community nurse to focus solely on the faith leaders within their district. The faith leaders are self-insured and the district identified that it is both difficult and expensive to locate replacement faith leaders when one becomes ill. Preventive health care measures are much more cost effective than having the faith leader in the hospital. Health coaching takes place via telephone calls or Skype meetings. The faith community nurse may prepare courses for the faith leaders on health maintenance, disease prevention, and early detection through recommended annual screening (Lightowler, personal communication, May 21, 2018).

12.9 Documentation Is Important

Maintaining a written account of care provided is a requirement of all professional nurses, including faith community nurses (American Nurses Association, 2017). Aggregated data abstracted from this documentation can demonstrate to the faith community, the health system, and funders the value of this nursing specialty. The faith community nurse must comply with all state and federal requirements for documentation including ensuring documentation is completed and that records are kept confidential using a secure system.

Although faith communities are not specifically included in the *Health Insurance Portability and Accountability Act* (HIPAA), as defined by the HIPAA Omnibus Rule, faith community nurses are obligated by the *American Nurses Association Code of*

Ethics (American Nurses Association, 2015) to ensure personal health information is kept confidential (U.S. Department of Health and Human Services, 2013). As a result, any private health information is kept confidential. At times, this can cause tension as faith communities and faith leaders may not understand why the faith community nurse is limited in what can be shared. To promote a two-way flow of sharing of information to benefit the health of the member, the health system may provide faith community nurses with a HIPAA-compliant release of information form to use as they work with health systems, agencies, and service providers in the community.

Faith community nurses collaborating with a health system typically use some form of electronic health record. This can range from a homegrown *Excel* spreadsheet to programs designed for this nursing specialty by health systems, such as the *Henry Ford Macomb* or *Pittsburgh Mercy Parish Nurse and Health Ministry* documentation programs. These nationally recognized documentation programs incorporate the *North American Nursing Diagnoses Association* (NANDA), *Nursing Intervention Classification* (NIC), or *Nursing Outcomes Classification* (NOC) systems. Although individual nurses may initially express resistance to using these classification systems, the benefit of using a standardized nursing taxonomy is the ability to measure outcomes based on interventions used by the nurse.

The most common measurable outcomes for health system's faith community nursing programs include the following:

- Client reported ability for self-care management of health.
- Reduction in medical errors due to clarification of medical and medication orders.
- Reduction in emergency room visit, inpatient days, urgent care visits, ambulance runs, and clinic encounters.
- Enhanced independent living and quality of life (Office of Disease Prevention, 2018).
- Increased compliance with primary care provider visits and patient reported increased knowledge of health resources.

One health system's faith community nursing program annual report demonstrated a cost avoidance impact of over $5 million dollars due to the work of the faith community nurses practice. The goal of calculating these savings is to demonstrate the value these faith-based ministries deliver with the hope that the financial and other support provided by the health system and faith communities will be maintained and perhaps enhanced (Hansen, personal communications, November 3, 2017).

12.10 Local, State, and National Initiatives

It is important that faith community nurses evaluate outcomes associated with initiatives and programs in which they are engaged. Some results from reported initiatives include:

- Noticeable increase in patients with a health care directive; in one community, faith community nurses collaborating with faith communities, senior centers, and other locations increase the rate from only 17% to 43% within 2 years (Parker, personal communication, May 23, 2018).

- By collaborating with physical therapy faculty from a local university, quantitative measures determined *Faithfully Fit Forever (FFF)* sessions improved balance, strength, flexibility, and endurance of participants (Johnson, personal communication, December 6, 2015).
- Nationally, the *Stepping On* program has been proven to reduce falls by over 30% among participants (National Council on Aging, 2015). A follow-up survey conducted with 35 individuals participating in North Dakota sessions in 2017 revealed positive changes in behavior including completion of eye exams and a home safety assessment, selecting safer footwear, working with a pharmacist to learn about medication side effects, and demonstrating techniques for safe transfers, ambulating, using stairs, and climbing curbs (Strommen, personal communication, May 3, 2018).
- Faith community nurses engaged in the *Diving into Good Blood Pressure (DIG)* program measured a 43% improvement in blood pressure and better compliance with prescribed medications or a change in medication regime (Blue, personal communication, June 20, 2018).
- Participants in the *Better Choices, Better Health®* chronic disease self-management program increased their physical activity level, reported better health, described higher levels of energy, and increased knowledge of how to manage the symptoms of their chronic health conditions (Swanson, personal communication, May 21, 2018).
- Congregants and community members who participate in the *Diabetes Prevention Program (DPP)* increased their physical activity and ate more healthfully. They reported having more confidence sustaining a more active, healthier lifestyle (Brown, personal communication, October 30, 2017). Participants in a community-based programs lost more than 7% of their body weight, had greater reductions in their impaired fasting glucose and HbA1C levels, improved systolic and diastolic blood pressures, and improvements in total cholesterol and low-density lipoprotein cholesterol levels (Hill, Peer, Oldenburg, & Kengne, 2017).
- District faith leaders coached by the faith community nurse reported making progress toward their personal health goals. A 3.8% of them reported completing their goal, 57% reported lower stress levels, 52% have improved HgA1C levels, 69% are eating more fruits and vegetables, and 48% report improved sleep habits (Lightowler, personal communication, May 21, 2018).

12.11   Transformation of Faith Community Nursing Through Technology

Every specialty in nursing needs to adapt to the knowledge accessibility now available through technology. The specialty of faith community nursing is no different. Numerous changes have occurred in the way that technology has impacted how prevention, health assessment, and health care delivery are provided. This change has occurred in a relatively short period of time. The challenge is to find ways to make digital technology accessible to engage and empower patients. The internet has become the sole source of health information for many. Beyond that, new applications of health technology are here. An example is the wearable fitness trackers that fit on the wrist like a watch that measures calories burned, sleep quality, blood pressure, heart rate, respirations, mood, energy levels, plus more. Other electronic devices that are up and coming are a medication tapering instrument that adjusts the dosage of medication to align to a specific genetic code. In addition, there are wireless in-home monitors that can determine if a person has bathed based on the in-home humidity, assess quality of sleep based on patient movement during the night, and identify when a person has fallen before they push a life alert button (Ni, Hernando, & de la Cruz, 2015).

12.12 Benefits of Faith Community Involvement

There is mutual benefit to the faith community nurse, the faith community, and the health system from collaborating to make this ministry available. Faith community nurses appreciate having access to the resources of the health system including, but not limited to, continuing education to help them meet licensure requirements. Most content is approved by the *American Nurses Credentialing Center's Commission on Accreditation* (ANCC) which provides affirmation that the information in the sessions is current and relevant to their nursing specialty, but also reflects evidence-based practice. Some health systems offer clinical pastoral education (CPE) to faith community nurses to help develop the major attribute of the practice, which is integration of faith and health (Ziebarth, 2014). Using theological reflection, the nurses in this training learn how to deliver relationship-centered care using transformational communication to promote healing (Hammer-Luken, personal communication, May 24, 2018). Monthly networking meetings allow these nurses to learn about programs and services provided by their fellow faith community nurses. This networking is especially important to nurses who are new in the ministry as they transition from traditional care settings to the faith community setting.

Faith community leaders get an orientation regarding the faith community nurse, assistance with preparing a role description, and guidance on the development of a health cabinet. Some health systems even offer scholarships, grants, or other financial resources to help the faith community start a faith community nursing program.

Through the faith community nurse program, the health system can build and sustain relationships with thousands of community members. Strong relationships between faith leaders and health system leaders promote trust among the faith community's members regarding the care and services provided by the health system. Since these nurses and faith leaders see health system patients every week, they have the ability to alert the health system to impressions of the community member as to unmet health needs. The faith community nurse makes the health system visible to members of the faith community and can follow up with a patient after discharge home. The innovative, autonomous practice of faith community nursing can also provide sources of evidence for several of the components of a Magnet® survey.

12.13 Conclusion

With shared mission and vision faith communities and health care organizations create powerful partnerships to benefit the individual and the community. Demonstrated effectiveness of such a partnership was seen through evidence-based practice approaches that included meeting community needs; role of a faith community nurse in life transitions; engaging faith community nurses in innovative ways; local state and national initiatives; transformation of faith community nursing through technology; and benefits of faith community involvement.

References

Additional Requirements for Charitable Hospitals; Community health needs assessments for charitable hospitals; Requirement of a Section 4959 excise tax return and time for filing the return, 79 Fed. Reg. 78953. (2014, December 31).

American Hospital Association. (2018). *Arkansas Children's Hospital works with community partners to address food insecurity.* Retrieved from https://www.aha.org/news/insights-and-analysis/2018-01-23-arkansas-childrens-hospital-works-community-partners-address

American Nurses Association. (2015). *Code of ethics for nurses, with interpretive statements.* Silver Spring, MD: Nursesbooks.org.

American Nurses Association and Health Ministries Association, Inc. (2017). *Faith community nursing: Scope and standards of practice* (3rd ed.). Silver Spring, MD: Nursesbooks.org.

Anderson, H. (1990). The congregation as a healing resource. In D. Browning, T. Jobe, & I. Evison (Eds.), *Religious and ethical factors in psychiatric practice* (pp. 264–287). Chicago, IL: Nelson-Hall.

Artiga, S., & Hinton, E. (2018). *Beyond health care: The role of social determinants in promoting health and health equity.* San Francisco, CA: Kaiser Family Foundation. Retrieved from https://www.kff.org/disparities-policy/issue-brief/beyond-health-care-the-role-of-social-determinants-in-promoting-health-and-health-equity/

Bolwerk, C. A. (2016). Parish nurses offer HOPE in serving rural populations. *Michigan In Touch.* Retrieved from http://michiganintouch.com/healthy-workers/parish-nurses-offer-hope-serving-rural-populations/

Brady, T. J., Murphy, L., O'Colmain, B. J., Beauchesne, D., Daniels, B., Greenberg, M., et al. (2013). A meta-analysis of health status, health behaviors, and health care utilization outcomes of the chronic disease self-management program. *Preventing Chronic Disease.* https://doi.org/10.5888/pcd10.120112. Retrieved from https://www.cdc.gov/pcd/issues/2013/pdf/12_0112.pdf

Butcher, L. (2017). If housing is healthcare, should insurers pay? *Hospitals & HealthNetworks.* Retrieved from https://www.hhnmag.com/articles/8116-if-housing-is-helath-care-should-insurers-pay

Casey, D., & Cull, T. (2018). Successful interventions, positive outcomes: Understanding the impact of social determinants of health. *American Journal of Managed Care.* Retrieved from from http://www.ajmc.com/contributor/medecision/2018/01/successful-interventions-positive-outcomes-understanding-the-impact-of-social-determinants-of-health

Centers for Disease Control and Prevention. (2017). *People with disabilities.* Retrieved from https://www.cdc.gov/ncbddd/disabilityandhealth/people.html

Erie   United   Methodist   Alliance.   (2017).   Faith   community   nurses   help   homeless.
    Go-Erie.com.   Retrieved   from   http://www.goerie.com/entertainmentlife/20180504/
    faith-community-nurses-help-homeless
Harris, M. D., & Longcoy, R. (2016). Collaborative efforts in the community: Faith community
    nurses as partners in healing. *Home Healthcare Now, 34*(3), 146–150. https://doi.org/10.1097/
    NHH.0000000000000350
Health Research & Educational Trust. (2016). *Creating effective hospital-community partnerships
    to build a culture of health.* Chicago, IL: Health Research & Educational Trust. Available from
    http://www.hpoe.org/Reports-HPOE/2016/creating-effective-hospital-community-partner-
    ships.pdf
Hill, J., Peer, N., Oldenburg, B., & Kengne, A. P. (2017). Roles, responsibilities and characteristics
    of lay community health workers involved in diabetes prevention programmes: A systematic
    review. *PLoS One, 12*(12), e0189069.
Hussein, T., & Collins, M. (2016). Why big health systems are investing in commu-
    nity health. *Harvard   Business   Review.*   Retrieved   from   https://hbr.org/2016/12/
    why-big-health-systems-are-investing-in-community-health
Institute for Healthcare Improvement. (2018). *The IHI triple aim.* Retrieved from http://www.ihi.
    org/Engage/Initiatives/TripleAim/Pages/default.aspx
Morris, G. S., & Miller, S. M. (2014). Collaboration in the gap: A new day for faith com-
    munity nursing. *Journal of Christian Nursing, 31*(2), 112–116. https://doi.org/10.1097/
    CNJ.0000000000000064
National Council on Aging. (2015). *Issue brief: Funding for elder falls prevention.* Retrieved from
    https://www.ncoa.org/wp-content/uploads/Falls-Funding-Issue-Brief-8-15.pdf
Newport, F. (2015). Frequent church attendance highest in Utah, lowest in Vermont.
    Soc   Policy   Issues.   Retrieved   from   https://news.gailup.com/poll/181601/frequent-
    church-attendance-highest-utah-lowest-vermont.aspx?utm_source=Social%20
    Issues&utm_medium=newsfeed&utm_campaign=tiles
Ni, Q., Hernando, A. B. G., & de la Cruz, I. P. (2015). The elderly's independent living in smart
    homes: A characterization of activities and sensing infrastructure survey to facilitate services
    department. *Sensors, 15*, 11311–11362. https://doi.org/10.3390/s150511312
Office of Disease Prevention and Health Promotion. (2018). Health-related quality of life and well-
    being. In *Healthy people 2020.* Retrieved from https://www.healthypeople.gov/2020/about/
    foundation-health-measures/Health-Related-Quality-of-Life-and-Well-Being
Parham,   T.   (2018).   Faith   community   nurses   help   health   body,   mind   and   soul.
    Interpreter   online.   Available   from   http://www.umc.org/news-and-media/
    faith-community-nurses-help-heal-body-mind-and-soul
Pew Research Center. (2014). *Religious landscape study.* Retrieved from https://www.pewforum.
    org/religious-landscape-study/region/midwest/
Rosenberg, C. E. (1995). *The care of strangers: The rise of America's hospital system.* Baltimore,
    MD: Johns Hopkins University Press.
Sussman, D. (2018). Who goes to church? *ABC News.* Retrieved from https://abcnews.go.com/US/
    story?id=90372&page=1
U.S. Department of Health and Human Services. (2013). Modifications to the HIPAA privacy,
    security, enforcement, and breach notification rules under the health information technology
    for economic and clinical health act and the genetic information nondiscrimination act; Other
    modifications to the HIPAA Rules; Final rule, 78, Fed. Reg. 5566 (Jan. 25, 2013) (to be codi-
    fied at 45 C.F.R. pts. 160 & 164).
Ziebarth, D. (2014). Evolutionary conceptual analysis: Faith community nursing. *Journal of
    Religion & Health, 53*(6), 1817–1835.
Ziebarth, D. (2016). Wholistic health care: Evolutionary conceptual analysis. *Journal of Religion
    & Health, 55*, 1–24. https://doi.org/10.1007/s10943-016-0199-6

From the Perspective of the Public Health Department

13

Wendy Zimmerman and Jennifer Cooper

> *If you pour yourself out for the hungry and satisfy the desire of the afflicted, then shall your light rise in the darkness and your gloom be as the noonday. And the Lord will guide you continually, and satisfy your desire with good things, and make your bones strong; and you shall be like a watered garden, like a spring of water Isaiah 58:10-11, Revised Standard Version.*
>
> *When "i" is replaced by "we," even "illness" becomes "wellness" Malcolm X, 2018.*

13.1 The Changing Landscape of Health Care

The very words "health care" are changing. The word "health" is about creating conditions in which people can be healthy and where the healthy choice is the easy choice. The word "care" is now less about providing care and more about building self-efficacy and skills that support self-care. As the meaning of these words is changing, so too must those entities responsible for promoting, protecting, and restoring the health of our nation. Trends with the US population are shifting, evidenced in a growing aging population (e.g., baby-boomers), a more ethnically diverse population, and those living longer with multiple chronic conditions. Within these trends, there is also the concern of health disparities that still exist within certain groups.

W. Zimmerman (✉)
Parish Nursing Program, Meritus Health, Hagerstown, MD, USA
e-mail: Wendy.zimmerman@meritushealth.com

J. Cooper
Department of Nursing, Hood College, Frederick, MD, USA
e-mail: cooper@hood.edu

© Springer Nature Switzerland AG 2020
P. A. Solari-Twadell, D. J. Ziebarth (eds.), *Faith Community Nursing*,
https://doi.org/10.1007/978-3-030-16126-2_13

The Affordable Care Act (ACA) was signed into law in 2010, which has led to many changes in health care. With the implementation of the ACA in 2014, approximately 23 million Americans gained coverage (National Association of County and City Health Officials (NACCHO), 2016). Despite efforts to reform health care through increases in coverage, a gap continues to exist between the expansion of health care and achieving health (NACCHO, 2016). Additionally, the ACA has moved health care delivery from a fee-for-service (quantity) to a value-based (quality) model of reimbursement, making a focus on optimizing health and the non-clinical factors that impact health more of a determinant than only reacting to illness. The Association of State and Territorial Health Officials (ASTHO) Center for Population Health Strategies describes how "health and wellness are significantly impacted by factors outside of the health care and public health delivery systems" (ASTHO, 2018a). These factors are the social determinants of health, or the non-clinical factors that can impact health, such as economics, education, politics and policy, and safety. Finally, non-profit hospitals must maintain their tax-exempt status by conducting community health needs assessments every 3 years.

Each of these trends calls for greater consideration of the needs of the community at large and non-clinical factors that impact health, achieving health and health equity, and providing quality care. "Public health promotes and protects the health of people and the communities where they live, learn, work and play" (American Public Health Association (APHA), 2018a). It is this space—communities where people live, learn, work, and play and pray—where the role of public health is defined within the changing landscape of health care. Local health departments are charged to fill the role of the "Community Chief Health Strategist," meaning that they play the leading role in providing foundational public health services (FPHS) aimed at preventing disease, disability, and death in our communities. This model of FPHS includes the minimal services that must be available in all state and local health departments, which include communicable disease control, chronic disease and injury prevention, environmental public health, maternal, child, and family health, and access to and linkage with clinical care (Public Health National Center for Innovations, 2018).

Public Health 1.0, 2.0, and 3.0 is a framework that has been used to illustrate the evolution of the health care system as it is impacted by internal and external pressures. The era of Public Health 1.0 (1800s–1950s) was linked to medicine and combating infectious diseases that existed at that time. Public Health 2.0 (1950s–2000) responded to an increased life expectancy and resulting rise in chronic diseases. Our nation is now moving into Public Health 3.0, which is centered on optimizing the health of individuals and populations, accountable care, and understanding how environment and social issues impact health (Halfron et al., 2014).

13.2   Public Health Infrastructure

Public health is mandated and funded by the U.S. government and is best understood through the infrastructure of public health at the federal, state, and local levels. Public health oversight at the federal level is primarily provided by the U.S.

Department of Health and Human Services (USDHHS) and, more specifically, by the Centers for Disease Control and Prevention (CDC). One CDC strategic direction includes public health and health care collaboration and a key practice of the community chief health strategist is to "collaborate with a broad array of allies—including those at the neighborhood-level and the non-health sectors—to build healthier and more vital communities" (CDC, 2012).

There are 51 state public health agencies in the U.S.A. and the District of Columbia. The ASTHO represents public health agencies and professionals within the agencies. The National Association of County and City Health Officials (NACCHO) represents the 2800 local public health agencies and professionals in U.S. counties and cities. State and local public health departments are structured as either centralized, decentralized, shared, or mixed. The differentiation is important, as infrastructure impacts financing, activities, and performance (ASTHO, 2012):

1. Centralized: = or >75% of the state's population is served by local health units that are led by employees of the state, and the state retains authority over many decisions relating to the budget, public health orders, and the selection of local health officials.
2. Decentralized: = or >75% or more of the state's population is served by local health units that are led by employees of local governments, and the local governments retain authority over many decisions relating to the budget, public health orders, and the selection of local health officials.
3. Shared: = or >75% or more of the state's population is served by local health units that meet one of these criteria: where local health units are led by state employees, local government has authority over many decisions relating to the budget, public health orders, and the selection of local health officials; OR, where local health units are led by local employees, the state has many of those authorities.
4. Mixed: combination of centralized, shared, and/or decentralized arrangements within the state.

In many communities, local health departments provide safety net services to those who are low-income or who are uninsured, especially in the absence of community clinics. This means that the health department provides direct care services, regardless on an individual's ability to pay. As public health is called to move to the provision of the FPHS and away from the provision of direct care services, this leaves fewer options for care in communities.

With the changing landscape of health care and the existing public health infrastructure and role of public health, the question becomes, can public health support the needs of the public and move toward public health 3.0? Despite the need for public health services, it remains underfunded, and therefore not an equal partner within the health care delivery system. Only three percent of total health care spending goes to public health prevention programs, and as of 2016, 18% of the U.S. gross domestic product was spent on health (Peterson Center on Health Care & Kaiser Family Foundation, 2017). This upward spending has remained higher than other developed countries since the 1970s. Inadequate funding for public health is noted in a decrease of just over one billion dollars in the CDC budget from 2005 to 2012, which equated to an average of just under $20/per person in 2012. The decrease in the CDC budget has led to cuts to state and local funding for public health departments, and almost all 50 states have reported loss of approximately 45,000 total positions since 2008 (Trust for America's Health, 2013).

13.3   From the Perspective of Public Health

In their professional role in non-traditional settings, faith community nurses help to support the needs of the public and the services offered by public health. But are they recognized by public health as a partner? While there is still work to be done to build and showcase these partnerships, the relationship and potential of public health and faith communities has been cited by national organizations. The APHA organizes a Caucus on Public Health and the Faith Community that "seeks to support the value of faith as a key to the delivery of effective community health services" (APHA, 2018b). In partnership with the Interfaith Health Program at Emory University's Rollins School of Public Health, ASTHO (2014) compiled a resource guide of model faith community and public health practices within the U.S.A., focused on preventing the flu. Lastly, within the national *Million Hearts® initiative in 100 Congregations*. This campaign works to build awareness within faith communities about preventing cardiovascular disease (USDHHS, 2018).

Faith community nurses provide a greater continuum of care, serving as a trusted provider to those who may not trust the health care system or governmental health services. They also promote health equity. While the benefit of personal presence is often lost within the health care system, it is consistently practiced within the whole person model of faith community nursing. The very nature of the faith community is to spread a message of hope. Faith community nurses can serve as the bridge between or beyond health care and public health to provide services to promote health and prevent disease, with a whole person perspective (American Nurses Association and Health Ministries Association, 2017). The value of the faith community nurse role is who they are and the ability they have to reach members of a faith community. A great number of people in a community can be reached when several faith communities located in a county, city, or state have a faith community nurse present, who is leading health promotion and prevention initiatives in partnership with the health department.

Specifically, faith community nurses aid public health efforts by providing health education and messaging to members of their faith community, offering vaccine clinics, and participating in disaster planning and preparedness activities. Faith community nurses can also serve as a link between school nurses, who see the many needs of children and families. Building an academic-practice partnership between schools of nursing and faith community nurses has a two-fold benefit; nursing students receive an experiential learning opportunity in the community and faith community nurses can receive support from nursing faculty and students in identifying and serving the many needs of their communities.

13.4 From the Perspective of the Faith Community and the Faith Community Nurse

There are many things that motivate faith community nurses in this ministry of whole person health. Many nurses talk about feeling the divine "calling" of this specialty practice, or a sense of vocation. Being able to combine professional nursing practice with the spiritual dimensions of care is often mentioned. The independence and autonomy of practice is also a key driver, along with a slow-paced, high-touch, low-tech, approach to care.

The reasons a faith community embraces this ministry vary. The type of programming provided may be shaped by the professional expertise and gifts of the faith community nurse and the team that supports this ministry. A faith community nurse's passion for social justice may encourage programming to support single parents or to provide meals for the homebound or school aged children over the weekend. The clergy and faith community leadership will certainly be interested in the expanded ministry that is offered to individuals and families. Practical help to those experiencing a health crisis or a complex health issue is of tremendous benefit. Health ministry also offers an opportunity for outreach. Hosting a yoga class or a 12-step program often results in someone from outside the faith community, finding a social network and a place to belong.

As faith communities join with other community agencies or health organizations, outside the four walls of the faith community, it's important to understand the strengths, needs, and motivations of the faith community nurse and the faith community membership (McNamara, 2014). The Rev. Dr. Gary Gunderson has devoted his career to making connections between faith and health. He identifies eight areas where faith communities excel (Gunderson, 1997, 2000), thus bringing these strengths to any partnership. These inherent qualities are the strength to: accompany, convene, connect, frame or tell stories, give sanctuary, bless, pray, and endure.

Faith communities reflect a web of interconnections where strong, enduring relationships are cherished and valued. The ability to connect and convene is evident even in a simple congregational dinner or coffee hour. Faith communities have physical buildings where people gather. Individuals show up in each other's lives, when struggling with care giving situations or chronic health conditions, to accompany, to pray, to bless. Safe places are created and sanctuary is offered, when those battling with issues such as mental illness or addictions are welcomed and embraced. Stories of healing and endurance are told when a physical cure is not possible. Spiritual and emotional strength become the primary focus, as a final and complete healing is accomplished through death.

As faith community nurses and faith communities assess their needs, motivations, and assets (American Nurses Association and Health Ministries Association, 2017), it is essential to note some practical realities when opportunities for partnering arise. Some faith communities may wish to maintain their independence from any government organizations, finding that this might negatively affect perceptions among their membership (Stajura et al., 2012). In rural areas, faith communities may be resistant to signing any formal documents between organizations, while more urban faith communities may require it, but have strong opinions on what the agreement will be titled, for example, Memoranda of Understanding (MOU), covenant, or contract.

So, why would a faith community even consider partnering with a public health agency? For the faith community nurse, local health departments have resources and programs that support health ministry. Smoking cessation programs, some direct services for the underserved, and addictions resources are just a few examples. A faith community may be interested in a regional community health problem, like teen pregnancy, as they find their county has a higher incidence in the state. They can deal with this independently, at the faith community level, but if they want to have a greater impact, partnering with the local or state health department, the local school district, and other faith communities, would influence a more systemic change, by dealing with the root of the problem.

Lastly, as funding opportunities for health-related programs are shrinking, grant applications that demonstrate a multi-organizational approach are much more likely to be awarded funds. Local health departments are natural conduits for state and federal funds, which would not be available to individual faith communities or faith community nurses.

13.5 Addressing the Separation of Church and State

Over the past two decades, there has been a renewed commitment to strengthen partnerships between faith communities and government programs (ASTHO, 2014). In 1997, the Centers for Disease Control (CDC) collaborated with the Interfaith Health Program to sponsor a forum on "Engaging Faith Communities as Partners in Improving Health." Additionally, the George W. Bush administration created the Office of Faith-Based and Community Initiatives, which continues in a reconfigured form in the Obama and Trump administrations, now recognized as the White House Faith and Opportunity Initiative (Exec. Order, 2018).

Phrases like "separation of church and state" and "first amendment considerations" are heard often in discussions when faith communities and government agencies partner. The first amendment of the US Constitution says that, "Congress shall make no law respecting an establishment of religion, or prohibiting the free exercise thereof (U.S. Constitution, amend I)." The amendment has two provisions concerning religion: the Establishment Clause and the Free Exercise Clause. The Establishment Clause prohibits the government from "establishing" a religion. Historically, "establishing" meant prohibiting a state-sponsored religious faith, such as the Church of England and the Christian faith.

First amendment considerations should always be respected when a faith community partners with any government entity. This is especially true when funding is being provided by a local, state, or federal government agency. This should not discourage these partnerships, but it is important that government resources be kept separate from those used for religious purposes.

The Supreme Court provides a three-part test that offers guidance for government agencies working in collaboration with communities of faith:

1. The statute or other government action must have a secular purpose
2. The principal effect of the action or statute must neither inhibit nor advance religion
3. The statute or government action cannot foster excessive government entanglement with religions (ASTHO, 2014).

For instance, if a faith community nurse is organizing a flu clinic and is collaborating with the local health department to administer the vaccine, any health department funds or services must be directly focused on the secular purpose of the flu clinic, and not any form of religious promotion. Or in response to areas where health disparities are prevalent, bringing needed public health resources through trusted faith leaders is possible if the focus rests solely on the health topic and not on advancing any specific religious belief.

There was successful litigation in 2004 against the Office of Rural Health located at Montana State University, and the Montana Faith-Health Cooperative, where federal funds were used to provide support to small, faith-based and community-based organizations, to expand their capacity of social and health service programs for the needy and underserved (Zimmerman, 2006). Some of the funds were used to support foundational education for faith community nurses and health ministers. The ruling, by the federal district court for the State of Montana, stated there was a violation of the Establishment Clause, by providing direct and preferential funding to faith community nursing, thus subsidizing and endorsing the activities of the Montana Faith-Health Cooperative. Funding to faith community nursing and health ministry education was terminated and the defendants chose not to appeal the ruling.

It may be helpful to think of the terms, "faith-placed" instead of "faith-based," as a way to guide collaboration and keep the focus on the defined health initiative and away from those things that might promote religion or a specific faith tradition.

13.6   Looking Beyond the Faith Community: Successful Faith Community and Public Health Collaborations in US Communities

13.6.1 Key Components to Successful Collaborations

Successful collaborations contain some key elements that encourage success (Gunderson, Peachey, Sharp, & Singh, 2018):

- Partnerships can only move at the "speed of trust"
- Build relationships to build trust—everything revolves around relationships
- Engage partners at the beginning of the process
- Identify common interests to build trust
- Involve people that reflect the community that is being served
- Work with community members to identify needs then collaborate with health care to offer or refine those services

- Faith-based organizations may be the only entity that can draw partners together
- Focus on the wider good instead of self-interest
- Develop a strategy for handling conflict
- Power is not a dirty word; consider the approach of: power with, instead of power over.

Another successful strategy in multi-organizational partnerships requires an awareness of their inherent differences. Some of these differences are contrasted in Table 13.1 (Gunderson et al., 2018).

Partnerships are more successful when these differences are addressed openly and intentionally at the onset of the partnering dialogue. Shared learning provides opportunities for collaborative thinking followed by structure and support, as partnerships mature.

To promote successful collaboration, it is also important to look at the capacity of the faith community nurse and the faith community. With a lone, unpaid faith community nurse, working a few hours a week, the capacity for partnership is very different than a team of unpaid faith community nurses, or a paid faith community nurse working full or part-time. Capacity is also influenced by whether the faith community nurse is functioning within an institutional framework, with the support of a faith community nurse manager or coordinator, versus working independently without institutional support. Urban and rural locations can influence the availability of potential partners as well as the financial and in-kind resources available within a faith community.

13.6.1.1 Examples of Successful Collaborations

One simple and very common type of collaboration is accomplished when a faith community nurse assists the local public health department to "push out" valuable health information. The faith community nurse can provide meeting space, help recruit an audience, and assist with hosting the event. The local health department

Table 13.1 A Comparison of Perspectives: Faith Community and Public Health

From the perspective of the faith community	From the perspective of public health
Interested in the individual person and value personal presence	Interested in generalized populations
Want to help but may be unsure how to best contribute	Looking at evidence-based practice
Relationships are very important	Goal oriented, looking at the macro level
Value resources such as trust, caring, respect	Tangible resources are important
Motivated by faith, service, social justice	Motivated by population health data
May be suspicious and hesitant to partner with government organizations	May not think of faith communities as potential partners
Use faith-based language; love, spirit, resilience	Use clinical language; outcomes, cohesion, population health
Health = body, mind, spirit	Health = health care
Measure outcomes by telling stories	Measure outcomes with data

provides the speaker or clinical expert to present the health information, help with advertising, and bring any printed materials that may be needed. Faith community nurses all over the country are active in this way, delivering health information related to opioid addictions and substance abuse, disaster preparedness, behavioral health education, parenting classes, healthy eating, dental care, the *Living-Well* evidence-based programming for chronic disease management, diabetes, caregiving, cancer, and HIV (Self-Management Resources, 2018). Federally qualified health centers (FQHC) may also have staff that would be available for these types of presentations.

Another way that faith community nurses "push out" valuable health information is by consulting websites sponsored by local, state, or federal agencies. These are often the most credible and unbiased sources. The best known federal sponsored websites are: the National Institutes for Health (NIH), Centers for Disease Control and Prevention (CDC), Health Resources and Services Administration (HRSA), Substance Abuse and Mental Health Services Administration (SAMHSA), Food and Drug Administration (FDA), Administration on Aging (AoA), National Heart Lung and Blood Institute (NHLBI), and Medline Plus. A simple on-line search can access any of these resources.

The Centers for Medicare and Medicaid (CMS) specifically support faith based and community partnerships (Centers for Medicare and Medicaid Services, 2018) by offering regular webinars and toolkits related to Medicare, Medicaid, the Health Insurance Marketplace, and Children's Health Insurance Program (CHIP). These health resources address ethnic and faith diversity (Centers for Medicare and Medicaid Services, 2018).

Health fairs are frequently facilitated by faith community nurses as they partner both public and private agencies to assist with screenings and early identification of disease. Some health fairs actually provide needed services to the underserved in the form of: dental care; lab work for blood sugar or cholesterol; immunizations; medication review; vascular screenings or breast cancer screenings. A key component of any health fair needs to include mechanisms for referral and follow-up in order to maximize continuity of care and facilitate participant accountability.

Faith community nurses also have the opportunity to build and be active participants in multi-agency health improvement projects. Here are examples of successful faith community nurse and public health collaborations that have patiently navigated their role differences and have impacted outcomes in communities across the U.S.A.

13.6.2 Improving Hypertension in Maryland

The ASTHO *Million Hearts State Learning Collaborative* launched in October 2013 and to date has supported 22 state health departments working to integrate public health and health care to address hypertension (ASTHO, 2018b) and meet the national Million Hearts goal to prevent one million hearts attacks and strokes by 2022 (U.S. Department of Health and Human Services, 2018). As part of the

ASTHO Million Hearts State Learning Collaborative in 2014 and 2015, Maryland received funding from this initiative and formed a collaboration between the local health department, health system, and faith community nurse network (FCNN) to address undiagnosed and uncontrolled hypertension in Washington County, MD (Cooper & Zimmerman, 2016). The FCNN of Meritus Health, in Hagerstown, MD was invited by the Washington County Health Department to assist with the initiative. The FCNN, founded in 1996, had established partnerships with over 100 unpaid, professional faith community nurses, practicing in 50 faith communities. The network is supported by a part-time, paid faith community nurse program manager.

An MOU was signed where the local health department would provide funding for patient education materials, digital blood pressure (BP) monitors, office supplies, a stipend for each participating faith community, and salary support for the faith community nurse program manager. The faith community nurses would identify congregants, who were hypertensive or at risk for hypertension. Each participant would be given a digital BP monitor to use over a three-month period of time. In addition, participants would choose one to two lifestyle areas, related to BP control, with education and coaching from the faith community nurse.

Twenty-five faith community nurses, representing fifteen faith communities, volunteered to participate from April–June, 2014. Fifty-one congregants completed the project, with forty-two showing a statistically significant improvement in systolic and/ or diastolic BP over the project period. Six out of seven lifestyle areas also showed statistically significant improvement. Stress management was the lifestyle area that was chosen for improvement by the participants (Cooper & Zimmerman, 2017).

Many faith community nurses reflected on how their participants had "ah-ha" moments, where they could see how their stress was directly correlated to higher BPs. Prayer, meditation, relaxation breathing, exercise, and coloring were the most common interventions employed to reduced stress, and thus improve BPs. One participant lost thirty pounds and gained stamina by exercising during the project period. This enabled him to travel overseas on a once in-a-lifetime business trip, which he would not have been able to do previously. The client credits this project and his faith community nurse for his success.

Some challenges in this collaboration included a very short time line for program planning and for funds to be spent. Creating a new mechanism to shift funds from the health department to the hospital was needed, as public funds were handled differently than previous grant awards from non-profit entities. Trust issues at times were a challenge as well as obtaining the preferred equipment, due to bid requirements. It was the established relationship of the two lead players that kept the project moving.

The State Health Department did the data analysis of the first project period, which helped with the visibility of the project and promoted the value of faith community nurses, at the state level. Minor changes were made to the project and it was repeated in 2015 with similarly successful results (Cooper & Zimmerman, 2017). This FCNN continues to employ the coaching strategies they learned during this project, along with some of the lifestyle educational materials and self-assessment form. The project and documentation forms have been shared with other faith community networks and public health departments across the nation.

13.6.3 Promoting Health Education and Access to Resources in Texas

The model created in Texas brings together faith community nurses, health ministry leaders, and state public health resources, reaching out to Texans with health care needs (Pattillo, Chesley, Castles, & Sutter, 2002). In fall 1996, the commissioner of the Texas Department of Health (TDH) through its Volunteer Health Corp identified faith community nursing/health ministry as a means to expand the mission of the health department. Representatives of TDH began working with the Central Texas Health Ministry Coalition, which interacted with many faith community nurses and health ministers. As a result of the coalition, nine central Texas organizations, including TDH, signed a MOU to collaborate in the health ministry movement. The MOU continues to be signed by the health department and the Texas Health Ministries Network (THMN). The Central Texas Health Ministry Coalition has expanded to become the THMN, which supports faith community nurses and health ministers throughout Texas.

The TDH, now titled the Department of State Health Services (DSHS) provides office space and access to computers for two unpaid faith community nurses. These two collaborate with DSHS staff to disseminate current health information and resources. The faith community nurses promote health education for individuals interested in health ministry, respond to questions, and have developed a database to disseminate vital health information. A newsletter called *The Spirit of Texas* is edited quarterly with contributions from faith community nurses/health ministers and includes timely health information from DSHS. Over 600 are reached by this newsletter.

Through the DSHS library, a comprehensive bibliography of health ministry resources was created, including a calendar of educational activities (Texas Department of State Health Services, 2018). In consideration of the vastness of Texas, THMN membership decided to meet three times per year in the areas of the state: Houston/Beaumont, Austin/San Antonio, and Dallas/Ft Worth. Topics are presented by local experts and recent topics include Responding to Family violence: A Toolkit for faith community nurses and Congregations and Asset Based Community Development in the Specialty of Parish Nursing (Carlson, 2018; Chesley, 2018).

13.6.4 Faith-Based Coffee in Washington State

Another impactful partnership between public health agencies, faith community nurses, local schools, and faith communities takes place in Vancouver, Washington. In 2011, the local Division of Children and Family Services (DCFS) Department was looking for ways to increase support for youth and families involved in their foster care system. In considering their potential partners for collaboration, faith community nurses and their faith communities arose as key initial partners. This initial effort was successful in hosting foster nights out, clothing drives, and foster parent recruitment nights.

In 2012, Clark County Public Health Department was looking at chronic disease statistics and health disparities, specifically for youth and families living in central Vancouver, an area of their community where children were more at risk to adverse childhood health outcomes. Building off the success of DCFS's Faith-Based Coffee pilot in 2011, Faith-Based Coffee (FBC) became a forum for gathering stakeholders and volunteers in the community, focused on improving family resilience and building a broader base of community support (National Association for the Education of Homeless Children and Youth, 2018).

The concept of Faith-Based Coffee includes monthly meetings that take place in a dedicated faith community. Coffee is served, snacks are provided, and guest speakers present on a local health disparities topic related to children and families. Time is allotted for discussion and networking. Those attending these monthly meetings take back the information to their faith community or volunteer organization, where structured teams have evolved to address the needs that arise. The primary location where faith communities are mobilized is through their local community schools in the Vancouver School District. Long-standing partnerships have been in place between faith organizations and schools, but the FBC has formalized the process and expanded the capacity for addressing local needs.

In 2015, Clark County Public Health replicated the Faith-Based Coffee model to support children and families in Evergreen School District. Some of the leadership team consists of representatives from the health department, the school district, faith community nurses, clergy, mentoring organizations, child protective services, juvenile justice, and the department of social and health services. Based on group feedback and input, the leadership team determines which topics are offered at the monthly FBC meetings. Topics have included adverse childhood experiences (ACE), immigration updates, homelessness/affordable housing, food insecurity, mentoring, foster care, preventing child abuse and neglect, early learning, interpersonal violence, equity, and restorative justice. In response to these presentations, faith communities have: mobilized efforts to provide student mentoring and tutoring; contributed to the housing relief fund; fostered caring relationships with male students through men's basketball nights; sponsored teen parenting workshops; hosted barbeques prior to sporting events; stocked food and clothing pantries, facilitated after school programs; implemented summer meals programs, and supported teachers by providing morning coffee and remodeling classrooms.

While certain outputs can be measured, i.e., the number of volunteers, funds donated, and resources provided, hard outcomes have been difficult to capture. They are also interested in expanding their partnerships with a more diverse faith representation. Faith-Based Coffee received the Promising Practice Award from the National Association of County and City Health Officials (NACCHO) in 2015. Faith community nurses have been involved in all levels of partnership to be present, to plan, and to connect.

13.6.5 Serving the Underserved in Connecticut

The Faith Community Nurse Program (FCNP) of St. Vincent's Medical Center (part of Ascension Health), in Bridgeport, Connecticut began in 1989 with only five faith communities and has since expanded to approximately 80 faith communities and a team of 250 faith community nurses. The FCNP has served as a resource for the CT Department of Health outreach planning in the greater Bridgeport area. The FCNP now leads point-of-care testing for the state via a mobile bus, collecting data on blood pressure, blood glucose, hemoglobin A1c, and waist circumference to track the health of the population. Point of care testing allows for diagnostic testing in the field, whether that is in a mobile unit or in the home (National Institutes of Health, 2013). The benefit of point-of-care testing is that it reaches the client where they are and provides data that providers need for monitoring, as well as rapid diagnosis and treatment. As of early 2018, 268 people had been seen through this mobile program. Similarly, the FCNP has offered a "Know your Numbers" (blood glucose, body-mass index, and blood pressure) program in soup kitchens and food pantries. As a result of this work, the FCNP now had data that allowed them to recommend the need for and lead a change in the way food is donated and distributed at the soup kitchens and food pantries. In partnership with Schools of Nursing, the faith community nurse program piloted "SWAP" (Supporting Wellness at Pantries) in 2017. Food on the shelves is categorized using a "stop light system" or red, yellow, and green, to indicate the nutritional value of foods. This awareness not only assists those supplied by the pantries, but also has changed the way people donate food to the pantry. The FCNP also leads an annual Medical Mission at Home program that draws over 300 people for point of care testing, foot-washing by clergy, new socks and shoes, and podiatry care.

One of the Connecticut FCNPs greatest challenges has been to see faith community nursing beyond a ministry only within the faith community, but also to the greater community. Overall, this program is a model that helps to generate revenue for the health system.

13.6.6 Community Outreach in Wisconsin

In Wisconsin, the Monroe Clinic is part of the area health care system, and provides outreach through faith community nurses, who are led by a paid faith community nurse coordinator. The outreach by faith community nurses began in 1997 and is focused on providing health education and advocacy in the community. Like Maryland, Wisconsin was one of 22 states to receive funding from the ASTHO *Million Hearts State Learning Collaborative*. The Green County Health Department partnered with the Monroe Clinic to provide community blood pressure screenings. The health department included the work on this project as part of their strategic plan for accreditation readiness. Additionally, they were the first local public health department to gain access to *EPIC*, the electronic health record that is also accessible to the faith community nurse program at the Monroe Clinic. The ability to communicate through the *EPIC* system has provided a community-clinical linkage between the health department, clinic, and health system that allows for bi-directional referrals to health care providers for greater continuity of care.

13.7   International Faith Community Nurse Programs

The majority of international faith community nurse programs are funded by faith-based organizations. Catholic Charities support faith community nurses in South Africa and the Lutheran denomination provides funding for faith community nurses in India and Palestine (Daniels, 2018). Very few programs partner with government organizations. In some countries, there is tension between faith-based organizations and the government, especially where the faith tradition represents a religious minority. One example of a faith community and public partnership in the United Kingdom (UK) is described here. The title Parish Nurse (PN) is used primarily as the professional designation for a faith community nurse in the United Kingdom.

13.7.1 Transitional Care in the United Kingdom

One parish nurse in the United Kingdom has had tremendous success with a transitional care pilot program launched in partnership with a hospital that was part of their National Health System (NHS) that ran from August to December 2016 (Stephenson, 2017). The parish nurse, paid by her faith community, was able to follow ten patients, post discharge from the hospital. In the United Kingdom, as part of the NHS, district nurses and social workers follow those who are discharged from the hospital. This is a free service to the patient, but visits are limited in frequency and both the nurses and social workers are thinly stretched. The parish nurse, on the other hand, had the freedom to visit more frequently and was able to respond more quickly, to refer to the district nurse, hospital, or general practitioner (GP), as needed.

Under an MOU, the faith community agreed to support the parish nurse in this project and the time it required, as all of the patients were not members of that faith community. Any needed durable medical equipment was provided by the NHS trust and clinical supervision and support was provided to the parish nurse by a hospital-based registered nurse. The parish nurse visited the patients regularly to do basic checks and to assess their general welfare. The parish nurse offered emotional and spiritual support, monitored blood pressure, checked weights, assessed the home environment for fall risk, offered nutritional or medication information, but any direct clinical care was referred to the district nurse.

By the end of the pilot project, one patient was re-admitted to the hospital, one was upgraded to GP care, while the others were able to manage independently, with either the same level of services or fewer services than at the onset. Two patients, who already identified themselves as Christians, had started attending church again. The nurse executive from the NHS hospital reported this aspect of the pilot, "I think it was a really positive thing for those people, because all of a sudden they are surrounded by people who support and care for them when they might otherwise have been very isolated." The hope is that more faith communities will be encouraged to support faith community nurses and that the NHS will consider further collaborations with private sector services, like parish nursing.

Approximately 100 parish nurses are practicing across the United Kingdom, with about 25–30% being paid, the rest being unpaid. These parish nurses are supported by eight regional coordinators from Parish Nurse Ministries United Kingdom who provide professional supervision, support, education, training, and development.

13.8   Leadership Strategies and Impacting Change in the Future

Deborah Patterson, former Executive Director of the International Parish Nurse Resource Center, in St. Louis, MO, discusses eight areas of FCN practice, where FCNs can make an important contribution as an advocate: (1) help obtain access to care, (2) serve as a health navigator, (3) serve as a patient advocate in the health care system, (4) work to acquire needed services in a community, (5) mobilize for the health of neighbors, (6) raise awareness of legislative issues related to health, (7) advocate for environmental health concerns, and (8) work for others in developing countries (Patterson, 2007).

The first four roles are common interventions in a faith community nurse's practice. When considering partnership and collaboration outside the boundaries of the faith community, mobilizing for the health of the neighbors and raising awareness of health-related legislative issues require an enhanced level of leadership. Faith community nurses in Texas and Louisiana have joined with their parishioners to respond to and better prepare for the future, after hurricanes Katrina and Harvey. These broad reaching endeavors often involve systemic change, and are more like running a marathon than a sprint. They take time, involve risk, and require us to focus on the wider good instead of self-interest. A faith community nurse may start with a faith community initiative, but the work of a faith community nurse director, manager, or coordinator may be required to move the initiative forward with a broader focus.

Faith community nurses in Ohio joined the efforts of the Greater Cleveland Congregations to influence health care policy with the expansion of Medicaid in 2013 (National Academies of Sciences, Engineering, and Medicine, 2018). Regardless of political affiliation, teaching people how to participate in government, attend lobby days, write letters to elected officials, participate in canvassing or public demonstrations, all help to bring about legislative change.

Joining with Health Ministries Association (HMA), the interdisciplinary membership organization for faith community nurses gives faith community nurses a professional voice in the dynamic profession of nursing, along with state nursing associations. As we face the future challenges of, increasing the number of paid faith community nurses, validating value added service with both tangible and intangible outcomes, and attracting younger nurses, we will secure the connective tissue of faith and health that we know and love in this specialty practice.

13.9   Conclusion

A common theme among public health and faith community nurse collaboration is the focus on prevention and health promotion, social justice, and providing services to low-income, uninsured, and migrant populations. This work is paramount in an existing health care delivery system that is influenced by political forces and population shifts and trends. Therefore, it is important for faith community nurses and public health to seek out each other in partnership, understanding their unique and complementary focus, to achieve greater health outcomes.

References

American Nursing Association & Health Ministries Association. (2017). *Faith community nursing scope and standards of practice*. Silver Spring, MD: American Nurses Association. Nursesbooks.org

American Public Health Association. (2018a). *What is public health?* Retrieved from https://www.apha.org/what-is-public-health

American Public Health Association. (2018b). *Caucus on public health and the faith community*. Retrieved from https://www.apha.org/apha-communities/caucuses/caucus-on-public-health-and-the-faith-community

Association of State and Territorial Health Officials. (2012). *State public health agency classification: Understanding the relationship between state and local public health*. Retrieved from http://www.astho.org/Research/State-and-Local-Public-Health-Relationships/

Association of State and Territorial Health Officials. (2018a). *Center for population health strategies: Information for state and territorial health officials*. Retrieved from http://www.astho.org/Programs/Clinical-to-Community-Connections/ASTHO-CPHS-Overview_FINAL/

Association of State and Territorial Health Officials. (2018b). *State learning collaborative to improve blood pressure control*. Retrieved from http://www.astho.org/Million-Hearts/State-Learning-Collaborative-to-Improve-Blood-Pressure-Control/

Association of State and Territorial Health Officials & Interfaith Health Program at Rollins School of Public Health at Emory University. (2014). *Public health and faith community partnerships: Model practices to increase influenza prevention among hard-to-reach populations* (pp. 1–16). Spring.

Carlson, R. (2018). *E-mail communication*.

Centers for Disease Control & Prevention. (2012). *Becoming the chief health strategist: The future of public health*. Retrieved from http://phsharing.org/wp-content/uploads/2016/09/Plenary-CDC.pdf

Centers for Medicare and Medicaid Services. (2018). *Faith based partners*. Retrieved from https://www.cms.gov/Outreach-and-education/Outreach/Partnerships/FaithBased.html

Chesley, D. (2018). *E-mail communication*.

Cooper, J., & Zimmerman, W. (2016). The evaluation of a regional faith community network's million hearts program. *Public Health Nursing, 33*(1), 53–64.

Cooper, J., & Zimmerman, W. (2017). The effect of a faith community nurse network and public health collaboration on hypertension prevention and control. *Public Health Nursing, 34*(5), 444–453.

Daniels, M. (2018). *E-mail communication*.

Exec. Order No. 13831, 83 FR 20715. (2018).

Gunderson, G. R. (1997). *Deeply woven roots*. Minneapolis, MN: Fortress Press.

Gunderson, G. R. (2000). Emergent wholeness: Congregations in community. *Word & World, 19*(4), 360–367.

Gunderson, G., Peachey, K., Sharp, J., & Singh, P. (2018). *Faith-health collaboration to improve community and population health: A workshop conducted at Shaw University*, Raleigh, NC.

Halfron, N., Long, P., Chang, D., Hester, J., Inkelas, M., & Rodgers, A. (2014). Applying a 3.0 transformation framework to guide large-scale health system reform. *Health Affairs, 33*(11), 2003–2011.

Malcolm, X. (2018). Retrieved from https://www.azquotes.com/quote/811613

McNamara, J. (2014). *Stronger together: Starting a health team in your congregation* (pp. 25–33). Memphis, TN: Church Health Center.

National Academies of Sciences, Engineering, and Medicine. (2018). Faith-health collaboration to improve population health. In *Proceedings of a workshop – In brief*. Washington, DC: The National Academies Press. https://doi.org/10.17226/25169

National Association for the Education of Homeless Children and Youth. (2018). *Faith- based coffee model: Engaging the faith community and social service agencies*. Retrieved from http://webcache.googleusercontent.com/search?q=cache:jcvcqu2Xz78J:naehcy.org/wp-content/uploads/2018/01/Implementing-the-Faith-Based-Coffee-Model.pptx+&cd=7&hl=en&ct=clnk&gl=us

National Association of County and City Health Officials. (2016). *Statement of policy: The local health department as community chief health strategist*. Retreived from https://www.naccho.org/uploads/downloadable-resources/15-11-LHD-as-Community-Chief-Health-Strategist.pdf

National Institutes of Health. (2013). *Fact sheet: Point-of-care diagnostic testing*. Retrieved from https://report.nih.gov/nihfactsheets/ViewFactSheet.aspx?csid=112

Patterson, D. L. (2007). Eight advocacy roles for faith community nurses. *Journal of Christian Nursing, 24*(1), 33–35.

Pattillo, M., Chesley, D., Castles, P., & Sutter, R. (2002). Faith community nursing: Parish nursing/health ministry collaboration model in central Texas. *Family & Community Health, 25*(3), 41–51.

Peterson Center on Health Care & Kaiser Family Foundation. (2017). *Total health spending*. Retrieved from https://www.healthsystemtracker.org/indicator/spending/health-expenditure-gdp/

Public Health National Center for Innovations. (2018). *Foundational public health services*. Retrieved from https://phnci.org/fphs

Self-Management Resources. (2018). *E-mail communication*.

Stajura, M., Glik, D., Eisenman, D., Prelip, M., Martel, A., & Sammartinova, J. (2012). Perspectives of community and faith-based organizations about partnering with local health departments for disasters. *International Journal of Environmental Research and Public Health, 9*(7), 2293–2311.

Stephenson, J. (2017). *Nursing director back church-based community nurse scheme*. Retrieved from http://www.nursingtimes.net

Texas Department of State Health Services. (2018). *Calendar*. Retrieved from www.dshs.state.tx.us/library/nursing.shtm

Trust for America's Health. (2013). *Investing in America's health: A state-by-state look at public health funding and key health facts*. Retrieved from http://healthyamericans.org/report/105/

U.S. Constitution. Amend. I.

U.S. Department of Health and Human Services. (2018). *Million hearts*. Retrieved from https://millionhearts.hhs.gov/

Zimmerman, W. (2006). The public private partnership: Expansion of the ministry. In P. A. Solari-Twadell & M. A. McDermott (Eds.), *Faith community nursing, development, education, and administration* (pp. 83–92). St. Louis, MO: Elsevier Mosby.

Part IV

Changing the Understanding of Health: Professional Organizational Perspectives

Historical Perspective and Organizational Development of Faith Community Nursing

14

Lisa M. Zerull and P. Ann Solari-Twadell

14.1 Early Organizational Roots of Nursing

For centuries religious women have formed groups for the purpose of caring for the vulnerable and the sick carrying out the healing ministry of their faith. Following the Judeo-Christian traditions, countless women followed the example of Jesus' ministry—healing, teaching, and praying with primary emphasis on spiritual and compassionate care. In so doing, the women shared common purpose and formal education that combined religion and medicine with nursing to benefit those in need from birth through death. Much more was accomplished by organizing in groups than as individuals. There are many historical examples of denominationally based groups of women involved in nursing and healing. Two such groups of women are introduced in this chapter—the Roman Catholic, Sisters of Charity, St. Vincent de Paul, and the Lutheran Deaconesses. Both worked out of the faith community setting promoting whole person care including care of the body and mind as well as the spirit.

In 1633, St. Vincent de Paul was successful in the revival of organized nursing care for the sick by founding the Roman Catholic Sisters of Charity (Kalisch & Kalisch, 2004). Louise de Marillac worked closely with St. Vincent de Paul to develop what was first called the "Ladies of Charity", which focused on the care of the sick. Madame de Marillac recommended that these providers be prepared with a basic education in home-based care. In 1633, St. Vincent de Paul supported the development of a school of nursing in Paris which was managed by Madame de Marillac (Seymer, 1933, pp. 56–59). Eventually, de Marillac and Vincent de Paul collaborated on the development of what is known today as the *Daughters of Charity*

L. M. Zerull (✉)
Winchester Medical Center-Valley Health System, Winchester, VA, USA
e-mail: lzerull@valleyhealthlink.com

P. A. Solari-Twadell
Marcella Niehoff School of Nursing, Loyola University Chicago, Chicago, IL, USA
e-mail: psolari@luc.edu

© Springer Nature Switzerland AG 2020
P. A. Solari-Twadell, D. J. Ziebarth (eds.), *Faith Community Nursing*,
https://doi.org/10.1007/978-3-030-16126-2_14

described as "a community of religious women who would create a life of religion in the world" (McNamara, 1996, p. 482). This religious order was the first to be non-monastic. In other words, the *Daughters of Charity* would live with one or two other *Daughters* renting lodging in a community, rather than being part of a religious community which lived separate from and all together separate from other members of the secular community (Solari-Twadell & Egenes, 2006).

In order to provide spiritual formation for the *Daughters*, Vincent de Paul provided regular lectures for these community-based women care givers. The lectures were formulated into the *Rules for the Sisters of the Parish* (Leonard, 1979, p. 1210). Although originally developed in the 1600s, the rules for Roman Catholic parish sisters provide a historical foundation for faith community nurses today regardless of differing faith traditions.

Another example of religious women trained as nurses was the Lutheran Deaconess movement which begun in 1836 with the Kaiserswerth Institutions in Germany. With a strong vision for better care, and in particular nursing care of persons in need, Lutheran clergy Theodor Fliedner and his wife created an organization of women formally trained as nurses in hospitals, homes for the elderly, and in the community setting (Fliedner, 1870). Deaconess education combined religion, medicine, Materia Medica (aka pharmacology), nursing, and general studies of math and writing. In return, the Lutheran Deaconesses were required to maintain an association with the larger organizing body called the "Motherhouse" receiving ongoing instruction, participation in rituals of faith, fellowship, and support. Deaconess nurses were well educated to minister to individuals and families attending to care of the body, mind, and spirit. With early success, the care soon expanded into several branches of deaconess nursing including the care and instruction of children, global mission work, older adult care, and parish work (Nightingale, 1851).

During this same period, multiple protestant denominations such as Methodists, Anglican, Presbyterians, and Baptists as well as Roman Catholics were also active in institutional work in hospitals, orphanages, homes for the aged, and other church supported institutions such as schools and mission stations (Bliss, 1952). It is the parish work of nurses based in the faith community setting in the 1800s that has common parallels to contemporary faith community nurses today.

14.2 Professional Nursing Organizations

Organization of nurses as professionals has strong international history beginning with the World's Fair in Chicago. As part of the fair buildings in 1893, there was a Woman's Building. One of the exhibits "under the charge of Mrs. Bedford Fenwick" from Great Britain who was responsible for the beginning of the "Royal British Nurses Association initiated in 1887," was the "nursing section". Mrs. Fenwick "was interested in meeting other trained nurses wherever they might be."

Thus, she "suggested to the World's Fair Officials that there be a space In the Woman's building for American Nurses to meet" (Jamieson & Sewall, 1954, pp. 394–395). The remainder is history. Early nurse leaders not only met and established the foundation for nursing professional organizations in the U.S.A., but also formed the foundation for today's *International Council of Nurses*. Similarly, the *American Nurses Association* initiated in 1911 was the result of the early *Nurses Associated Alumnae of the United States and Canada* (Jamieson & Sewall, 1954, p. 410).

The reasons that contemporary nurses join professional nursing organizations are many: (1) be informed; (2) receive education; (3) network with others; (4) to mentor or receive mentoring; (5) define and promote excellence in practice; (6) attend local, regional, national, and international gatherings; (7) engage in certification; (8) contribute, develop, and have access to resources specific to a specialty nursing practice; (9) advance a specialization within nursing; and (10) influence health policy. Nurses frequently cite one, several, or all reasons for choosing membership in one or several professional nursing organizations.

The importance of nursing's contributions and impact on quality, patient-centered care is in the spotlight (Greiner & Knebel, 2003). The enactment of the *Affordable Care Act* in the U.S.A. (U.S. Department of Health & Human Services, 2010) and the release of the Institute of Medicine's report *The Future of Nursing: Leading Change, Advancing Health* (Institute of Medicine, 2010) focus on the profession of nursing's valuable contributions and tremendous potential to transform the quality of care. It is well known that nurses are the key to quality care in all of the settings in which they work. The *Institute of Medicine's* history of recommending improvement in health care and reforming health professions has resulted in stimulating positive change. The *Institute of Medicine's* previous reports include *To Err is Human: Building a Safer Health System* in 1999, *Health Professions Education: A Bridge to Quality* in 2003, and *Keeping Patients Safe: Transforming the Work Environment of Nurses* in 2004 (Institute of Medicine, 1999, 2003, 2004). Collectively, the Institute of Medicines priorities of patient safety and promoting quality care, in addition to the *Future of Nursing* report (2010), provide the evidence base for making the case that nurses should be at the forefront of systemic change in health care. Another strong argument for the profession of nursing leading this change is the public's high regard for the profession (Gallup Poll, 2017). When combined with nursing's history of leading social change as well as the education and skill bank developed by each nurse, the nursing profession is uniquely positioned to assume a major role in the transformation of the health care system (Jones, 2010; Mendes, 2010; p. 2012).

14.3   Professional Nursing Organizations Supporting Faith Community Nursing

Similar to Theodor Fliedner's establishment of the Lutheran Deaconesses and Vincent de Paul's founding of the Daughters of Charity in the 1800s, Rev. Dr. Granger Westberg is widely known as the founder of contemporary parish nursing now known as faith community nursing in the 1980s. After conducting a pilot program with a nurse working out of his Lutheran congregation, Westberg immediately recognized the value of promoting whole person health out of the faith community setting, and it was nurses who were central to this care (Westberg, 1985, 1987).

Rev. Granger Westberg was indeed a catalyst for change in healthcare. He wanted to move away from the increasing emphasis on illness treatment which was costly and burdensome. Rather Westberg championed a focus on health promotion as cost effective and with more favorable outcomes for individuals, families, communities, and health systems. See Box 14.1 presenting Westberg's verbatim on "Why Churches Should Get Back into Health Care." In particular, his vision of a faith community as an important setting of health promotion with the nurse in a primary role was the spark to ignite a movement that has continued to expand for more than three decades (Westberg, 1987). A timeline of the evolution of faith community nursing from 1983 to 2018 is presented in Box 14.2. Much has been accomplished over time in addition to the synergy and favorable outcomes resulting from partnerships formed between secular and religious organizations.

Box 14.1 Westberg's Verbatim on "Why Churches Should Get Back Into Health Care"

Let me suggest ten statements that could be accepted by churches of all denominations. They could be a first step in formulating, some basic propositions: from these, the several denominations might begin to develop a strategy for encouraging health living.

1. Health is intimately related to how a person "thinketh in his heart."
2. Health is not to be "our chief end in this life"—only a possible by-product of loving God and one's neighbor as oneself.
3. Health is closely tied to goals, meanings, and purposeful living—it is a religious quest.
4. Illness is often present in a life that is empty, bored, without purpose, or aims.
5. Our present disease-oriented medical care system must be revised to encourage modeling and teaching wellness.
6. Our present separation of body and spirit must go, and an integrated, wholistic approach must be put in its place.
7. There is a difference between mere existence and a life lived under God, responsive to the promptings of His spirit.
8. The body functions at its best when a person, who is the body, exhibits attitudes of hope, love, faith, and gratitude.
9. True health is closely associated with creativity, by which we as people of God participate with Him in the ongoing process of creation.
10. The self-preservation instincts of a person can be happily blended with the innate longing to love and to help others.

Source: Peterson, W.M. (Ed.). (1982). *Granger Westberg verbatim: A vision for faith & health.* St. Louis, MO: International Parish Nurse Resource Center.

Box 14.2 Timeline Parish/Faith Community Nursing

1983	Granger Westberg pilot program with a nurse running a wellness clinic out of the faith community setting—Our Saviour Lutheran Church, Tucson, AZ
1984	Parish Nurse Program partnership begun with six faith communities and Lutheran General Hospital, Park Ridge, IL
1986	Lutheran General Hospital establishes a Parish Nurse Resource Center to share resources about health ministry and parish nursing with others
1987	First Westberg Parish Nurse Symposium held
	Granger Westberg publishes book *The Parish Nurse*
	Parish Nurse Resource Center becomes the *National* Parish Nurse Resource Center
1989	Health Ministries Association (HMA) formed in Iowa as a non-profit membership organization for parish nurses and others active in health ministry
1991	Marquette University offers eight-day parish nurse education program titled the *Wisconsin Model*—a curriculum later modified to become the *Foundations of Faith Community Nursing* course
	First annual HMA Meeting and Conference held in Northbrook, IL
1995	Lutheran General merges with Evangelical Health Systems Corporation to create Advocate Health Care
	National Parish Nurse Resource Center becomes the *International* Parish Nurse Resource Center (IPNRC)
1997	American Nurses Association (ANA) recognizes parish nursing as a specialty practice
1998	First scope and standards for parish nursing practice released by the HMA and ANA
1998	Parish Nurse Preparation Curriculum published by the IPNRC
1999	Parish Nurse Coordinator Curriculum published by the IPNRC
	Death of Granger Westberg (July 1913–February 1999)
2002	IPNRC transfers assets from Advocate Health System to the Deaconess Foundation, St. Louis, MO
2004	World Forum for FCN is formed with 22 members from Australia, Canada, South Korea, Swaziland, and the U.S.A.
2005	ANA/HMA revise and publish scope and standards
	Title changed from *parish* to *faith community* nurse
2006	Parish Nursing Ministries UK formed to promote and support
2011	IPNRC assets transferred from Deaconess Foundation, St. Louis, MO to the Church Health Center, Memphis, TN
	The 25th Annual Westberg International Parish Nurse Symposium held
2012	ANA/HMA revise and publish faith community nurse scope and standards—2nd edition
	Parish Nursing Ministries UK becomes the Resource Centre for the European network of faith community nurses
2013	The nurse membership organization of Faith Community Nursing International formed
2014	American Nurses Credentialing Center (ANCC) launches FCN certification through portfolio
	Foundations of Faith Community Nursing curriculum revised

2015	First in a series of FCN Position Statements released by the IPNRC—*How is Faith Community Nursing the Same or Different than Other Nursing Specialties?*
	Knowledge Ministry Platform for FCN (online) introduced by IPNRC
2016	IPNRC renamed Westberg Institute
	30th anniversary of the Annual Westberg International Parish Nurse Symposium held in Chicago, IL
2017	ANA/HMA revise and publish FCN scope and standards—3rd edition
	The Westberg Institute takes the Westberg Symposium "On the Road" to multiple locations in the U.S.A. and internationally
	FCN certification by portfolio no longer offered by the American Nurses Credentialing Center (ANCC, 2017)
2018	Documented 31 countries active with FCN

Source: Zerull, L.M. (Ed). (2018). FCNs active around the world. Perspectives 17(2), 8–9.

Careful review of the timeline for faith community nursing reveals how small groups provided an early infrastructure of education and support and then grew into multiple larger organizations as the demand for information and resources increased (Solari-Twadell, 2002). In 1984, Westberg gained administrative support for a hospital-based group of parish nurses associated with Lutheran General Hospital, now Advocate Healthcare (Westberg & McNamara, 1987). As highly sought after speaker, Westberg energetically promoted faith community nursing to faith leaders and nurses around the U.S.A. It was no surprise that Lutheran General Hospital was deluged with inquiries about how to start parish nurse programs. In response to the high interest, a *Parish Nurse Resource Center* was begun in 1986 followed by an informational symposium held in 1987 (Westberg & McNamara, 1987). The early resource center shared their knowledge and experience on how to begin a parish nursing practice. As demands for more information about parish nursing increased from across the country, the center added the word *"National"* to the Resource Center's title. To reach an even larger audience around the globe prompted the name to change yet again in 1995 to *International Parish Nurse Resource Center* (Solari-Twadell & McDermott, 2006). Still in existence today, the faith community nurse resource center, *Westberg Institute*, is part of *Church Health* located in Memphis, Tennessee. The *Westberg Institute* provides global resources for education and health ministries. The newest title gives homage to Rev. Granger Westberg's many contributions to faith community nursing (Campbell, 2016).

14.4 Interdisciplinary Collaboration

Westberg understood that in order to sustain the parish nurse movement, a membership organization needed to be developed. In 1989, the Health Ministries Association (HMA) was formed inviting faith leaders, nurses, and other health professionals involved in spiritual care, along with lay persons to join its membership (ANA/

HMA, 2017). With low numbers of parish nurses and most working as unpaid volunteers, in addition to many nurses having an unclear understanding of how a membership in HMA could benefit them, its membership remained small. Regardless of its membership size, the HMA worked with intent and diligence for eight years to have parish nursing recognized as a nursing specialty practice. HMA's vision, diligence, and persistence paid off. The American Nurses Association (ANA) recognized parish nursing as a distinct specialty practice in 1997. This recognition was soon followed by the first scope and standards for parish nursing practice published solely by the HMA in 1998 (ANA/HMA, 1998). Subsequently, HMA partnered with the ANA to publish the FCN scope and standards released in 2005, 2012, and the 3rd edition in 2017 (ANA/HMA, 2012, 2017).

The scope and standards are essential for the establishment of a specialty practice. Additionally, the contents provide a common understanding of the specialty practice for incorporation into educational curricula and job descriptions. In the 2005 scope and standards for practice, the title of parish nurse was changed to "faith community nurse." The title change encompassed the Judeo-Christian traditions yet was more inclusive of all faith traditions (ANA/HMA, 2005). There still remains some use of the title *parish nurse* by individuals, in select faith traditions, and in various locations around the world such as Europe and Zimbabwe.

Since the late 1980s, the HMA has been recognized as the first interdisciplinary organization for faith community nurses. A second membership organization was introduced in 2013 known as *Faith Community Nursing International—FCNI* (FCNI, 2018). The impetus for its creation was nurses desiring an "all-nurse" professional membership organization for faith community nurses—distinct from the broader and more diverse HMA membership. Another key goal of *FCNI* was to encourage further research within the specialty practice. Partnering with Western Kentucky University, *FCNI* created an online international journal widely available to its membership and a larger population of anyone having internet access. This wider access results in greater dissemination of research guiding practice along with open invitation to add to the *FCNI* body of knowledge. See Chapters 15 and 16 for more in-depth description of the HMA and *FCNI* as membership organizations.

14.5 International Expansion

For more than two decades, educators, researchers, faith leaders, and experienced faith community nurses have come together to create comprehensive curricula for both the foundational and advanced leadership preparation of nurses to the specialty practice. While several curricula are available for use with traditional classroom and online learning formats, the most frequently used, evidence-based and well-regarded resource is published by the *Westberg Institute*. Updates to the curriculum are planned every five years to remain current with the research and evidence for the faith community nurse specialty practice. Some adaptations to the curriculum allow for use in other countries taking into consideration differing cultures, language, and healthcare delivery systems. Based upon the numbers of nurses taking the *Foundations of Faith Community Nursing* course of the *Westberg Institute,* there are approximately 500 new faith community nurses each year (Zerull, 2016). The number is estimated even higher when adding the nurses who took other preparatory courses available around the world, thus making an exact number faith community nurses unobtainable without a shared database or collective summary.

Another international effort supported by the *Westberg Institute* is the World Forum. Formally organized in 2004, a faith community nurse staff member paid by the *Westberg Institute* and living abroad collaborates with representatives from various countries to develop new faith community nurse networks, promote faith community nurse education, and encourage the establishment of faith community resource centers for each continent. Active efforts are underway to promote the evidence-based faith community nurse curricula foundational and coordinator preparation in countries where they would not otherwise have a resource for education. Identifying contacts willing to work with *Westberg Institute* as well as translating the curricula from English to the primary language of the country requires considerable time and effort. This is an additional example of how much more can be accomplished together in collaboration when nurses identify the need and organize toward a common goal.

The global state of faith community nurse outreach is documented. There are now 31 countries around the world with documented faith community nurse initiatives (Zerull, 2018). In countries where faith community nursing is just beginning or has a small membership such as New Zealand or Swaziland, the Westberg Institute provides a wealth of rich resources that may not otherwise have been available. For example, through the use of available technology in the form of Skype, a *Foundations of Faith Community Nurse* course was offered with success to a group of Nigerian nurses. Another global communication tool supported by *Church Health* and the *Westberg Institute* is the *Knowledge Ministry Platform for Faith Community Nursing* (Swistak & Lemons, 2016). The platform uses the web-based technology of *Yammer* to form online chat groups for knowledge sharing and social media connections. The platform is an endless repository of knowledge in the form of research, feedback, webinars, groups, and resources (Lemons & Campbell, 2017, p. 15). Users have instant access to the latest news and announcements of activities, conferences, and publications along with offering a host of formal resources such as position statements for faith community nursing practice. There are now more than 1100 nurses engaged in using the platform with more than 80 interest groups to join based upon interest (Lemons & Campbell, 2017, p. 13). Some examples of platform interest groups include state, country, or denomination based; roles (e.g., educators and coordinators), activity (e.g., retreat or conference); special interest (e.g., research or curriculum); and a digital archive. The positive outcomes realized from groups of nurses coming together using available technology in creative ways are limitless.

14.6   Advocacy

In the past few years, seven position papers for faith community nurses were created by the *Westberg Institute*. Each position paper presented an "explanation, a justification, or a recommendation for a course of action that reflects nursing's stance regarding a practice concern" (Ziebarth, 2015). The position papers responded to frequent questions asked by faith community nurses by providing practice guidance and designed to be a more specific supplement to the scope and standards of practice.

Many faith community nurse networks across the U.S.A. are supported by health systems. Faith Community nurses working as partners with health care institutions need to be informed of the initiatives of the health care institution and acknowledge the sponsoring organizations mission, vision, and priorities. Thus creative endeavors connecting actions with favorable outcomes are necessary such as cost avoidance, risk reduction, the promotion of quality care, or advocating for individuals. An excellent example that can achieve most of the aforementioned outcomes is the promotion of documented advance directives in the community (Congregational Nurse Project of Northwest Ohio, 2005; Garrido, Idler, Leventhal, & Carr, 2013; Medvene, Base, Patrick, & Wescott, 2007).

Since only about 26% of Americans currently have a documented Advance Directive (ACEP, 2016) there is unique opportunity for faith community nurses to improve this statistic and advocate for individuals.The faith community nurse is a known and trusted health resource. The faith community is an ideal setting to complete the Advanced Directive *before* end of life decisions need to be made. Another positive outcome of a documented Advanced Directive is to relieve family members of decision-making burdens. The promotion of Advanced Directives is one excellent example of advocacy and the difference a faith community nurse can make for individuals, families, faith communities, and the larger regional community.

14.7   The Importance of Membership Organizations for Faith Community Nurses

Nurses, as the primary providers of health care to all communities in all settings, are key to the contribution and achievement of the Sustainable Development Goals (United Nations, 2015) developed through the United Nations (Box 14.3). Investment by nurses in their professional organizations is significant to this contribution if there is any chance at succeeding in addressing these goals. Although the stated goals seem lofty, each faith community nurse, by taking time to review, could identify how at least half of these goals pertain to their specific local community. Starting locally is an important way to succeed globally.

Overcoming challenges and pushing boundaries is certainly not foreign to faith community nurses. Each faith community nurse has been a pioneer forging a new

Box 14.3 Sustainable Development Goals
GOAL 1
End poverty in all its forms everywhere
GOAL 2
End hunger, achieve food security and improved nutrition, and promote sustainable agriculture
GOAL 3
Ensure healthy lives and promote well-being for all at all ages
GOAL 4
Ensure inclusive and equitable quality education and promote lifelong learning opportunities for all
GOAL 5
Achieve gender equality and empower all women and girls
GOAL 6
Ensure availability and sustainable management of water and sanitation for all
GOAL 7
Ensure access to affordable, reliable, sustainable, and modern energy for all
GOAL 8
Promote sustained, inclusive, and sustainable economic growth, full and productive employment, and decent work for all
GOAL 9
Build resilient infrastructure, promote inclusive and sustainable industrialization, and foster innovation
GOAL 10
Reduce inequality within and among countries
GOAL 11
Make cities and human settlements inclusive, safe, resilient, and sustainable
GOAL 12
Ensure sustainable consumption and production patterns
GOAL 13
Take urgent action to combat climate change and its impacts*
GOAL 14
Conserve and sustainably use the oceans, seas, and marine resources for sustainable development
GOAL 15
Protect, restore, and promote sustainable use of terrestrial ecosystems, sustainably manage forests, combat desertification, and halt and reverse land degradation and halt biodiversity loss
GOAL 16
Promote peaceful and inclusive societies for sustainable development, provide access to justice for all, and build elective, accountable, and inclusive institutions at all levels

GOAL 17
Strengthen the means of implementation and revitalize the global partnership for sustainable development

Source: United Nations (December, 2015). Getting started with the sustainable development goals December 2015: A Guide for Stakeholders. In *Full report of the Open Working Group of the General Assembly on Sustainable Development Goals* (UN Publication No. A/68/970). Retrieved from http://unsdsn.org/wp-content/uploads/2015/12/151211-getting-started-guide-FINAL-PDF-.pdf

understanding of health and a way of making decisions regarding health, encouraging incorporation of these ideas on a daily basis, and reinforcing behavior consistent with these ideas. Every decision faith community nurses take on and actualize is critical in making a difference. Faith community nurses need support and reenergizing to continue in their ministry. It is important that each faith community nurse has the ability to network, exchange ideas, and advance their understanding and practice. This is where the value of belonging to a professional nursing organization can reap benefits as the capacity for advancing as a professional is built in to the nature of a professional nursing organization.

Faith community nurses are innovative and have the potential to impact health policy, practice, and health outcomes. Given the whole person perspective from which faith community nurses practice, their ministry and work is consistent with *Healthy People 2020* (Institute for Public Health, 2016) and the *Sustainable Development Goals* (United Nations, 2015). At the local and regional levels faith community nurses can be part of nurse-led initiatives related to issues facing different communities. Faith community nurses can also demonstrate how a faith community nurse working inter-professionally with others can motivate and stimulate collaboration working through small groups of people, forming powerful partnerships across professions, while bringing about meaningful and permanent change.

More than 30 years ago Rev. Granger Westberg paired his vision of change in healthcare with the unique contributions of a faith-based nurse: "the parish nurse movement offers an opportunity to totally transform healthcare as we know it today" (Deaconess Board, 1903; Peterson, 1982, p. 11; Zerull, 2010). Faith community nurses are agents of change resourcing the public's understanding of a different way of integrating health, encouraging good health and well-being, as well as leading the understanding of how communities and health care systems are affected by factors such as poverty, public policy, climate change, economic growth, and education. It is time for faith community nurses everywhere to join in the vision that this "grass roots" movement is part of the solution to quality health care. This decision to be engaged in the process of health policy development "calls" for further risk taking.

The risk entails breaking out of the historical and stereotypical ideas that a faith community nurse is limited to providing services to a single faith community. Faith community nurses are educated, experienced professionals central to the health of nations. Faith community nurses are a valuable part of enabling communities to improve and reach equitable quality of life and health care access for all. Faith community nurses can be strong voices providing innovative leadership.

The 2030 agenda proposed as part of the *1992 Rio Declaration* provides a shift from a growth-based economic model to new thinking that aims at sustainable and equitable economies and societies, as well as greater public participation in decision-making (United Nations, 1992). This agenda "aims to replace unsustainable consumption and production patterns with sustainable lifestyles and livelihoods that benefit all. Central to the agenda is the understanding that a healthy, well-functioning environment is crucial for humankind to prosper" (United Nations, 2015).

Historically, there appears to be some confusion about membership when the faith community nurse has multiple choices of professional nursing organizations supporting faith community nursing. The following chapters relay a more in-depth history of contributions and descriptions of current initiatives of the *Westberg Institute*, the *HMA*, and *FCNI*. Ultimately, the faith community nurse must make the decision of how to become a part of the whole and support professional practice in faith community nursing.

Much has been accomplished in the past three decades with the evolution of faith community nursing. Notably, faith community nursing is a recognized specialty nursing practice, complete with scope and standards for practice, active research and professional organizations. Opportunity for greater collaboration among the membership organizations of *HMA* and *FCNI*, as well as stronger partnerships with the *Westberg Institute*, creates strength through collaboration. Increased collaboration yields benefits for this expanding and maturing nursing specialty practice. Faith community nurses are invited to participate in this "call" to action. In addition to promoting whole person health, the faith community nurse is invited to join one or both faith community nurse membership organizations, i.e., *HMA* or *FCNI*, and become an active member. As a professional nurse, there is a responsibility to engage with the profession, remain current with practice changes by linking to regional faith community nursing networks, support national and international faith community nurse initiatives, all will advance the specialty practice of faith community nursing.

References

American College of Emergency Physicians (ACEP). (2016). *Nearly two-thirds of Americans don't have living wills—Do you?* Retrieved from http://newsroom.acep. org/2016-03-21-Nearly-Two-Thirds-of-Americans-Dont-Have-Living-Wills-Do-You

American Nurses Association and Health Ministries Association (ANA/HMA). (1998). *Scope and standards of practice of parish nursing practice.* Washington, DC: American Nurses Publishing.

American Nurses Association and Health Ministries Association (ANA/HMA). (2005). *Faith community nursing: Scope and standards of practice*. Silver Spring, MD: American Nurses Association.

American Nurses Association and Health Ministries Association (ANA/HMA). (2012). *Faith community nursing: Scope and standards of practice* (2nd ed.). Silver Spring, MD: American Nurses Association.

American Nurses Association and Health Ministries Association (ANA/HMA). (2017). *Faith community nursing: Scope and standards of practice* (3rd ed.). Silver Spring, MD: American Nurses Association.

American Nurses Credentialing Center. (2017). *Faith community nurse certification no longer available*. Retrieved from http://www.nursecredentialing.org/faithcommunitynursing

Baltimore Lutheran Deaconess Motherhouse, A Handbook 1903, ELCAA, ULCA 61/8/1 Handbook/Catalogue, Lutheran Deaconess Motherhouse and Training School, 1903, box 1, folder 1, 5.

Bliss, K. (1952). *The service and status of women in the church*. London: SCM Press.

Brenan, M. (2017). *Nurses keep healthy lead as most honest, ethical profession. Gallup poll social series*. Retrieved from https://news.gallup.com/poll/224639/nurses-keep-healthy-lead-honest-ethical-profession.aspx?g_source=CATEGORY_SOCIAL_POLICY_ISSUES&g_medium=topic&g_campaign=tiles

Campbell, K. P. (2016). IPNRC becomes the Westberg Institute. *Perspectives, 15*(2), 1.

Congregational Nurse Project of Northwest Ohio. (2005). *The role of faith communities and congregational nurses in advance directives*. Adapted from Respecting choices: Facilitator's manual. Gundersen Lutheran Medical Foundation, La Crosse, WI. Retrieved from http://www.wcnet.org/~lfulcher/pages/page14.html

Faith Community Nursing International. (2018). Retrieved from https://www.fcninternational.org/

Fliedner, T. (1870). *Some account of the deaconess work in the Christian church*. Kaiserswerth: Sam Lucas.

Garrido, M. M., Idler, E. L., Leventhal, H., & Carr, D. (2013). Pathways from religion to advance care planning: Beliefs about control over length of life and end-of-life values. *Gerontologist, 53*(5), 801–816. https://doi.org/10.1093/geront/gns128

Greiner, A. C., & Knebel, E. (Eds.). (2003). Committee on the health professions education summit. In *Health professions education: A bridge to quality*. Washington, DC: National Academies Press.

Institute for Public Health. (2016). *Healthy people 2020 and the sustainable development goals*. Retrieved from https://publichealth.wustl.edu/healthy-people-2020-and-sustainable-development-goals/

Institute of Medicine. (1999). In L. T. Kohn, J. M. Corrigan, & M. S. Donaldson (Eds.), *To err is human: Building a safer health system*. Washington, DC: National Academies Press. Retrieved from http://www.nationalacademies.org/hmd/~/media/Files/Report%20Files/1999/To-Err-is-Human/To%20Err%20is%20Human%201999%20%20report%20brief.pdf

Institute of Medicine. (2003). *Health professions education: A bridge to quality*. Washington, DC: National Academies Press.

Institute of Medicine. (2004). *Transforming the work environment of nurses*. Washington, DC: National Academies Press.

Institute of Medicine. (2010). *The future of nursing: Leading change, advancing health*. Washington, DC: National Academies Press.

Jamieson, E. M., & Sewall, M. F. (1954). *Trends in nursing history: Their relationship to world events*. Philadelphia, PA: W.B. Saunders.

Jones, J. M. (2010). *Nurses top honesty and ethics list for 11th year [news release]*. Princeton, NJ: Gallup. Retrieved from http://www.gallup.com/poll/145043/Nurses-TopHonesty-Ethics-List-11-Year.aspx

Kalisch, P. A., & Kalisch, B. J. (2004). *American nursing: A history* (4th ed.). Philadelphia, PA: Lippincott, Williams & Wilkins.

Lemons, S., & Campbell, K. (2017). Westberg Institute announcements: 1,000 members. *Perspectives, 16*(3), 13, 15.

Leonard, J. (1979). *The conferences of St Vincent DePaul to the daughters of charity (Translated from the French)*. London: Collins Liturgical Publications.

McNamara, J. K. (1996). *Sisters in arms: Catholic nuns through two millennia*. Cambridge, MA: Harvard University Press.

Medvene, L. J., Base, M., Patrick, R., & Wescott, J. (2007). Advance directives: Assessing stage of change and decisional balance in a community-based educational program. *Journal of Applied Social Psychology, 37*(10), 2298–2318. https://doi.org/10.1111/j.1559-1816.2007.00259.x

Mendes, E. (2010). *In US, more than 8 in 10 rate nurses, doctors, highly [news release]*. Washington, DC: Gallup. Retrieved from http://www.gallup.com/poll/145214/Rates-Nurses-Doctors-Highly.aspx

Nightingale, F. (1851). *The institution of Kaiserswerth on the Rhine, for the practical training of deaconesses*. London: London Ragged Colonial Training School.

Page, A. (Ed.). (2012). Committee on the work environment for nurses and patient safety. Keeping patients safe. *President's Message* (95)5.

Peterson, W. M. (1982). *Granger Westberg verbatim: A vision for faith & health*. St. Louis, MO: International Parish Nurse Resource Center.

Seymer, L. R. (1933). *A general history of nursing*. New York: MacMillan.

Solari-Twadell, P. A. (2002). *The differentiation of the ministry of parish nursing practice within a congregation*. Doctoral Dissertation. Retrieved from Abstracts International. (63(06), 569A UMI No 3056442).

Solari-Twadell, P. A., & Egenes, K. (2006). A historical perspective of parish nursing: Rules for the sisters of the parishes. In P. A. Solari-Twadell & M. A. McDermott (Eds.), *Parish nursing: Development, education, and administration*. St. Louis, MO: Mosby/Elsevier.

Solari-Twadell, P. A., & McDermott, M. A. (Eds.). (2006). *Parish nursing: Development, education, and administration*. St. Louis, MO: Mosby/Elsevier.

Swistak, A., & Lemons, S. (2016). Church health's knowledge ministry platform for faith community nursing community. *Perspectives, 15*(1), 6–7.

U.S. Department of Health & Human Services. (2010). *Affordable care act and the health care and education reconciliation act*. Retrieved from https://www.hhs.gov/healthcare/about-the-aca/index.html

United Nations. (2015). *Getting started with the sustainable development goals December 2015: A guide for stakeholders*. Full report of the Open Working Group of the General Assembly on Sustainable Development Goals (UN Publication No. A/68/970). Retrieved from http://unsdsn.org/wp-content/uploads/2015/12/151211-getting-started-guide-FINAL-PDF-.pdf

United Nations General Assembly. (1992). *Rio declaration on environment and development*. A/CONF.151/26 (Vol. I). Retrieved from http://www.un.org/documents/ga/conf151/aconf15126-1annex1.htm/

Westberg, G. E. (1985). Presentation on 12 September 1985, Westberg Collection, Loyola University at Chicago University Archives, Box 1, folder 3, p. 1.

Westberg, G. E. (1987). Why a nurse on the staff of a church. In *Parish nurse news: A newsletter* (p. 1). Park Ridge, IL: Parish Nurse Resource Center.

Westberg, G. E., & McNamara, J. W. (1987). *The parish nurse: How to start a parish nurse program in your church*. Park Ridge, IL: Parish Nurse Resource Center.

Zerull, L. M. (2010). *Nursing out of the parish: A history of the Baltimore Lutheran deaconesses 1893–1911*. Doctoral dissertation. Retrieved from ProQuest. (ATT 3436021).

Zerull, L. M. (2016). Foundations of faith community nursing graduates. *Perspectives, 15*(1), 12–13.

Zerull, L. M. (2018). FCNs active around the world. *Perspectives, 17*(2), 8–9.

Ziebarth, D. (2015). Introducing IPNRC position statements. *Perspectives, 14*(2), 1.

The Westberg Institute: An Evolution of the International Parish Nurse Resource Center

15

P. Ann Solari-Twadell and Maureen M. Daniels

15.1 Supporting the Development of Faith Community Nursing

The development of the *Parish Nurse Resources Center*, Lutheran General Hospital in 1986 was in response to a need. The first six original parish nurses working in three Lutheran, two Roman Catholic, and one Methodist faith community were receiving numerous requests from those interested in beginning parish nurse programs. Reverend Granger Westberg was like "Johnny Appleseed" spreading the news and excitement about this innovative ministry that included registered nurses as part of the staff of local faith communities retrieving the health ministry of the church. Reverend Westberg would get people excited about the church and health in one location, and then he was off to another speaking engagement in another state. Those with questions sought out the six original nurses. To relieve the first nurses of this additional work, a resource center was initiated where those interested in parish nursing could get questions answered, receive information regarding start up, and seek resolutions to problems. The intention was that the "resource center" would decrease frustration on the part of those interested in starting program and provide some standardized responses to questions with no intention of being a membership organization. This was intentional to avoid politicizing and encouraging splintering of the resources of a young movement.

P. A. Solari-Twadell (✉)
Marcella Niehoff School of Nursing, Loyola University Chicago, Chicago, IL, USA
e-mail: psolari@luc.edu

M. M. Daniels
Westberg Institute for Faith Community Nursing, Church Health, Memphis, TN, USA

© Springer Nature Switzerland AG 2020
P. A. Solari-Twadell, D. J. Ziebarth (eds.), *Faith Community Nursing*,
https://doi.org/10.1007/978-3-030-16126-2_15

15.2   Parish Nurse Resource Center

The functions of the *Parish Nurse Resource Center* were: (1) organizing and conducting educational programs; (2) serving as a reference center for people who
wanted information; and (3) consulting with nurses, pastors, churches, hospitals,
agencies, and religious denominations who were interested in beginning parish
nurse programs. The *Parish Nurse Resource Center* quickly began developing a life
of its own. Soon phone calls were coming to 312-696-8773, which spelled 'my
nurse'. By January 1987, the director of the center was spending 80% of her time on
the work of the resource center, when the position was only designated as half-time.
As parish nursing grew to include sites in, and resources from, and for other countries, the name of the center was changed first to the *National Parish Nurse Resource
Center*, and then to The *International Parish Nurse Resources Center* (IPNRC)"
(Westberg, 2013, p. 236). During this time, the *Westberg Symposium* was developed, with the center sponsoring 15 of the international educational conferences
with printed proceedings in the Chicago area. In addition, quarterly issues of
Perspectives, the newsletter of the resource center, were published and sent out to
the "Friends of the Center" and other interested parties. The Basic Parish Nurse
Curricula for parish nurses, coordinators, and educators was developed and fran-
chised to sites nationally and internationally. The proceedings of the Westberg
Symposium, issues of *Perspectives*, and the beginnings of the various curricula as
well as other writings of Rev Granger Westberg are housed in the Archives of the
Cudahy Library on the Lake Shore Campus of Loyola University Chicago.

As Lutheran General Health System merged with Evangelical Health System in
the Chicagoland area to form Advocate Health Care, the demands of health care
financing drew the organization to sharpen its mission more directly on the delivery
of acute care services. After supporting and financing the IPNRC for 16 years,
Advocate Health Care sought a new home for the resource center.

15.3   Deaconess Foundation

In 2002, the IPNRC was relocated to the Deaconess Foundation, St Louis Missouri.
Rev. Deborah Patterson became the new director. The Deaconess Foundation was
funded through the sale of Deaconess Hospital in St. Louis. The leadership of the
foundation welcomed the IPNRC as Deaconess Foundation was compatible with
the long history of providing parish nursing services in the St. Louis and surrounding areas. The Basic Preparation Curricula, *Perspectives*, Westberg Symposium and
many of the resources continued to be provided along with consultation through the
support of the Deaconess Foundation. Through the efforts of Alvyne Rethemeyer,
Sheryl Cross, and Maureen Daniels, who were originally parish nurses in the
Deaconess Network, the work of the resource center thrived.

During the 10 years that IPNRC was in St. Louis, the *Perspectives* newsletter
continued, the *Westberg Symposium* was held annually with available proceedings,
and the Basic Preparation Curriculum was updated in 2009 with a new module

format, a new conceptual model, more learning and teaching tools, and a separate instructional section for faculty. At this time the curriculum name was changed to the *Foundations of Faith Community Nursing*. In 2011, a second printing of the curriculum was made when the name of *parish nurse* was changed to *faith community nurse*, following the Faith Community Nurse Scope and Standards revision of 2005 (IPNRC, 2011, pp. 8–12). Additionally, the 2000 Coordinator/Manager Curriculum was significantly revised in 2012 and titled *Faith Community Nurse Coordinator Curriculum* along with a supporting *Faith Community Nurse Coordinator Manual*. This new manual offered new forms and tools. Twelve Supplemental Modules for additional education were also written in 2005 and eleven more in 2007. Other accomplishments during this time period included connections made with several national and governmental organizations on public policy, consultation on faith community nurse and health ministry issues, reaching out to faith community nurse coordinators nationally, and also relationships with other countries initiating and growing faith community nurse programs were strengthened.

With the strengthening of international relationships came the development of the *World Forum*. International faith community nurses and other interested in international aspects of health and healing connections had been attending the *Westberg Symposium* in order to learn about the practice. In addition, many who were from other countries came to present about their faith community nursing experience and learning in their faith communities. Because of this, a group of international faith community nurses presented a proposal to the Board of Deaconess Ministry at the 2004 Symposium and discussed the need for more international outreach and education. The result was the creation of the *World Forum*. The vision for the *World Forum* was to create an opportunity for education and best practices, ideas, and theology, as well as resources and networking for parish nurses around the world. Today there are 31 countries participating in the *World Forum*. The 31 countries are divided into seven geographic regions of the world—U.S.A., Canada, Central and South America, Europe, Africa, Asia, and Australia/New Zealand. A staff person from IPNRC was assigned to coordinate this international effort in 2008. The *Westberg Institute* has remained committed to the *World Forum*.

In 2010–2011, when the Deaconess Foundation in St. Louis made the decision that the IPNRC was no longer consistent with their mission, there was a search to find a new home for the IPNRC. Where should it go, to whom would it next belong? Who or what was in a position to nurture its future development? Many concerns were presented and the maintenance of the IPNRC was a concern of the faith community nurse professionals who had relied on the IPNRC for almost 30 years. The Board of Directors of Deaconess Parish Nurse Ministries LLC was diligent in their seeking a fit for the future of the IPNRC. There were basically three choices—one become independent on its own, second, partner with another organization as it had done in Chicago and St. Louis, or third, and least desirable, was to close.

The IPNRC was not able to become independent as expenses exceeded revenue. Proposals were initiated to have expenses covered through revenue, but there was no satisfactory solution that could accomplish the goal of financial independence. The third option was so undesirable that it was not considered, unless absolutely no other choice was available. In the meantime, other organizations were considered. Deborah Patterson, the former Executive Director of Deaconess Parish Nurse Ministries LLC, had an association as a contributing editor to the "Church Health Reader," a resource of the *Church Health Center*. In Chapter 11 it was noted that after thoughtful consideration, the *Church Health Center* Board of Directors agreed to take on the IPNRC and its mission and ministry to the faith community nurses.

15.4   Purpose of the Church Health Center

The *Church Health Center*, now called *Church Health*, is the "United States largest privately funded, faith-based health care organization. Since 1987, *Church Health* has expressed its vision under the broad categories of medical, wellness and outreach. Added to this is a fourth category of knowledge or thought leadership as part of the *Church Health* structure (Sheehan, Bisognano, & Waller, 2014, p. 42)".

Dr. Morris presented the development of *Church Health* as part of Chapter 11 in this book. Rev. Gary Gunderson stated, "…data in Memphis shows that patients going to the hospital from covenant congregations and churches with intentional relationships with the hospital, have half the mortality rate as similar, carefully matched patients and stay out of the hospital 39 percent longer on average. The patient benefits by staying well and active much longer… we see (these results) even in these very tough communities (Ranson, 2012, p. 17)."

A natural outgrowth of *Church Health's* ministry was the development of resources in print materials, books, and related tools for health promotion. The *Church Health Reader* is one of the primary resources that is published providing "inspirational and innovative resources drawn from knowledgeable sources and offers practical ways to create happier, healthier communities (Davis, 2017, p. 2)."

Another development from the *Church Health* was the "Knowledge Ministry." This ministry started as knowledge or thoughtful leadership. Faith Community Nursing became the very first online social media and knowledge sharing platform developed by *Church Health*. Participants enrolled in the platform share knowledge, mobilize, and grow community. (https://westberginstitute.org/fcn-knowledge-sharing-platform) Westberg Institute (n.d.-a, b) "Sharing knowledge—both what we know and what we need to learn—becomes a platform for grounded decisions and quality improvement insights at the intersection of faith and health (Sheehan, 2014, p. 3)."

In summary, the purpose of *Church Health* began from the vision and inspiration of Rev. Granger Westberg's early ideas. Westberg's model of whole person health care connecting body, mind, and spirit through blending of faith and health delivering care outside the medical system with community help drives the work of *Church Health* today (Peterson & Westberg, 1982). While Rev. Westberg moved onto working with parish nurses suggesting a professional model of health ministry in congregations, *Church Health* has focused on not only health ministry development in faith communities, but also creating whole person health care resources available to all through local faith communities in the Memphis, Tennessee area.

The Mission Statement is *"Church Health* seeks to reclaim the Church's biblical commitment to care for our bodies and our spirits" with the core purpose being "To improve health and well-being so that people can experience the full richness of life." The values of *Church Health* are: (1) we are welcoming to people of all beliefs and respectful of their individual needs; (2) we are compassionate, nurturing the health, well-being, and dignity of each other and those we serve; (3) we are collaborative, seeking and sharing best practices, and respecting the mutual contributions we make in fulfilling our mission; (4) we are innovative, challenging ourselves and our partners to improve the way we work and serve; (5) we are passionate in the pursuit of our mission; (6) we serve all equally, with integrity and openness, breaking down barriers that build injustice. (Church Health Website. *Mission Statement, Purpose, Core Values.* Retrieved from: https://churchhealth.org/about-church-health/.) Not only are the mission and values of *Church Health Website* (n.d.) consistent with faith community nursing, but also there is a history of both organizations providing resources to fuel a change in the understanding of health, the importance of collaboration, use of evidence, and a history of working with policy makers.

15.5 International Parish Nurse Resource Center and Faith Community Nursing

Faith Community Nursing with its foundation being health of body, mind, and spirit was a natural fit with *Church Health* mission of "wholeness in, with and through the community of faith..." (https://westberginstitute.org/history-mission/) Westberg Institute (n.d.-b). Faith community nursing also related closely to the *Church Health's* mission to reclaim "the Church's biblical commitment to care for our bodies and our spirits" (https://churchhealth.org/about-church-health/; Zerull, (2013)) and the interest and "call" is to serve "the whole person in the context of their community (westberginstitute.org/history-mission)."

There are historically some differences in the two organizations. The IPNRC focused on a professional model of health ministry while *Church Health* was more supportive of the lay health promoter model. Another difference is the international focus of the *IPNRC*. While *Church Health* was more focused on local and national resourcing, the *IPNRC* had partnerships with many all over the world. However, the similarities were more substantial than the differences. Interviews with two of *Church Health's* leadership team, also part of the original contacts with St. Louis before and after the move, agreed that faith community nursing was "a natural fit" with the mission and ministry of *Church Health*. It fits so well with the ministry of *Church Health* with churches, "it was a no-brainer (Sturdivant, personal communication, May 7, 2018)." The matching of *Church Health* with the *IPNRC* was envisioned to offer opportunity for both entities. At the 2011 *Westberg Symposium* held in St. Louis, the announcement about the move of the *IPNRC* to Memphis was made. Dr. Morris came to the Westberg Symposium and spoke about the willingness of *Church Health* to assume the operation of the *IPNRC*.

In 2016, the *IPNRC* was renamed the *Westberg Institute*. The four principles that *Church Health* continues to support with the development of the *Westberg Institute* in encouraging the further development of faith community nursing are: (1) *Church Health* is fundamentally about health and faith communities, as is faith community nursing; (2) *Church Health* values nurses and the nursing profession as nurses are at the heart of health ministry; (3) *Church Health* was attracted to *IPNRC* because of its health resource center. *Church Health* had already integrated resource development and production; and (4) *Church Health* will support health ministry in its broadest sense and seek to be supportive of anyone who is committed to health ministries in faith communities. "Rev. Granger Westberg planted a seed that *Church Health* considers a sacred obligation to grow and see flourish. I look forward to the development of faith community nursing in remarkable ways in the years to come." (Morris, 2012, p. 13).

In 2014 prior to the opening of the *Westberg Symposium* a meeting was held of the IPNRC staff, Church Health Center leadership, and other faith community nursing leaders, coordinators, and educators. This group brainstormed about how to make the name of the *IPNRC* more relevant to current practice, keep the connection to its historical roots, and yet reflect the great growth and expansion of the ministry. This included aligning with the new title for the practice as defined in the Scope and Standards new revision. Several other meetings in 2015 with the *Faith Community Nurse Educational Advisory Team* and other faith community nurse leaders and nurses, were held to continue this discussion about the services of the *IPNRC* including a potential name change. The word *institute* was identified by many and reflected more of the research work being done, along with the education, consultation, and resource development. Consideration was also given to honoring Rev. Granger Westberg and his life's work in wholistic health. So the name *Westberg Institute* was chosen. Later that year a marketing company reviewed all the aspects of the proposed name change and implications for the future. Then the *Church Health Center* leaders agreed to change the name to *Westberg Institute for Faith Community Nursing* (Campbell, 2016).

Additionally, the *Health Ministries Association* with *American Nurses Association* had decided to replace the name of *parish nurse* with *faith community nurse* in the 2005 revision of the Faith Community Nursing Scope and Standards of Practice, to be more inclusive of all the faith traditions served. It followed that having a resource center that had the name "parish nurse" in it was not matching the growth and maturity of the ministry.

15.6   Church Health Priorities for International Parish Nurse Resource Center/Westberg Institute

From the beginning of the *IPNRC* integration into *Church Health*, the priority was to continue the services and programs that had been the core work of *IPNRC* from the beginning. Reverend Stacy Smith (2012, pp. 2–3) noted in the first *Perspectives* published from *Church Health Center* "Our priority has been to continue the services you had come to expect while further acquainting ourselves with you and you with us." Discussion included plans to upgrade many of resources, build advisory groups of knowledgeable, expert faith community nurses to discuss issues of education, professionalism, teamwork, and international outreach. Some of this has been achieved. Some of these goals are still in process.

Today, significant work has been put into continuing to ensure that what originally was the *Basic Preparation for Parish Nurses* and the coordinators and educators curricula are contemporary and comprehensively modified. There are regular meetings for faith community nurse educators to ensure that the process and content of the foundations course are delivered in a manner consistent with the philosophy of faith community nursing. The *Westberg Symposium* is now sponsored in multiple locations across the U.S.A. to encourage more faith community nurses to be able to attend. Early on, the value of the *Westberg Symposium* was recognized by *Church Health.* Sturdivant, commented on the collegiality of faith community nurses. "They feel a great 'calling' and understanding of religious faith and this ministry (Sturdivant, personal communication, May 7, 2018)." Another comment regularly heard at the 2016 *Westberg Symposium* in Chicago was that the "spirit in the room where the faith community nurses had prayed and shared was palpable, that the Holy Spirit was present." It is commonly heard in faith community nursing circles, that faith community nurses are willing to share their work, tools they have found, resources and practices, along with their successes. Everyone is so willing to help each other. That bonding is indeed real and based on shared beliefs.

There is a great benefit to faith community nurses being able to access resources of *Church Health* such as the "Model for Healthy Living," some of the spiritual resources, such as "Stations of the Cross—Mental Illness," or "Holding Hope: Grieving Pregnancy Loss" during Advent, or some of the nutrition information, or "Congregational Health Promoter" training curriculum. Also, access to the "knowledge ministry" work with the "knowledge platform" is a significant resource for faith community nurses to promote community, information sharing, and collegial support (https://westberginstitute.org/fcn-knowledge-sharing-platform, *Westberg Institute*, n.d.-a, b). These tools are contemporary means to aid faith community nursing, and also spark ideas of how to create one's own unique tool for their faith communities and communities at large. Additionally, the staff at *Church Health*, who work with these tools and programs, are available and open to answering questions, as well as developing other community resources to assist faith community nurses to address newly identified problems and concerns.

Challenges for this partnership are not new. Finances have been a challenge for faith community nursing since it began in Chicago. The financing of the resource center has always been a "mission activity" with little expectation of the resources covering the bottom line. Going forward this mindset of "mission" needs to change as *Church Health* has to cover its expenses. Historically, many faith filled organizations and foundations gave many years of support to parish nursing and now faith community nursing like Advocate Lutheran General and Deaconess Foundation, and now *Church Health.* Financial support for this work will continue to be a concern until faith community nursing is recognized for the value of the role in addressing a changing health care environment and ongoing health care reform nationally and internationally.

Another challenge is raising the importance and contribution of the faith community nurse, not only within the *Church Health* structure, but also with health care system leadership, insurance companies, and decision makers engaged in health care reform. Early in the acquiring of the *IPNRC*, a simple survey of all the faith community nurse coordinators connected to *IPNRC*, about 226 then, was completed. Results showed that 149 of the surveyed programs were still sponsored by hospitals/health care systems. It was a concern that 34% of the hospitals had dropped their programs (Daniels, 2010). Without sustainable faith community nursing programs the future of this ministry is challenged being networked into the continuum of care. As a response, *Church Health* and *Westberg Institute* initiated research on the "Transitional Care" program utilizing faith community nurse networks and corresponding hospital systems. The research in process is intended to document a difference in the care given clients through the integration of faith community nurses. More information is provided in Chapter 11 of this book on the progress made with this research project. The government in the U.S.A. is currently financially supporting transitional care, and other related prevention programs that can easily be employed through faith community nursing (see Chapter 13).

15.7　United States

There is no identified way to track how many faith community nurses are practicing in the U.S.A. Being unable to identify all faith community nurses also compromises knowing other useful demographics, such as location of service, educational background, hours worked, and types of service offered. There is also no clarity on how many health care systems are supporting or resourcing faith community nurse programs. Research completed in 2002 did identify that parish nursing was present in every state (Solari-Twadell, 2002). However, it is not clear whether all those programs have sustained over time.

15.8　Summary and Recommendations

The *Westberg Institute* is a key partner organization to further the specialty practice of faith community nursing. It has the advantages of all the health promotion resources, staff, and the knowledge platform of *Church Health* to make great contact with and promote sharing of knowledge and support of faith community nurses with each other and other related professionals. It has the advantage of the connections that *Church Health* has made over many years to advance faith community nursing's needs and talents. It has had the largest number of subscribers (it is not a membership organization), and the advantage of the ownership of the faith community nursing curricula offering the profession a highly developed, reviewed, updated, and produced standardized course on a regular schedule. It has had the benefit of well-qualified faith community nurse leaders involved. Along with the curriculums, the *Westberg Institute* also supports national and international conference, position papers, and online electronic platform for the needs of the faith community nurse. The challenge as stated earlier is the lack of financial support to sustain the *Westberg Institute* with *Church Health*. There is definitely need for collaboration among those organizations that have a stated goal of advancing faith community nursing in order to advance and mature the ministry of faith community nursing with one voice.

References

Campbell, K. (2016). IPNRC becomes the Westberg Institute. *Perspectives, 15*(2), 1.

Church Health Website. (n.d.). *Mission statement, purpose, core values.* Retrieved from https://churchhealth.org/about-church-health/

Daniels, M. (2010). *Summary data from IPNRC coordinator's database.* Unpublished.

Davis, R. (2017). Front material. *Church Health Read, 7*(4), 2.

IPNRC. (2011). *Introduction. Foundations of faith community nursing curriculum.* Second printing (pp. 8–12)

Morris, S. (2012). Why health ministry? *Church Health Read, 6*(4), 19–21.

Peterson, W., & Westberg, G. (Eds.). (1982). *Granger Westberg verbatim: A vision for faith and health* (p. 57). St. Louis, MI: International Parish Nurse Resource Center.

Ranson, S. (2012). Faith in the future. *Church Health Read, 2*(3), 17.

Sheehan, A. (2014). The Church Health Center and Faith Community Nursing relationship: Mutuality, connection, and sharing to move together toward the future. *Perspectives, 13*(4), 1, 3.

Sheehan, A., Bisognano, M., & Waller, R. (2014). The Church Health Center and Faith Community Nursing relationship: Mutuality, connection, and sharing to move together toward the future. *Perspectives, 4*(4), 42–45.

Smith, S. (2012). A time of transition. *Perspectives, 2012,* 2–3.

Solari-Twadell, P. A. (2002). The differentiation of the ministry of parish nursing practice within a congregation. Doctoral Dissertation. *Retrieved from Abstracts International 63* (06), 569A. (UMI No. 3056442)

Westberg, G. (2013). The work of the Rev. Granger Westberg. *Perspectives, 12*(1), 1.

Westberg Institute. (n.d.-a). *Faith community nurse knowledge-sharing platform.* Retrieved from https://westberginstitute.org/fcn-knowledge-sharing-platform

Westberg Institute. (n.d.-b). *Mission statement and history.* Retrieved from https://westberginstitute.org/history-mission/

Zerull, L. (2013). Scriptural charge for faith-based care. *Perspectives, 12*(1), 3.

Health Ministries Association

16

Alyson J. Breisch and Marlene Feagan

16.1 Health Ministries Association: An Interdisciplinary Membership Organization for Faith Community Nurses

Shortly after the formation of the *Parish Nurse Resource Center* there was concern as to how this enterprise would continue to be funded over time. Although Lutheran General Health System had agreed to support a pilot project on parish nursing, the development of a resource center was not even a consideration when the pilot of the nurses in the churches was initiated. No one, except for maybe Reverend Granger Westberg, anticipated how this "grass roots" movement would take off among faith communities, pastors, nurses, and lay leaders. Certainly, the risk taking and creative nature of the President of Lutheran General Health System, George Caldwell, did not envision how quickly Westberg would be electrifying different parts of the country, religious denominations, nurses, and faith communities on this new innovative nursing role, whole person health, and the role of the faith community in health. Soon after the pilot through Lutheran General was initiated, the need for information on starting up such a health ministry spreads nationwide and stimulated the need for information and resources. Thus, as noted in Chapter 15, a need was created for resources. The concern over long-term financing for supporting the *Parish Nurse Resource Center* stimulated the development of an Advisory Committee for the Parish Nurse Resource Center. The first meeting of the Advisory Committee was on Monday, April 13, 1987. The inaugural members of the Advisory Committee were: Rev. Granger Westberg, Rev. James Wylie, Corporate Vice President of Church Relations, Lutheran General Health System, Kay Litherland, Vice-President for Nursing, Lutheran General Hospital, Dr. Mary Ann McDermott,

A. J. Breisch (✉)
Faith Community Nursing Consultant, Breisch Health Education, PLLC, Durham, NC, USA

M. Feagan
Health Ministries Program, St. Elizabeth Healthcare, Fort Thomas, KY, USA
e-mail: marlene.feagan@stelizabeth.com

© Springer Nature Switzerland AG 2020
P. A. Solari-Twadell, D. J. Ziebarth (eds.), *Faith Community Nursing*,
https://doi.org/10.1007/978-3-030-16126-2_16

Chair of Community Health Nursing, Loyola University Chicago, Rev. Larry Holst, Director of Pastoral Care, Lutheran General Hospital, and Ann Solari-Twadell, Director, Congregational Health Resources/Parish Nurse Resource Center (Parish Nurse News, 1987). The purpose of the Advisory Committee was to oversee the activities of the *Parish Nurse Resource Center* and make recommendations to the development and growth of the center. It was not long after that initial meeting that additional members were added to the Advisory Committee. Rev. David Carlson, Iowa Lutheran Hospital, Jan Striepe, RN, MSN, Parish Nurse, also from Iowa and Judith Ryan RN, PhD, Executive Director, American Nurses Association rounded out the additional membership of the Advisory Committee.

The first recommendation of the Advisory Committee was to create a specialty nursing organization for parish nurses. The small numbers of parish nurses at that time imposed a challenge to the organization's development: many of these nurses were in unpaid positions and had stronger affiliation with their religious denominations than interest in formation of a specialty nursing organization. However, Reverends Westberg and Carlson did sense that a broader-based organization that included membership of hospitals, clergy, seminaries, and lay people would create a more financially solid base from which to support the organization. The *Health Ministries Association* was voted upon and initiated at the *Annual Westberg Symposium* in 1988. In 1989, a three year Kellogg Foundation Grant supported the development of the *Health Ministries Association*, and it was incorporated as a nonprofit membership organization in Iowa in 1989 with offices provided by Iowa Lutheran Hospital.

The *Health Ministries Association* provided communication and networking among faith community nurses, health ministers, and clergy. Rev. Carlson, the Director of Iowa Lutheran Hospital's Pastoral Services Department, became one of *Health Ministries Association's* two Executive Co-Directors. Mary Ellen Dykstra, RN was the other Co-Director, at the time the *Health Ministries Association* was incorporated demonstrating the interdisciplinary nature of this new organization (Westberg & McNamara, 1990).

Reverend Westberg's vision for two components to promote whole person health, an educational resource center and a complimentary professional association for those involved in health ministries, is evident in the ongoing growth of both of these organizations. As noted in a letter he wrote to Rev. Carlson, Westberg expressed thanks for the association which provided "new impetus to the whole Parish Nurse movement" (G. Westberg, personal communication, December 2, 1996, Source: Letter to David Carlson). Today, these two separate organizations continue their original missions. The *Parish Nurse Resource Center* continues to be housed in institutions that accept its vision and are in a position to support the ongoing development of the center financially. The *Health Ministries Association* is a financially solvent organization that continues to experience growth through outreach and collaboration with denominations, community agencies, government entities, and healthcare systems.

It is important to note that the *Health Ministries Association* from its inception has been an interdisciplinary professional membership organization. This is important in that health promotion and pastoral care in faith communities involves an active interdisciplinary team, the pastoral leadership, laity, and staff. Health ministries that incorporate the educational and occupational backgrounds and diverse skills of team members facilitate the process of integrating health and healing into the life of the faith community.

Today, the *Health Ministries Association* represents "a convergence of health promotion and religious beliefs" which "…encourages, supports and empowers leaders who integrate faith with the promotion of health and wholeness in local communities." The "membership of the *Health Ministries Association* is made up of health ministers, faith community nurses, clergy, chaplains, faculty, and program leaders who have developed and provide health ministries in diverse faith communities (www.hmassoc.org, 2018)".

Over the past 30 years, the *Health Ministries Association* developed chapters and more recently regional networks. Communication to members includes a dedicated section of the organization's website, a bimonthly electronic newsletter, and social media pages. The *Health Ministries Association* annual meeting and conference provides networking opportunities and educational programs on current trends and research outcomes. Committees of the constituent groups—faith community nurses, health leaders, program leaders, and spiritual leaders—communicate regularly with the Board of Directors, leadership, and other members through conference calls, social media, and personal interactions.

The *Health Ministries Association* serves as a national multi-faith organization for faith communities involved in health ministries; membership is open to laity, clergy, faith community nurses, and other health professionals. The *Health Ministries Association* aspires to engage, educate, and empower people of faith to be passionate and effective leaders for creating healthier communities. Its mission is to encourage, support, and empower leaders in the integration of faith and health in their local communities. Since the late 1980s, the *Health Ministries Association* has published several "how to" manuals and resources related to starting health ministries. The most recent publication, *The Health Minister Role: Guidelines and Foundational Curriculum Elements*, 2nd Edition, incorporates models from seminaries and faith-health initiatives from national centers (HMA, 2018).

The *Health Ministries Association* is recognized by the *American Nurses Association* (ANA) as the professional membership organization for faith community nurses and is charged to define the scope and standards of this nursing specialty practice. The document, *Faith Community Nursing Scope and Standards of Practice*, 3rd Edition, co-published by the *American Nurses Association* and *Health Ministries Association* addresses the essential aspects of this practice (HMA & ANA, 2017). While primarily for faith community nurses and other nurses, the organization also is aimed at connecting other health care providers; spiritual leaders, families and members of faith communities; along with employers, insurers, policymakers, and regulators.

The *Health Ministries Association* has "Organizational Affiliate" status with the *American Nurses Association* giving the *Health Ministries Association* representation at the *American Nurses Association's* annual Membership Assembly with voting privileges. The *Health Ministries Association* serves as the voice for the U.S.A. faith community nurses in partnerships with the *American Nurses Association*, state boards of nursing, and other nursing specialty organizations. The *Health Ministries*

Association actively collaborates with the *Westberg Institute*; the *Journal of Christian Nursing*; the National Council of Churches Health Task Force; Mental Health First Aid; the National Council on Aging; and other regional, denominational, and national faith-health organizations. The *Health Ministries Association* has collaborated with governmental agencies including the Centers for Medicare and Medicaid Services, and the Office of Women's Health to support health education and access to care. Further information may be found at www.hmassoc.org

16.2 Certification for Faith Community Nurses

In 2007, the *Health Ministries Association* began ongoing work with the *American Nurses Association Credentialing Center* (ANCC) to develop a process by which faith community nurses could receive certification through a portfolio. The *Health Ministries Association* provided financial support, nurse experts, and reviewers during the development phase and continued during the certification process. In August 2014, the *Health Ministries Association* and the *ANCC* announced that a certification process by portfolio was available for the specialty practice of faith community nursing. This collaboration with the *ANCC* to develop the portfolio process and subsequent certification in faith community nursing was a major accomplishment for the Health Ministries. This process of certification not only validated faith community nursing as a specialty but also achieved recognition among colleagues in the broader nursing community and increased their awareness of the contributions of faith community nurses to promoting whole person health.

On October 9, 2017, the *Health Ministries Association*, along with six other nursing specialties, were informed that the Commission on Certification was going to discontinue the portfolio process of certification. The complexity of validation of the portfolio process for smaller nursing specialty practices was unsustainable by the *ANCC*. Effective November 17, 2017 certification by portfolio was suspended and no further applications were processed. The *Health Ministries Association* continues to work with the *ANCC* and the other nursing specialties impacted by ANCC's decision to seek alternative initiatives to promote professional practice. From 2014 to 2017, 146 faith community nurses successfully completed this certification process through ANCC (www.hmassoc.org, 2018). Faith community nurses who completed certification will be able to maintain this recognition by meeting ANCC's renewal requirements.

16.3 Membership Benefits

As a membership organization the *Health Ministries Association* provides many benefits to its membership that include:

- Bimonthly *Health Ministries Association* Today e-newsletter,
- Representation for specialty of Faith Community Nursing to the *American Nurses Association*:

- Defining Scope and Standards of Professional Practice,
- Developing Position Statements relevant to faith community nursing practice,
- Voting privilege as an Organizational Affiliate,
- Faith Community Nurse Mentor Program,
- *Health Ministries Association* committees: Scope and Standards Work Group, Marketing Guidance Committee, Spiritual Leadership committee, and Program Leadership Committee,
- Faith Community Nursing Society for members who are certified faith community nurses,
- Discounted rates for *Health Ministries Association* annual conference,
- Discounts on selected publications, products, and continuing educational opportunities,
- Ongoing professional development,
- Posting of member-sponsored educational events and activities on the *Health Ministries Association* website, and
- Constituency Group meetings and communications.

16.4   International Perspective: Health Ministry

The term "Health Ministry" takes on a very different meaning in countries other than the U.S.A. The Ministry of Health was the first health body in the United Kingdom that could be properly regarded as a department of government. It was created by the Ministry of Health Act 1919 and consolidated under a single authority of the medical and public health functions of central Government. Local medical services were expanded by war efforts and led to the establishment of the National Health Services in 1948. In 1968, the Ministry of Health and the Ministry of Social Security were dissolved and their functions transferred to the Department of Health and Social Security, which was divided 20 years later into the Department of Social Security and Department of Health (Segen's Medical Dictionary. © 2012 Farlex, Inc. All rights reserved). Most executive governments in the world are divided into departments or ministries. In most countries, other than the U.S.A., there is a department or Ministry responsible for health.

The functions of Ministry of Health in countries internationally have a range of responsibilities that are addressed through its body. The Ministry of Health may formulate health policy and set standards for provision of health care in a country providing strategic direction for health services. The use of traditional alternative medicine may be guided by a Ministry of Health in a given country. In addition, the monitoring or evaluation of health care may be managed by the Ministry of Health. Food, drugs, and health service delivery and practice may be regulated providing a framework for the development and management of health services.

References

Health Ministries Association. (2018). *The health minister role: Guidelines and foundational curriculum elements* (2nd ed.). Dayton, OH: Health Ministries Association.
Health Ministries Association (HMA). (2018). Retrieved September 15, from www.hmassoc.org

Health Ministries Association (HMA) and American Nurses Association (ANA). (2017). *Faith community nursing scope and standards of practice* (3rd ed.). Silver Spring, MD: Nursebooks. org.

Parish Nurse News. (1987). *Advisory committee for Parish Nurse Resource Center meets.* St. Louis, MO: Parish Nurse Resource Center.

Segen's Medical Dictionary. © 2012 Farlex, Inc. All rights reserved. Retrieved September 16, 2018

Westberg, G., & McNamara, J. (1990). *The parish nurse: Providing a minister of health for your congregation.* Minneapolis, MN: Augsburg.

Faith Community Nurses International

17

Andrea Mercer West and Beverly Siegrist

17.1 Professional Organizations

There are over 180 specialty nursing organizations which serve professional nurses from a state, national, and international perspective (Nurses.org, 2019). There are also several professional organizations for faith community nursing which serve their constituents from a state or regional, national, and international perspective. Examples of these organizations are:

- State or regional secular organizations, such as the *Faith Community Nurses Association of Oklahoma.*
- National denominational organizations, such as *Evangelical Lutheran Parish Nurse Association.*
- National secular interdisciplinary organization, such as the *Health Ministries Association* (HMA).

What was perceived as missing in supporting the faith community nursing constituents was an international secular "professional" organization that would represent "only registered nurses practicing in the specialty of faith community nursing."

A. M. West (✉)
FCNI, Centennial, CO, USA

B. Siegrist
University Distinguished Professor School of Nursing, Western Kentucky University,
Bowling Green, KY, USA
e-mail: Beverly.siegrist@wku.edu

© Springer Nature Switzerland AG 2020   243
P. A. Solari-Twadell, D. J. Ziebarth (eds.), *Faith Community Nursing*,
https://doi.org/10.1007/978-3-030-16126-2_17

17.2 History of Faith Community Nurses International

Conversations on the need for a professional organization solely for faith community nurses began in the early 2000. There was a constituency of faith community nurses that felt that faith community nurses should be the driving force for this nursing specialty practice and not influenced by other health care professionals. This group supported the ideal expressed by Klass, (1961) which states, "the internal governance of a profession must lay with its own membership" (p. 699). This idea took a while to actualize, but the phrase was understood strongly by some faith community nurses. The idea of a specialty nursing organization whose membership was registered professional nurses practicing in the specialty practice of faith community nursing only was believed to be viable.

In 2013, seven parish nurses met in at a retreat center to explore the possibility of a professional organization solely for faith community nurses. Those in attendance represented a variety of locations, faith traditions, and individual practices across the U.S.A. The discussion was led by a facilitator who guided the discussion into the various aspects of formulating a professional organization. The decisions made at the retreat set the underpinnings of the *Faith Community Nurses International.*

Faith Community Nurses International was the name selected to reflect the goal of expanding the boundaries to a worldwide presence. At the initial meeting, a phone conversation was held with a representative of the *Australian Faith Community Nurses Association*. With encouragement from leadership in faith community nursing from another country, the organizers moved forward to include an international focus. The Vision Statement for the organization was written to reflect this scope: "to connect, support, and promote the global community of Faith Community Nurses".

As the group explored the idea of a professional specialty nursing organization for faith community nursing, six Guiding Principles were developed. They are:

1. We invite a shared intelligence and promote a sense of ownership—every faith community nurse can contribute.
2. Compassion, excellence, caring, and gratitude are hallmarks of all efforts.
3. Respect for faith and service as a basis for professional practice, we recognize that interfaith practices and beliefs are essential to growing our specialty.
4. Care of the spirit, education, and lifelong learning are underpinnings of our professional responsibilities.
5. Integrity, honesty, and transparency are the basis for organizational business practices and services to members.
6. We support faith community nurses in their efforts to provide excellence in professional practice through promotion of *American Nurses Association Scope and Standards of Practice* (Faith Community International Board Meeting Minutes, October 30, 2015).

As the Guiding Principles were developed, the group envisioned specific goals that would reflect these six Guiding Principles. The seven goals for the organization were then established. These seven goals are:

1. Advance faith community nursing as a nursing specialty.
2. Connect faith community nurses worldwide.
3. Promote financial sustainability of the specialty.
4. Support research in faith community nursing.
5. Provide continuing education programs for faith community nurses.
6. Develop an online, peer-reviewed nursing journal.
7. *Advocate* for faith community nurses locally, nationally, and internationally (FCNI Board Meeting Minutes, October 30, 2015).

Every organization requires a "home," a place that would be recognized as the site for the organization. *Faith Community Nurse Network,* Minneapolis was designated as the office location. Staff from *Faith Community Nurse Network* served as support for the beginning activities of Faith Community Nursing International. Launching a new specialty nursing organization takes significant perseverance, fortitude, and frequent meetings. The original group members volunteered for specific assignments directed to the development of the organizational structure. Between August and November meetings of 2013, several persons withdrew from their responsibilities in the organization due to personal and professional time constraints. This left three of the original charter members to continue the work. These three faith community nurses developed a list of activities, which included (a) contracting with a pro bono lawyer about Articles of Incorporation, (b) submitting a 501(c) 3 Non-Profit Application, (c) proposing presentations for the *Westberg Symposium,* (d) submitting a grant application to *Wheat Ridge Ministries,* (e) creating a brochure, (f) preparing a membership application form, and (g) developing bylaws.

At the *Westberg Symposiums,* 2014 and 2015, new members for *Faith Community Nurses International* were actively recruited. From the new members that joined the organization at that *Westberg Symposium,* a Bylaws Committee was formed. Bylaws were sent to the membership for a vote in May 2015 and were accepted and signed by the acting president, on July 31, 2015.

The membership application used to market the purpose and goals of this new organization asked the members to identify their interests. An e-mail was sent to all those indicating an interest in "leadership." This email recruited those who noted an interest in "leadership" on their membership form, asking them to serve on the *Board of Directors* (BOD) of the new organization. The responses from this email effort yielded six additional members for the BOD of the organization. These newly selected members were invited to a retreat, which was held in Minneapolis, October 29 through November 1, 2015. The charter members of the BOD for the *Faith Community Nurses International* were: Wanda Alexander, Donna Callaghan, Susan Dyess, Alice Murphy, Tamara Otey, Susan Richards, Beverly Siegrist, Judy Shackelford, and Andrea West. Board members were assigned to committee functions as specified in bylaws of the organization.

Like all organizations in the twenty-first century, developing and maintaining a website is a high priority. The board met with a website developer and a preliminary layout was decided upon with specific duties assigned to various board members. Through this website *Faith Community Nurses International* was able to reach out to members of the organization using mass media. This has been essential to the ongoing success of the organization since 2016 when the website became operational.

One important function of a professional organization is adding to the knowledge base of the practice. To this end, a free, online, peer-reviewed journal for faith community nurses was discussed. *Western Kentucky University School of Nursing* agreed to provide the platform for this journal, which had its inaugural edition published in the spring of 2015. The *International Journal of Faith Community Nursing* (IJFCN) has continued to date. This journal may be accessed via the *Faith Community Nurses International* organization website. Publication of research pertinent to faith community nursing has provided a means for the *Faith Community Nurses International* to enhance the education of its members and other nurses interested in faith community nursing as a specialty practice.

In the second year of the organization, the membership grew to over 100 members from 28 states. *Faith Community Nurses International* continued to host a display regarding this specialty nursing organization at the Westberg Symposium. The work of the Standing Committees began to function as members were recruited and goals developed. Other tasks that were completed over time included completing and printing of the final membership brochure; being in dialogue with the *Church Health Center* through the staff person responsible for faith community nursing; and responding to the draft of the Third Edition of *Faith Community Nursing Scope and Standards of Practice* (ANA & HMA, 2017).

Faith Community Nurses International Board of Directors is made up of faith community nurses from across the United States. Monthly meetings are held via *Zoom Conferencing* through Widener University, School of Nursing. This platform allows face-to-face dialogue for the business of this membership organization.

17.3 Mission, Vision, and Goals

The initial Vision Statement, Mission Statement, and Goals remain as written and are currently used to guide the organization. Progress on all stated goals of the organization is ongoing as *Faith Community Nurses International* moves from its initial development phase.

17.3.1 Goal 1: Advance Faith Community Nursing as a Nursing Specialty

Faith community nursing is a specialty nursing practice aligned with other specialty nursing organizations such as Public Health Nursing and the Holistic Nurses Association. Faith community nurses, however, have a unique set of knowledge and skills that have been developed post formal nursing education. As this specialty practice continues to grow and mature, it is important to maintain a common educational experience and help practicing faith community nurses deliver whole person health care that promotes well-being of the individual while supporting the health of the faith community.

The literature documents the growth and expanse of faith community nursing research and practice. However, there is limited documentation about our value to both nurses and the community (Mock, 2017). Professional organizations, such as *Faith Community Nurses International*, are focused on the support, health, and growth of faith community nurses through education, dissemination of research, and identification of best nursing practices employed by faith community nurses.

17.3.2 Goal 2: Connect Faith Community Nurses Worldwide

The *International Council of Nursing* (ICN, 2018) established *Connecting Nurses*, which is an online forum developed in 2016 to assist nurses in sharing ideas and high quality innovation. The *ICN* states that learning about different cultures, their needs, and our commonalities help the nurses to provide a deeper, richer, and higher quality patient care. The *ICN* created a *You Tube* video, *Connecting Nurses: Every Raindrop Deepens the Ocean* (ICN, 2014). *Faith Community Nurses International* like the *ICN* believes that global nursing organizations are a method of connecting nurses.

17.3.3 Goal 3: Promote Financial Sustainability of the Specialty

An issue that continues to impact this specialty practice is financial sustainability. Merton (1958) suggests an organization should be concerned with the "economic and social welfare of practitioners in the profession, for if the membership organization does not do so, who will?" (p. 50). Faith community nurses work in paid and unpaid positions in a variety of practice arenas. Faith community nurses may be employed by a faith community, health care systems, or other health care or community-based agencies. *Faith Community Nurses International* strives for integration of faith community nurses into the staff of local faith communities with financial remuneration. This is imperative if there will be significant numbers of faith community nurses who will be able to participate in the financial sustainability of a professional faith community organization. This is a long-term goal which is believed to be significant to the advancement of the specialty of faith community nursing.

17.3.4 Goal 4: Support Research in Faith Community Nursing

Merton (1958) states that professional organizations "have the further function of advancing research in its field, either directly through research agencies of the association or, more often, indirectly through help to other individuals and groups in the profession (p. 53)." A Research Committee was developed to provide members of *FCNI* with more information and education regarding the research process. The *FCNI* Research Committee promotes and supports faith community nursing practice through research by:

- Providing direction in identifying faith community nursing evidence-based practice information to support the development of scholarly work;
- Providing resources related to the development, implementation, and evaluation of faith community nursing-related research projects;
- Establishing a network of faith community nurses interested in research that can provide guidance and mentorship to its members;
- Develop strategies to increase the awareness, application, and advancement of evidence-based practice in faith community nursing (American Nurses Association and Health Ministries Association, Inc, 2017).

The Research Committee has developed a newsletter which can be found on the *Faith Community Nurses International* organization's website. The purpose of this newsletter is to share information and connect with members who are interested in research and research findings related to faith community nursing. The committee has engaged in research having completed an online survey about the member's practice as faith community nurses. Research studies on faith community nursing are summarized from a variety of nursing journals including the *International Journal of Faith Community Nursing*. In addition, grant opportunities are also included on the *Faith Community Nurses International* website. This is intended to encourage collaboration and initiation of grant funded faith community nursing projects. The research committee members are available to assist those who are interested in the research process. The Research Committee has sponsored the Faith Community Research Forum at past international faith community symposiums.

17.3.5 Goal 5: Provide Continuing Education Programs for Faith Community Nurses

Faith community nurses often begin by attending a basic preparation or *Foundations in Faith Community Nursing* course that builds on previous formal nursing education. The faith community nurse blends professional nursing practice with the intentional care of the spirit. *Faith Community Nurses International* began continuing education programs that provide the participant with continuing education credits using online webinar technology. The content of the first educational webinar was selected from a research study that identified topics of interest for faith community nurses participating in continuing education programming. The Education Committee strives for presentation of quarterly continuing education programs.

17.3.6 Goal 6: Develop an Online, Peer-Reviewed Nursing Journal

Merton (1958) states that one of the responsibilities of a professional organization is the establishment of a professional journal "devoted to the reporting and spreading of new knowledge" (p. 53). The *International Journal of Faith Community Nursing* is a free, online, peer-reviewed journal for those interested in faith community nursing. The Western Kentucky University Libraries through WKU TopSCHOLAR® continues to provide the platform for the journal (WKU Libraries, 2018). The *Faith Community Nurses International*, Board of Directors determined that the selection of an open-access free journal would help promote the practice of faith community nursing from an international perspective. Articles published in *International Journal of Faith Community Nursing* address primarily the following categories:

1. Research from nursing or related disciplines that provide evidence of the effectiveness and economic contribution of faith community nursing practice;
2. Studies on nursing evidence-based interventions or related disciplines that document important outcomes and insights for faith community nurses and their practice; and,
3. Critical reviews of social-change research, programs, or theories that generate new ideas for research and practice (International Journal of Faith Community Nursing, 2018).

A section of the *International Journal of Faith Community Nursing* was added with evidence-based practice education and guidelines (e.g., best-practices in care of hypertension patients, helping patients in the congregation with depression), following comments and recommendations from practicing nurses faith community nurses (International Journal of Faith Community Nursing, 2018).

WKU TopSCHOLAR® allows the inclusion of an interactive world map that provides the numbers of readers by country in real time. This feature allows for the identification of the number of readers who have accessed the journal in the past 30 days (WKU Libraries, 2018). A review of the summative statistics from the *International Journal of Faith Community Nursing* is provided to the editor every 3 months including most downloaded articles (International Journal of Faith Community Nursing, 2018). This is helpful not only for the authors, but also for the editors and the editorial board. Figure 17.1 is a snapshot of the map identifying the readership of one of the published articles in the journal. The map documents that readers are found in many of the states in the U.S.A. and many different locations in the world.

One of the journal's challenges is getting authors to submit manuscripts for review and inclusion in each issue. The editors of the journal document that many letters of inquiry describe reports of projects. However, publishable worthy faith community nursing content is often difficult to bring to publication. Another barrier noted by the editors is the lack of skills in research development, writing and

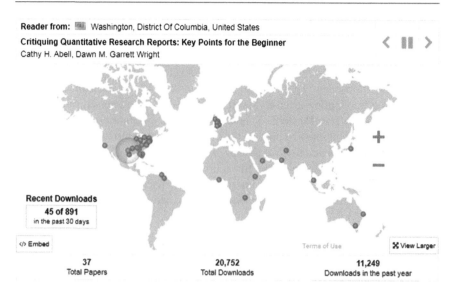

Reader from: Washington, District Of Columbia, United States

Critiquing Quantitative Research Reports: Key Points for the Beginner
Cathy H. Abell, Dawn M. Garrett Wright

Recent Downloads
45 of 891
in the past 30 days

</> Embed   Terms of Use   ✕ View Larger

37   20,752   11,249
Total Papers   Total Downloads   Downloads in the past year

Fig. 17.1 IJFCN international readership map snapshot. Capture of a moment from the IJFCN international readership map. Retrieved from IJFCN. (2018). *IJFCN: Home page, 4*(1). Retrieved from https://digitalcommons.wku.edu/ijfcn/

reporting by faith community nurses. To help eliminate this barrier, a special edition of the journal was devoted to the use of research tools. These articles continue to be some of the most downloaded articles published in the journal. The Research Committee is also working to support individual faith community nurses on research methods and writing for publication.

17.3.7 Goal 7: Advocate for Faith Community Nurses Locally, Nationally, and Internationally

The word advocate means 'to plead the cause of another' (Salvage, 2016). Faith community nurses today are considered to be advocates for patients and the community. The role of advocate is identified in professional standards and competencies as a significant mandate of the professional nurse. Faith community nurses are advocates in many situations. The question is, then, who advocates for the faith community nurse? *Faith Community Nursing International* believes that this specialty nursing organization dedicated to the faith community nurse and the professionalization of the practice of faith community nursing is in a position to advocate for the faith community nurse. Mock (2017), found that many individuals and groups still do not know what constitutes faith community nursing practice. Developing an organization dedicated to the specific specialty practice of faith community nursing is essential to bring the information forward as to the value of faith community nursing in this time.

Mason et al. (2016), state "advocacy is time consuming and requires significant commitment (p. 34)." Additional advocacy barriers include lack of advocacy skill due to a dearth of information included in nursing education, lack of energy, and also fear. Faith community nurses especially have little time, resources, or energy for advocacy for the specialty practice. Logically, collective numbers result in a larger power base and support for advocacy efforts for a specialty practice. *Faith Community Nursing International* continues to grow advocacy support through education, networking, and research.

17.4 Conclusion

Faith Community Nursing International is an exclusive registered nurse professional organization for faith community nurses. As a specialty nursing organization dedicated to only the specialty nursing practice of faith community nursing, this membership organization is focused on the future growth, development, and maturation of faith community nursing. While many of the characteristics, e.g., a code of ethics and standards of practice for nursing, identified by Matthews (2012) are undertaken by the *American Nurses Association*, *FCNI* provides continuing education, research support, and an online peer-reviewed journal to those nurses engaged in the specialty nursing practice of faith community nursing. The journal is being accessed by international readers, thus extending the influence of this specialty nursing practice into the international arena. *Faith Community Nursing International's* vision to *connect, support, and promote the global community of faith community nurses* is being realized as this organization moves forward.

References

American Nurses Association and Health Ministries Association, Inc. (2017). *Faith community nursing: Scope and standards* (3rd ed.). Silver Springs, MD: Nursesbooks.org.

ICN. (2018). *What we do: Connecting nurses.* Retrieved from http://www.icn.ch/what-we-do/connecting-nurses

International Council of Nursing (ICN). (2014). *Connecting nurses: Every raindrop deepens the ocean.* Retrieved from https://www.youtube.com/watch?v=rnCcDMxHTM0&feature=youtu.be

International Journal of Faith Community Nursing (IJFCN). (2018). *IJFCN: Homepage.* Retrieved from https://digitalcommons.wku.edu/ijfcn

Klass, A. A. (1961). What is a profession? *Canadian Medical Association Journal, 85*(12), 698–701.

Matthews, J. H. (2012). Role of professional organizations in advocating for the nursing profession. *Online Journal of Issues in Nursing, 17*, 3. Retrieved from http://www.nursingworld.org/MainMenuCategories/ANAMarketplace/ANAperiodicals/OJIN/Tableofcontents/Vol-17-2012/No1-Jan-2011-Organization

Merton, R. K. (1958). The functions of the professional association. *American Journal of Nursing, 58*(1), 50–54.

Mock, G. S. (2017). Value and meaning of faith community nursing: Client and nurse perspectives. *Journal of Christian Nursing, 34*(3), 182–189. https://doi.org/10.1097/CNJ.0000000000000393

Nurses.org. Retrieved February 2019, from https://nurses.org/orgs.shml

Salvage, G. (2016). Advocacy in nursing and health care. In D. J. Mason, G. Deborah, F. H. Outlaw, & E. T. O'Grady (Eds.), *Policy and politics in nursing and health care, 7th edn* (pp. 22–30). St. Louis, MO: Elsevier.

WKU Libraries. (2018) *Library special collections information: TopSCHOLAR.* Retrieved from https://www.wku.edu/library/services/archives/info.php

American Nurses Association, Regional, State, and Denominational Faith Community Nursing Organizations

18

Deborah Jean Ziebarth and P. Ann Solari-Twadell

18.1 Early Beginning: Establishing Ongoing Support for Faith Community Nurses

Early in the development of faith community nursing, the importance of supervision, continuing education, spiritual reflection, and support was provided through the first Institutional Based Model at Lutheran General Hospital, Park Ridge, Illinois. Holst (1987), Responsible for the chaplaincy department, facilitated bi-weekly meetings for the parish nurses to "share experiences, solve problems, deal with organizational issues, receive clinical supervision, and be informed on medical/nursing trends" (p. 14). As time went on, the Kellogg Foundation was instrumental in funding other networking models of faith community nursing which included collaborative relationships and a more regional networking to provide "stipends, resources, equipment and educational preparation" for parish nurses (King, Lakin, & Striepe, 1993, p. 30). As the "grass roots" growth of parish nursing took place at a remarkable rate, models developed to fit the nature of the town, region, or state. These models did not always provide the needed resourcing for the new parish nurse. Today, networking is essential not only for viability of the faith community nursing program, but also for the ongoing development, supervision, and quality of the faith community nursing program.

International and national annual gatherings of faith community nurses resulted in three challenges being identified for faith community nursing by Ryan (2000), keynote speaker of the *Westberg Symposium*. These challenges were: (a) to the nursing profession to reclaim the spiritual dimension of health; (b) to the

D. J. Ziebarth (✉)
Nursing Program Chair, Herzing University, Brookfield, WI, USA
e-mail: dziebarth@herzing.edu

P. A. Solari-Twadell
Marcella Niehoff School of Nursing, Loyola University Chicago, Chicago, IL, USA
e-mail: psolari@luc.edu

© Springer Nature Switzerland AG 2020
P. A. Solari-Twadell, D. J. Ziebarth (eds.), *Faith Community Nursing*,
https://doi.org/10.1007/978-3-030-16126-2_18

healthcare system to provide whole person care; and (c) to the faith community to restore its healing mission. In this address, Ryan (2000) noted that "it is about connecting three institutional cultures—the nursing profession, faith community and healthcare to achieve the best whole person health possible for every individual."

Stixrud (2006) presents an emerging leadership role which naturally evolved to ensure the integrity and sustainability of the parish nurse network as part of the Northwest Parish Nurse Network in the Northwest region. This leadership role was identified as the "Parish Nurse Coordinator" (p. 285). The coordinator role assisted in further building the parish nurse network, providing necessary leadership, support, and education in order to begin other new parish nurse programs. As this new leadership role emerged, so did a specific Parish Nurse Coordinator Basic education course. The intent was to ensure that as other network leadership emerged, the new leader would be provided with the information, skills, and support to grow and sustain in their management of the newly formed parish nurse network.

With the development of the Parish Nurse Coordinator role becoming integrated into the fabric of managing parish nurse programs and networks, there was a natural opportunity for identifying what skills and information were important for the maturation of a nurse in the coordinator role. Burke and Solari-Twadell (2006) identified eight capacities that were important for the Parish Nurse Coordinator to foster. These capacities are: (1) appreciation for the power of prayer, (2) listening skills, (3) interest in the history and understanding of the culture of the faith community, (4) appreciation of politics, (5) clarifying expectations, (6) excellent communication skills, (7) good organizational skills, and (8) the ability to follow through in the midst of conflict (pp. 243–244). This leadership role demonstrated the intricacies of attempting to develop sustaining partnerships between "uncanny" partners—the health care institution, faith community, and the professional nurse.

With all partnerships, there needs to be clarification of what each partner is going to be responsible for in the relationship. Development of protocols, contracts, and written agreements evolved naturally to ensure clarity and sustainability of the new faith community nurse programs. The benefits of having a written protocol, agreement, or contract for any partnering faith community nurse program are to: (1) provide a consistent plan identifying the resources that would be committed by each party in developing and sustaining of the faith community nurse program; (2) establish a ground work for furthering relationship development between all parties; (3) identify what learning opportunities would be part of the developing and ongoing relationship; (4) provide a mutual vision for the development and sustainability of the faith community nurse program; (5) be informed of the commitment that is being made on the part of all involved, not just for the immediate time period, but long term; (6) encourage a team approach to the ongoing development and sustaining of the faith community nurse programs creating a mindset of collaboration; (7) create an opportunity for all involved to learn of the culture of each partner organization involved and to participate fully in the selection of the faith community nurse (Burke & Solari-Twadell, 2006, pp. 245–246).

18.2   Role and Relationship with the American Nurses Association

The *American Nurses Association* is no stranger to faith community nursing. Their organizational involvement initially was sought in the development of the standardized curriculum for faith community nurses (McDermott, Solari-Twadell, & Matheus, 1999, p. 273). In 1998, the *American Nurses Association* identified faith community nursing as a specialty practice and since that time the *American Nurses Association* has been integral to three editions of the Scope and Practice for Faith Community Nursing. The *American Nurses Association* relates to the nurses of different states through its constituent state nursing organizations. This relationship of the individual states with the *American Nurse's Association* led to the development of another model for organizing and networking among faith community nurses. This model was one where a specialty group was formed under the umbrella of the state nursing organization affiliated with the *American Nurses Association*.

18.3   An Example: Wisconsin Nursing Association and Faith Community Nursing

Since 2000, the *Wisconsin Nurses Association* recognized the need to support and nurture Wisconsin's faith community nurses. In 2001, the *Wisconsin Nurses Association* honored a request for faith community nurses to be recognized as a Special Interest Group. The Special Interest Group's title was initially the Wisconsin Parish Nurse Coalition and now is referred to as the *Wisconsin Faith Community Nurse Coalition*. The mission remains unchanged: "Uniting and nurturing the professional development and practice of faith community nursing within Wisconsin" (Ziebarth, 2010, p. 1). Since its inception, the *Wisconsin Faith Community Nurse Coalition* holds monthly meetings and an annual education day that brings together faith community nurses from all areas of the state and beyond. In addition, the *Wisconsin Faith Community Nurse Coalition* publishes articles in the *Wisconsin Nurses Association* quarterly newsletter. In a recent development, the *Wisconsin Faith Community Nurse Coalition* and the *Wisconsin Nurses Association* together hosted an annual *Foundations of Faith Community Nursing* course (Jacobs, 2014).

The *Wisconsin Faith Community Nurse Coalition* finalized a position statement of the role of the faith community nurse. The position statement states that "the faith community nurse possesses a valid state of Wisconsin nursing license and performs in accordance with the Wisconsin Nurse Practice Act and is guided by the Scope and Standards of Practice: Faith Community Nursing. The practicing faith community nurse will have completed a basic training course that uses a standardized faith community nurse curriculum that is not less than 35 contact hours. The faith community nurse maintains current knowledge of nursing practice and possesses an understanding of both legal and ethical issues as it is related to professional practice" (Wisconsin Nurses Association, 2003). To meet the stated requirements, the registered nurse who wants to work as a faith community nurse in Wisconsin must attend a basic faith community education course of their choice.

It was through the development of the faith community role description position statement that one of the faith community nursing faculty posed the question, who has the authority to say what is faith community nursing is in the state of Wisconsin? That question led to exploration of what faith community education programs existed in Wisconsin. In addition, this exercise led to the development of standards for faith community nursing education programs in the state of Wisconsin.

It was discovered that the spectrum of faith community nursing education in the state of Wisconsin was inconsistent. Those nurses interested in faith community nursing basic preparation were exposed to different educational experiences in faith community nursing depending on where in Wisconsin or elsewhere they engaged in a basic preparation program. There were a variety of academic institutions that provided a basic faith community nursing education program. These programs ranged from 2 to 5 days in length and consisted of 36–53 continuing education credits (Ziebarth, 2005). Three of the four programs used the *Westberg Institute's Foundations of Faith Community Nursing Course* (Jacobs, 2014). In addition, other out of state education venues were available to registered nurses via long-distance formats. With the differences in faith community nursing educational programs, a six year project was undertaken by the *Wisconsin Faith Community Nursing Coalition* to create standardized educational objectives for practicing faith community nurses in the state of Wisconsin. This project was supported by the *Wisconsin Nurses Association* in its formal relationship with the *Wisconsin Faith Community Nursing Coalition*, as a Special Interest Group (Ziebarth, 2015). To obtain a free copy of the booklet "Wisconsin Minimum Set of Basic Parish Nurse Education Outcomes and Behavioral Objectives," call the *Wisconsin Nurses Association*.

18.4 Health System Faith Community Nurse Networks

Large regional health systems that support faith community nurse networks are also an excellent resource for faith community nurses. Particularly, those regional health systems that span large rural areas where few other resources are available to support the work and development of the faith community nurse. Chapter 12 in this book expands on network arrangements and demonstrates how faith communities are resourced through a health care system network.

This partnership between faith communities, faith community nurses, and health care systems are a win–win for all. It is important as reiterated in different chapters in this book that standardized documentation systems are used to report out the work by faith community nurses and associated outcomes-hours, number of clients, cost savings, changes in health indicators, and decrease of hospital utilization through the faith community nurse program. Today with quality indicators based on the uniqueness of the client and community faith community nursing networks surface as an excellent model for investment on the part of a health care system.

18.5   Religious Denominational Networks

Early on, in the development of faith community nursing religious denominations initiated nurse consultants that would serve as a resource for their religious denomination on the development, preparation, and integration of faith community nursing into the denominations affiliated faith communities.

Given that Rev. Granger Westberg was a Lutheran clergy man, the Lutheran Church, Missouri Synod was one of the first denominations that initiated this role. Marcia Schnorr, RN, MSN was serving as a parish nurse in a Southern Illinois Missouri Synod Church when asked to assume this role in the late 1980s. She continues in this capacity today. The Lutheran Church Missouri Synod Church identifies "parish nursing" as an option under "Health Ministry" on the denominational website. The website states that, "The parish nurse is a registered nurse who is committed to—and, on a broad level, is an integral part of—this concept of health ministries. He/she works with the members of the health ministry committee or health cabinet, helping and enabling people of the congregation and the community to attain, maintain and/or regain optimal health." The website further states that "Parish nursing is a unique blending of professional nursing and spiritual caregiving. We recommend that the parish nurse attend a special preparation program for parish nursing. Opportunities for basic preparation and continuing education are available within the Lutheran Church Missouri Synod. You might consider the following sources of Lutheran parish nurse preparation at Concordia University Wisconsin, Mequon" (https://lcms.org/how-we-serve/mercy/health-ministry/parish-nursing/).

The Evangelical Lutheran Church in America (ELCA) supports a 501(c) 3 not-for-profit organization for parish nurses within that denomination. The stated mission of that non-profit is "to provide leadership in fostering the spiritual growth and development of Parish Nurses, promote the expansion of this ministry into more congregations, and strengthen the Parish Nurse presence within the Synods." The goals of this organization include the following:

- Assure Parish Nurses have a place at the Synod Council and are integrated into the practices and future development of the Church
- Enhance the spiritual development of ELCA and other Lutheran Parish Nurses
- Promote Parish Nursing within the ELCA and encourage the development of parish nursing programs within all ELCA and other Lutheran congregations
- Provide networking opportunities and forums for sharing programs, projects, and resources
- Support parish nurses in their ministries and encourage appropriate wage and benefit standards
- Promote wellness among congregations and our rostered leaders (https://elpna. org/nurses/research.php).

The Presbyterian Church United States of America, in a 2001 Statement, approved the *Resolution on the Ministry of Caregiving in Relation to Older Adults* which included the following directives:

1. Encourage the church to be diligent in being faithful to its covenantal responsibility to care for all its members, in fact as well as in faith, especially older adults, those with debilitating and/or fatal illnesses, and their caregivers.
2. Direct the General Assembly Council, Office on Older Adult Ministry, to make available resources that enable congregations to celebrate caregiving through conducting ceremonies and in the use of symbols, such as in healing services, liturgies, banners, stories, and others, in order to support the spiritual nurture of caregivers.
3. Affirm the *Parish Nursing* model for the ministry of caregiving and encourage local congregations to contact the Office of Health Ministries (U.S.A.) for resources on *Parish Nursing*.
4. Establish or strengthen the *Parish Nursing* model by partnering with community hospitals/other health care agencies to provide and/or strengthen the ministry of caregiving. [The 213th General Assembly, 2001, pp. 281–282]. The Presbyterian Health Network includes parish nurse ministry, presbytery and congregational health ministries and advocacy for health, healing, and wholeness (https://www.presbyterianmission.org/ministries/phewa/phn/).

The United Methodist Church certified its first lay parish nurse in 2017. Joy Eastridge from Kingsport, Tennessee served as a church nurse for over two decades before becoming the first certified lay minister with the specialization of United Methodist parish nurse. Joy was in her 12th year as parish nurse at First Broad Street United Methodist Church. She started the process soon after United Methodist parish nurses were given the opportunity to earn a certification in their specialized ministry in March, 2016. Discipleship Ministries offers a parish nurse specialization for nurses through the certified lay ministry process, in consultation with the General Board of Higher Education and Ministry (GBHEM) and the Global Health Division of the General Board of Global Ministries (GBGM). GBHEM offers deacons or elders who are also parish nurses a certification in parish nurse ministry. This process of certification for parish nurses provides a system of training, supervision, support, and accountability through the established certified lay minister program. By participating in such a process it builds a much stronger support system within and connection to The United Methodist Church.

Discipleship Ministries: Parish nurses are seen in the Methodist Church as part of the church's pastoral team, and the role of a parish nurse is to work with the pastor in a team approach based on the pastor's vision for the church. In her role as parish nurse Eastridge works with a congregational care team of about 15 people who implement a variety of church-wide events, like walking programs, blood drives, routine blood pressure checks, health fairs, and dental clinics (https://www.umcdiscipleship.org/resources/united-methodist-church-certifies-first-lay-parish-nurse).

Essential to the conversation of support for a faith community nurse is the acknowledgement of the role of the religious denomination and the resources that can be made available to the faith community nurse through this organizational structure. It is interesting to note that although there has been a change in title of this ministry from "parish nursing" to "faith community nursing" by the profession of nursing, the religious denominations maintain the original denotation of "parish nursing."

18.6   Conclusion

Those nurses who have been "called" to faith community nursing have many resources available to assist in their preparation, development, and ongoing professional maturation in this specialty nursing practice. It is essential that nurses in ministry not become isolated. Integral to the success in the role of faith community nursing is that of being "connected." Connection should not only include a denominational affiliation, but also a professional organization membership. Participation in these organizations will ensure, protect, and inform the nurse "called" to the professional practice and ministry of faith community nursing.

References

Burke, J. M., & Solari-Twadell, P. A. (2006). Parish nurse coordinator: Working with congregations and clergy in fostering the ministry of parish nursing practice. In P. A. Solari-Twadell & M. A. McDermott (Eds.), *Parish nursing: Development, education and administration* (pp. 283–295). St Louis, MO: Elsevier/Mosby.

Holst, L. (1987). The parish nurse. *Chronicle of Pastoral Care, 7*(1), 13–17.

Jacobs, S. (Ed.). (2014). *Foundations of faith community nursing* (3rd ed.). Memphis, TN: Church Health Center.

King, J. M., Lakin, J. A., & Striepe, J. (1993). Coalition building between public health nurses and parish nurses. *Journal of Nursing Administration, 23*(2), 27–31.

McDermott, M. A., Solari-Twadell, P. A., & Matheus, R. (1999). Educational preparation. In P. A. Solari-Twadell & M. A. McDermott (Eds.), *Parish nursing: Promoting whole person health within faith communities* (pp. 269–276). Thousand Oaks, CA: Sage Publications.

Ryan, J. (2000). Parish nursing a Kairos moment: Keynote address. In *Fourteenth Annual Westberg Paris Nurse Symposium: Weaving parish nursing into the new millennium*. September, 2000, Itasca, IL.

Stixrud, A. D. (2006). Building a parish nurse network: A case study. In P. A. Solari-Twadell & M. A. McDermott (Eds.), *Parish nursing: Development, education and administration* (pp. 283–295). St Louis, MO: Elsevier/Mosby.

Wisconsin Nurses Association. (2003). *Position statement: Role of the parish nurse*. Madison, WI: Wisconsin Nurses Association.

Ziebarth, D. (2005). *Comparison of Wisconsin parish nurse training programs*. Madison, WI: WPNC.

Ziebarth, D. (2010). *Wisconsin minimum set of basic parish nurse education outcomes and behavioral objectives* (pp. 1–69). Madison, WI: Wisconsin Nursing.

Ziebarth, D. (2015). Demonstration: Development of a minimum set of parish nurse educational outcomes and behavioral objectives. *International Journal of Faith Community Nursing, 1*(3), 4. http://digitalcommons.wku.edu/ijfcn/vol1/iss3/4

Part V

Changing the Health of Nations: Issues and Trends in Faith Community Nursing

Documentation and Storage of Records

19

Deborah Jean Ziebarth and P. Ann Solari-Twadell

19.1 Faith Community Nurse and Documentation

No matter what country, the culture and norms of a health care system and those of a faith community are very different. This is important to recognize and understand when discussing the significance of documentation and storage of health records for faith community nursing. It is interesting to think what life would be like today if the gospel writers in the Christian tradition did not document the life of Christ. This documentation provided by the Evangelists, Matthew, Mark, Luke, and John, furthers the understanding of the most significant truths that were inherent in Christian ministry today. Through generations, multiple cultures, and nations the documentation provided by these gospel writers has been essential to the longevity and value of many religions today. If there was no documentation from these early historians of faith, there would be no reference to healings, martyrdom, or even the crucifixion! One wonders if religion would be as central to life and personal development for some without this documentation. Faith community nurses today need to develop the tenacity and fortitude of these gospel writers and tell their experiences of whole person care through use of nursing diagnosis made, educational programs provided, anticipatory guidance offered, and ongoing evaluation of the client. Additionally, visits completed, nursing interventions successfully employed in caring for their clients and outcomes that resulted are equally important. Remember the old adage, "if it is not documented, it is not considered done."

D. J. Ziebarth (✉)
Nursing Program Chair, Herzing University, Brookfield, WI, USA
e-mail: dziebarth@herzing.edu

P. A. Solari-Twadell
Marcella Niehoff School of Nursing, Loyola University Chicago, Chicago, IL, USA
e-mail: psolari@luc.edu

© Springer Nature Switzerland AG 2020
P. A. Solari-Twadell, D. J. Ziebarth (eds.), *Faith Community Nursing*,
https://doi.org/10.1007/978-3-030-16126-2_19

19.2   Culture Differences

Faith communities are primarily volunteer organizations. From a historical perspective, the church had a primary role in fostering health. Even to the point of being the stimulus for the creation of hospitals to care for those in the community that could not do so for themselves. However, over time, the role of health and healing was abdicated by the professionalization of health care. Today, many people wonder why the church would be engaged in health. Doesn't the church have enough to do caring for the spirits and souls of people? Where would the church get the resources to be engaged in a ministry of health and healing with some faith communities having very few paid positions? In addition, record keeping is usually at a minimum in faith communities with few systems for collection of data, resources to develop those systems, and policies to guide any collection and storage of data.

However, faith communities can engage people through all stages of life, and over a life span as some people are baptized, married, and buried from the same faith community. Participation in a faith community provides friendship and a very important ingredient to health—relationships and a support system. Faith communities assist in "shaping values and practices unique to their own beliefs and identity. Inherent is this belief and identity is the understanding that faith communities are a catalyst for growth and change" (Solari-Twadell, 1997, p. 5). This is an ideal environment for encouraging a different understanding of health–health, not just health as the absence of illness, but health as gift, with a personal responsibility to make the best decisions on a daily basis to protect that gift.

Health care systems, on the other hand, are usually large organizations with many paid employees and today are run primarily from a business perspective. Documentation is necessary in all departments and levels of the organization. There are clear systems established for the capture of necessary data along with resources to support the latest electronic equipment and programs to aid in documentation requirements. In addition, there are usually clear policies and procedures that adhere to guidelines based in legal requirements. Although "health care systems" are promoted as places of health and healing, are they really? Most often health care systems are concerned with severe illness, acute care, chronic illness, death, and dying. Health care systems usually have big budgets and a profit margin. Both the health care system and the congregation tend to have a unique language. This language is quite different from a faith community that operates on less funds, fewer resources, a dearth of policies/procedures, and often, little margin.

This difference in operation and culture can be problematic or complimentary. It depends on how you frame the argument. Faith community nursing is unique in that the nurse can translate the language used in the health care system into the more lay language found in the faith community. The faith community nurse, as a faith filled leader, has a foot in each camp and can be the bridge that brings the best of both the faith community and health care system to collaborate in caring for the health and well-being of members of that faith community and community at large constituting a unique continuum of care.

The issue of documentation and storage of records, however, is foreign to most faith communities. Additionally, the policies and procedures required to ensure integrity of the documentation and storage of records over time are also often a stretch. However, both are necessary if the faith community nurse and faith community do not want to put themselves in jeopardy of violating legal requirements. Suggested policies and procedures are included in the previous text "Parish Nursing: Development, Education and Administration" in a chapter entitled "Policies and Procedures for the Ministry of Parish Nursing Practice" (Ziebarth, 2006a, pp. 257–267).

19.3 Faith Community Nursing Documentation

The research summary in the Documenting Practice (page 2) module of *Foundations of Faith Community Nursing* includes the following explanation which is foundational to this discussion:

"The ability of the faith community nurse to document appropriately and comprehensively is an indicator of the quality of the content regarding the nursing process, as well as demonstration of the practice (Wang, Hailey, & Yu, 2011). The content of the faith community nurse documentation contains the evidence of patient care and information critical for continuity and patient safety. In addition, the content of documentation is critical for tracking patient outcomes. Dyess, Chase, and Newlin's (2010) review of faith community nurse research in the areas of evaluation and documentation found a lack of outcomes. The study further found that only 7 out of the 25 faith community nurse articles reviewed had content related to documentation and evaluation. This insufficiency in documentation is a barrier to demonstrating the legitimacy and effectiveness of the practice as a specialty. To improve the quality of documentation content, several research studies emphasized the use of a standardized nursing language, documentation of education, use of electronic documentation of systems, application of nursing theory, and emphasis on standards of practice or guidelines" (Campbell, 2014; Dyess et al., 2010; Solari-Twadell & Hackbarth, 2010; Wang et al., 2011).

19.4 Documenting the Unique Nursing Role and Understanding of Health Promoted by Faith Community Nursing

The discussion around liability of the nurse working in the congregation began with the Summer 1991 issue of "Perspectives" which was then a quarterly publication of the *International Parish Nurse Resource Center*. McCammon and Lang discussed two broad categories and liability issues associated with both the faith community working with a health care system and the faith community acting solely with the nurse (McCammon & Lang, 1991). The significance of documentation in faith community nurse became an ongoing focus with the *11th Annual Westberg Symposium*,

Parish Nursing: Documenting the Journey held in 1997, being dedicated to this important practice issue. The keynote speaker was Dr. Joanne McCloskey who spoke on the importance of using standardized nursing language in documenting care rendered. At this meeting, Burkhart (1997) noted how currently the standardized languages lacked "interventions that apply to parish nursing practice." She then reported that as part of a Kellogg funded grant, parish nurses from *Advocate Health Care and Trinity Medical Center* developed and submitted new spiritual and community interventions to the Iowa Intervention Team at the University of Iowa (p. 121). This work of creating standardized spiritual care interventions was instrumental in supporting the faith community nurse to document not only the importance of the spiritual to health, but also the nature of the practice of the faith community nurse. In addition, the creation of the spiritual interventions provided all nurses the opportunity to document the spiritual care provided to patients at all levels of care.

Despite this early work, the universal incorporation of documentation as being integral to the faith community nursing practice on a day-to-day basis is not consistent and sometimes lacking. Depending on the organizational model of the faith community nursing practice, the incorporation of documentation can be a challenge. Faith community nurse programs that are part of a larger network have resources to pay into an established electronic documentation system offered nationally. Thus, these models will be more likely to report outcome data. This may create biases in the type of documentation collected and reported. Without having from all faith community nurses, it is difficult to advocate for inclusion of this specialty practice into the current health care system payment mechanisms. In addition, without documented outcomes it is almost impossible to meet with political representatives and present a convincing demonstration of the value and contribution a faith community nurse can make to the well-being of constituents, reduction in cost, not only due to early intervention, but also due to effective management of chronic disease. Registered nurses are chancing a violation of the Nurse Practice Act and the Scope and Standards of Faith Community Nursing (ANA & HMA, 2017), putting their nursing practice at risk. In addition, faith community nurses that do not document are in essence negating any opportunity to create the outcome data necessary to substantiate the value of the faith community nursing program or communicate the significance of their work.

19.5   Documentation: A Legal Obligation

Each registered nurse practices under the legal authority of each state's Nurse Practice Act and the Board of Nursing policies. Nurse Practice Acts are statutory laws enacted by state legislators, and the State Boards of Nursing and exist to safeguard the public. The Boards of Nursing have the ability and obligation to discipline any nurse they suspect of not acting in the best interest of the patient.

Documenting also protects the nurse against the risk of legal malpractice. Malpractice is negligence, misconduct, or breach of duty by a professional person that results in injury or damage to a patient. In most cases, it includes failure to meet a standard of care or failure to deliver care that a reasonably prudent nurse would deliver in a similar situation. The most common reasons that nurses have been sued for malpractice are failure to follow standards of care for their specialty practice, failure to communicate, or failure to document (Glabman, 2004).

The Westberg Institute published a position statement in regard to documentation. It states that,

> All nurses must document care provision to be compliant with laws and regulations regardless of specialty or compensation (paid or unpaid). Documentation is the written record of patient care in electronic or hard copy format. In all cases, the written record of professional nursing care delivered by a faith community nurse provides evidence of care provision at a point in time. Evidence of care provision includes what services or care the patient received; when services were rendered; the response or reaction the individual had to the services/treatment; who provided the services; and whether communication to other providers were carried out (Ziebarth, 2015).

19.6 The Documentation Record

Who Is the Custodian? Regardless of the model, there needs to be a written policy to clarify who, health care organization, faith community, or the faith community nurse, is the custodian of the documentation. In addition, a policy/procedure to address the maintenance and storage of the documentation record is essential. The *Westberg Institute* consulted with legal counsel for the *Wisconsin Nursing Association*, who recommended the following:

- When a faith community nurse is employed by a health care organization, the health care organization is the custodian of the documentation.
- When a faith community nurse is in a formal, contractual partnership with a health care organization, but not employed by it, there needs to be a determination of who is the custodian of the documentation. If the health care organization is not the custodian of the documentation, then custodianship falls to the faith community nurse.
- When a faith community nurse is working without a formal partnership with a health care organization and is working in or with a faith community, whether in a paid or unpaid position, he or she is responsible to maintain and store the documentation. When there is a change in a faith community nursing position, the documentation can be transferred to a new faith community nurse with the permission of the client (Ziebarth, 2015).

19.7 Maintenance and Storage of Documentation

Regardless of the model, there needs to be a written policy/procedure to address the maintenance and storage of the record. The faith community nurse's documentation, whether electronic or hard copy, is required to be safely stored for 7 years. If paper, documentation should be safely stored/filed under lock/key. If electronic in nature, all documentation should be stored on a password protected file on the computer's hard drive or on an encrypted USB jump drive and protected in a locked cabinet or file drawer only accessible to the faith community nurse. It is important to note that patient information in any nursing documentation needs to be available to the patient upon request (Ziebarth, 2015).

After 7 years, the patient documentation generated by a faith community nurse should be destroyed. The documentation can be destroyed by shredding or burning. Simply throwing papers in the trash bin is not sufficient. If electronic in nature, deleting the files on the hard drive or destroying the encrypted USB jump drive where the files were stored will be a necessity. If necessary, it may be helpful to consult a technology specialist regarding the best method to permanently destroy the electronic footprints of patient's files (Ziebarth, 2015).

What to Document? Per *Faith Community Nursing the Scope and Standards of Practice* (ANA & HMA, 2017), and the State Boards of Nursing, the nurse needs to document: (a) assessment, (b) planning, (c) implementation and interventions, (d) outcome, and (e) evaluation on each patient. Basically these steps are what we know as the nursing care plan. There is significant support for new nurses online in regard to writing nursing care plans. A review of the steps may be helpful to the new faith community nurse. A good website for assistance is NRSNG: 5 Steps to Writing a Nursing Care Plan located at https://www.nrsng.com/writing-nursing-care-plan/.

Types of Documentation Tools The *Documenting Practice* module of the *Foundations of Faith Community Nursing Course* (Jacob, 2014) has several examples of documenting formats. One such electronic format is the *Henry Ford Macomb's* electronic documentation tool (Girard, 2013). It was developed for the faith community nursing practice using the Nursing Intervention Classification language, which collects and describes nursing interventions. The *Henry Ford Health System* in Michigan developed a password-protected website documentation system for faith community nurses (Brown, 2006). It is used by over 500 faith community nurses in 22 states (Yeaworth & Sailors, 2014). The Nursing Intervention Classification System is embedded to capture the nursing interventions employed by the faith community nurse. Creators of this documentation system chose the Nursing Intervention Classification System over other standardized languages, because the *Henry Ford Health System* uses the documentation system developed by Cerner. Cerner is an information system vendor that uses the taxonomies of North American Nursing Diagnosis Association, Nursing Intervention Classification System, and Nursing Outcome Classification for nursing documentation (Frederick & Watters, 2003). There is also a narrative component where faith community nurses can document electronically. There is a cost to use the system, which may present financial complications for some faith community nursing models. The advantage of a faith community nurse using a standardized documentation system is the use of standardized nursing languages. A "nursing language" is defined as a "common language, readily understood by all nurses, to describe care" (Keenan,

1999, p. 12). When a standardized nursing language is used to document practice, effectiveness of care delivered in multiple settings by different providers can be compared and evaluated (Bulechek, Butcher, Dochterman, & Wagner, 2013). Other benefits of using a standardized language for nursing documentation include increased visibility of nursing interventions, improved patient care, enhanced data collection to evaluate nursing care outcomes, greater adherence to standards of care, and facilitated assessment of nursing competency (Rutherford, 2008).

19.8 Showing the Value of Faith Community Nursing Through Documentation

Faith communities and health care organizations may want other documentation in addition to data located on the client's record. Altruistic and economic evidence may be requested. Using altruistic and economic data can communicate program effectiveness to health care organizations and faith communities, with both subjective and objective outcomes. Faith community nursing programs are at risk for elimination when funding sources are threatened. The collection and presentation of altruistic and economic evidence to assess the effectiveness of prevention health services may seem like extra work for the nurse, but may create the support and eliminate unnecessary and premature program termination (Ziebarth, 2016a, 2016b).

Altruistic Measurements: Storytelling Stories are both endearing and memorable. Patient stories can be very persuasive in showing a faith community nursing program's value. Stories can be included in monthly reports, but it is important to eliminate any patient identifiers before sharing. Stories are also used for "community benefit" reporting (Raden & Cohn, 2014). All not-for-profit health care organizations must justify their continuing tax-exemption as a charitable institution. This is done by demonstrating that they are providing "community benefit" activities that are intended to address community health service need that lead to improvement of health status (Brown, Coppola, Giacona, Petriches, & Stockwell, 2009; Raden & Cohn, 2014).

A "DIARY" format can be used to create patient stories (Rydholm, 1997, 2006; Ziebarth, 2004, 2006a, 2006b, 2016a, 2016b). It is similar to SOAP documentation. A Northwest faith community nursing program used the North American Diagnose Taxonomy, Nursing Intervention Classification System, and Nursing Outcome Classification system, which was created at the University of Iowa (Johnson, Maas, & Moorhead, 2000) to frame the acronyms in a DIARY format. The DIARY acronym stands for:

- "D" Data or facts of the problem
- "I" Interpretation (NANDA)
- "A" Action taken (NIC)
- "R" Responses (NOC)
- "Y" Yield

"Yield" is described as the outcome that pertains to the health care organization, community, or patient (Ziebarth, 2016a, 2016b). Guidelines for the use of "yield" include:

(a) When the "Yield" is directed to the health care organization, outcomes may include "Cost-Avoidance" or "Revenue-Producing" and can include: averted unnecessary emergency department visit, access to health care systems and/or physician office visit facilitated, averted hospitalization for specific chronic disease or population (ex. early dx. of diabetic foot ulcer or early assessment of Congestive Heart Failure in Medicare patients), and service recovery, which includes complaint resolution.

(b) When the "Yield" pertains to the community, the outcomes may include "Community Building" (using community assets or community individuals to support needs of a client) and "Community Advocacy" (when a service gap is identified for more than one client and resources are provided to fill that gap for the greater community) (Ziebarth & Miller, 2010). An example of community advocacy is starting a needed Obsessive Compulsive Disorder support group where one was not offered previously.

(c) When the "Yield" pertains to patients, it includes outcomes such as "Enhanced Independent Living" (for seniors, mentally ill, or disabled), "Medical Device Obtained," "Injury Prevention" (fall risk assessment completed and fall prevention intervention), and "Enhanced Quality of Life" (makes a significant positive difference). A DIARY shared monthly can support the "valuing" of the faith community nursing program (Ziebarth, 2016a, 2016b, p. 73).

Storytelling can be presented as the collection of "quality indicators" or "core principles." In one health care organizational sponsored faith community program, core principles collected for an annual evaluation were identified as:

- Serving targeted populations
- Focusing on key community health needs
- Creating community by building new capacity
- Meeting needs of both target markets and the health care organization
- Providing seamless continuum of client care
- Identifying direct links to clinical service available in the community
- Aligning annual employee merit goals specific to core principles

Storytelling can also be done through nominal number collection of patients, referrals, screenings, educational events, and attendance. The tool used to collect this data is completed by each faith community nurse monthly and presented annually to stakeholders by the faith community nurse program coordinator. One health care organization supported faith community nurse program asked their faith community nurse to collect the number of the following items:

- Patients that the nurse was case-managing,
- Patient contacts,
- Direct referrals from clients,

- Referrals to site,
- Referrals to MD,
- Referrals to other health care professionals,
- Referrals to community resources,
- Referrals to hospital programs,
- Events and program attendance (Screenings, Support Groups, Educational), and
- Other outcomes.

Other outcomes may include what is most important to the stakeholder. Ziebarth (2015) explains that other outcomes may include patient information such as:

- *Hospital/Emergency Room Avoidance*—management of unstable chronic illness which is usually a significant event causing a referral to a doctor and follow-up for assessment and/or meds, assessment and education for meds, advocacy, consistent assessment/surveillance for medication compliance, consistent surveillance or health maintenance, and early detection of other health problems.
- *Enhanced Independent Living*—for seniors, mentally ill, or disabled where there has been a medical device obtained, consistent surveillance of safety issues, risk management, resource networking: meals, transportation, lifeline, senior living options, home health, education related to safety and risk management, and financial advocacy/referrals.
- *Injury Prevention*—such as bike helmets, car seat safety education, safety education, risk management, and assessments/intervention related to safety, as well as Hospital Avoidance or self-management of illness,
- *Enhanced Quality of Life*—makes a significant positive difference through symptom management—decreased pain, spiritual support, successful resource networking, and successful financial advocacy/referral.
- *Medication or Medical Device Obtained*—client has received glasses, canes, hearing aid, glucometer, or wheelchair to enhance well-being.

Economic Measurements Some health care organizations want to collect data that show a monetary case for prevention activities. There are several ways to show that some prevention actions eventually can net a financial gain. Two measurements are net benefits and cost–benefit analysis.

Calculating a net benefit (Buxton et al., 1997; Dranove, 2003; McGuigan, Hozack, Moriarty, Eng, & Rothman, 1995; Ziebarth, 2016a, 2016b) can assist in presenting a monetary case for a faith community nursing program. Using this equation: $NB(x) = B(x) \, C(x)$ (NB = net benefits, x = FCN program, B = expected benefits associated with the program, and C = expected cost of program), the expected benefit and cost associated with the program may provide the economic evidence to convince stakeholders of considerable value. In calculating the benefits associated with a faith community nursing program, one might consider:

(a) Medical cost averted because an illness is prevented. This is done when the cost of a procedure or illness (myocardial infarction or stroke) is known in terms of medical service costs. This perspective is most often valued by the health care system, especially if the cost of the service is more than the reimbursable costs, which is most often the case. An example is a hospital's loss of reimbursements for Medicare patients that are readmitted shortly post discharge. If the faith community nurse can prevent a hospitalization or readmission of a Medicare patient, that saves money for the health care organization.

(b) Risk analysis has been computed by *Harvard University Center for Risk Analysis*. They have computed the cost per life year for 587 specific prevention interventions (Tengs et al., 1995). For instance, a mammography for a woman over age 50 is $1215 annually. The costs were originally estimating using 1993 dollars and were adjusted to 2010 dollars (Folland & Rocco, 2013). A pneumonia vaccination is $18,000 annually while influenza vaccine is $21,000 (p. 68).

(c) Monetary value of the "loss in production" diverted because good health is restored. Another viewpoint is "loss of income" is averted because death is postponed. The most commonly used calculation to do this is the "forgone earnings approach," which consists of estimating the earnings lost by an individual who dies prematurely or is disabled due to illness. These earnings are usually estimated by the "human capital method," by examining the earnings of comparable individuals. Loss in production is usually estimated at $100 a day or $100,000 per year, depending on age. Leisure time is estimated at half of this ($50 a day or $50,000 per year).

(d) Monetary value of the loss in satisfaction or utility (usefulness) averted due to a continuation of life or better health or both. Santerre and Neun (2012) stated that "This calculation is still quite controversial because how does one attach a dollar amount to less pain and suffering…" (pp. 88–92).

Cost–Benefit Analysis Can Be Used to Show a Monetary Case of an Intervention Based on Timing The timing of benefits is an important consideration when certain preventive health services are done in the community. Cost–benefit analysis can be used to show a monetary value based on timing of interventions. Cost–benefit analysis can also be used to decide the best option. Using the concept "discount rate" or "discounting" converts future costs into present value This accounts for the fact that people value present costs and benefits more than future costs and benefits (Santerre & Neun, 2012, pp. 89–90). The calculations find the monetary value, the future amount of money that has been discounted to reflect its current value, as if it existed today. Discounting is the opposite of compounding. The rate at which a future value is discounted is closely related to the rate at which present values are compounded, namely the interest rate. As we know from compounding, if the interest rate is 5%, then a dollar placed in the bank today will be worth $1.05 a year from now. This means that if the interest rate is 5%, $1.05 to be received next year is worth only $1.00 today. The standard formula is: PV = FS (fixed sum) divided by $1 + r$ (r being annual rate of interests). If FS equals 104 and r equals 4%, or 0.04, so PV equals 100 (Santerre & Neun, 2012, p. 193). Looking at two examples will help to understand how to use discounting to show a monetary value based on timing of an intervention.

(a) Polio and rubella vaccinations. The benefit of the immediate vaccine is felt in allowing children to live healthy that are not afflicted with polio. You would see an immediate drop in number of reported cases of polio and rubella.

(b) Education of a young married couple of the benefits of polio and rubella vaccination. The ultimate benefit of education will take time. Let's say that it required $20 = FS (1 h) to educate one couple, the $r = 4\%$ compounding discount annually. In 4 years (when the couple had their first child) the PV of the original $20 is worth $79.84 after 4 years in PV instead of $83.20. If the original $20 was invested at 4% the compounded yield would have been $83. What is unique about this example is that the young couple may have more than one child and the cost–benefit multiples. On the other hand, if the young couple chooses to ignore the education, the loss also multiples.

19.9 Conclusion

Faith community nurses are legally and ethically bound to document (a) assessment, (b) planning, (c) implementation and interventions, (d) outcome, and (e) evaluation on each patient. Prevention of health services have been the preferred option for promoting health and reducing disease rates. For many, this argument is reason enough to invest in prevention health services as a community, national, or global health initiative but for others, it is not. There are other altruistic and economic data that can be important to collect such as nominal numbers of patients, referrals, and events. In addition, certain interventions can be collected and measured.

Although foreign to faith communities, the development of policies and procedures that ultimately will protect the faith community nurse, faith community, and health care system is necessary and protects the interests of all parties.

References

American Nurses Association & Health Ministries Association, Inc. (2017). *Faith community nursing: Scope and standards of practice* (3rd ed.). Silver Spring, MD: Nursebooks.org.

Brown, A. (2006). Documenting the value of faith community nursing: Faith nursing online. *Creative Nursing, 12*(2), 13.

Brown, A. R., Coppola, P., Giacona, M., Petriches, A., & Stockwell, M. A. (2009). Faith community nursing demonstrates good stewardship of community benefit dollars through cost savings and cost avoidance. *Family & Community Health, 32*(4), 330–338.

Bulechek, G. M., Butcher, H. K., Dochterman, J. M. M., & Wagner, C. (2013). *Nursing interventions classification (NIC)*. St. Louis, MI: Elsevier Health Sciences.

Burkhart, L. (1997). How to code parish nursing practice using NANDA and NIC. In *Parish nursing: Documenting the journey* (pp. 115–126). Park Ridge, IL. Ed note: These proceedings can be found in the archives at Loyola University Chicago Cudahy Library: Advocate Health Care.

Buxton, M. J., Drummond, M. F., Van Hout, B. A., Prince, R. L., Sheldon, T. A., Szucs, T., et al. (1997). Modelling in economic evaluation: An unavoidable fact of life. *Health Economics, 6*(3), 217–227.

Campbell, K. (2014). Documenting practice. In S. Jacob (Ed.), *Foundations of faith community nursing* (3rd ed., p. 2). Memphis, TN: Church Health Center.

Dranove, D. (2003). *What's your life worth. Health care rationing … Who lives*. Upper Saddle River, NJ: FT Prentice Hall.

Dyess, S., Chase, S. K., & Newlin, K. (2010). State of research for faith community nursing 2009. *Journal of Religion and Health, 49*(2), 188–199.

Folland, S., & Rocco, L. (2013). *The economics of social capital and health: A conceptual and empirical roadmap*. Singapore: World Scientific Publishing.

Frederick, J., & Watters, M. (2003). Integrating nursing acuity, NANDA, NIC, and NOC into an automated nursing documentation system. *International Journal of Nursing Terminologies and Classifications, 14*(s4), 26.

Girard, S. (2013). *Henry Ford Macomb's Faith Community Health Program is in the national spotlight.* Mount Clemens, MI: Macomb News.

Glabman, M. (2004). The top ten malpractice claims. *Hospitals & Health Networks, 78*(9), 60–102.

Jacob, S. (Ed.). (2014). *Foundations of faith community nursing* (3rd ed.). Memphis, TN: Church Health Center.

Johnson, M., Maas, M., & Moorhead, S. (2000). *Nursing outcomes classification (NOC).* St. Louis, MO: CV Mosby.

Keenan, G. M. (1999). Use of standardized nursing language will make nursing visible. *The Michigan Nurse, 72*(2), 12–13.

McCammon, G., & Lang, D. (1991). Protecting the nurse. *Perspectives in Parish Nursing Practice, 1*(2), 1–2. Note: This document can be found in the archives of the Cudahy Library, Loyola University Chicago.

McGuigan, F. X., Hozack, W. J., Moriarty, L., Eng, K., & Rothman, R. H. (1995). Predicting quality-of-life outcomes following total joint arthroplasty: Limitations of the SF-36 health status questionnaire. *The Journal of Arthroplasty, 10*(6), 742–747.

Raden, B., & Cohn, G. (2014). Sweet charity: The truth behind hospital's community benefit windfall. *City Watch, 12*, 49. http://www.citywatchla.com/in-case-you-missed-it-hidden/7066-sweet-charity-the-truth-behind-hospitals-community-benefits-windfall

Rutherford, M. (2008). Standardized nursing language: What does it mean for nursing practice. *Online Journal of Issues in Nursing, 13*(1), 243–250.

Rydholm, L. (1997). Patient-focused care in parish nursing. *Holistic Nursing Practice, 11*(3), 47–60.

Rydholm, L. (2006). Documenting the value of faith community nursing: Saving hundreds, making cents—a study of current realities. *Creative Nursing, 12*(2), 10–12.

Santerre, R., & Neun, S. (2012). *Health economics* (6th ed.). Boston, MA: Cengage Learning.

Solari-Twadell, P. A. (1997). The caring congregation: A healing place. *Journal of Christian Nursing, 14*(1), 4–9.

Solari-Twadell, P. A., & Hackbarth, D. P. (2010). Evidence for a new paradigm of the ministry of parish nursing practice using the nursing intervention classification system. *Nursing Outlook, 58*(2), 69–75.

Tengs, T. O., Adams, M. E., Pliskin, J. S., Safran, D. G., Siegel, J. E., Weinstein, M. C., et al. (1995). Five-hundred life-saving interventions and their cost effectiveness. *Risk Analysis, 15*(3), 369–390.

Wang, N., Hailey, D., & Yu, P. (2011). Quality of nursing documentation and approaches to its evaluation: A mixed-method systematic review. *Journal of Advanced Nursing, 67*(9), 1858–1875.

Yeaworth, R. C., & Sailors, R. (2014). Faith community nursing: Real care, real cost savings. *Journal of Christian Nursing, 31*(3), 178–183.

Ziebarth, D. (2004, 2006). *Documentation tools: Outcome guidelines.* Waukesha, WI: Waukesha Memorial Hospital.

Ziebarth, D. (2006a). Policies and procedures for the parish nursing practice. In P. Solari-Twadell & M. McDermott (Eds.), *Parish nursing: Development, education, and administration* (pp. 257–282). St. Louis, MO: Elsevier Mosby.

Ziebarth, D. (2006b). Innovation betters community health. *Creative Nursing Management Journal, 12*(2), 6–7.

Ziebarth, D. (2015). *Position statement: Documentation. International parish nurse resource center.* Memphis, TN: Church Health Center.

Ziebarth, D. (2016a). *Transitional care interventions as implemented by faith community nurses* (pp. 1–138). Milwaukee, WI: University of Wisconsin Milwaukee, UWM Digital Commons.

Ziebarth, D. (2016b). Altruistic and economic measurements used for prevention health services. *Evaluation and Program Planning, 57*, 72–79.

Ziebarth, D., & Miller, C. (2010). Exploring parish nurses' perceptions of parish nurse training. *The Journal of Continuing Education in Nursing, 41*(6), 273–280.

Long-Term Sustainability of Faith Community Nursing Programs

20

P. Ann Solari-Twadell and Deborah Jean Ziebarth

20.1 Establishing a Solid Foundation for Faith Community Nurse Programs

Maintaining a faith community nurse program with the goal of the ministry "sustaining over time" requires planning upfront with that intention from the beginning of the program development. In other words, development of a faith community nurse program includes building in the understanding, structure, and resources that will foster sustainability of the faith community nurse program over time. Change is a constant in the world. Leadership, financial, personnel, health, denominational priorities, reports and documentation required, stakeholders, policies and procedures, job description, title, professional requirements, and relationships all can be altered over time. Insuring that a faith community nurse program sustains through pastoral change, faith community nurse program changes and financial demands of faith communities requires solid planning on the part of all invested partners and stakeholders from the inception of program development.

20.2 Vision and Mission Declaration

Being intentional in taking the time upfront to develop a faith community nurse ministry vision and mission statement engages all parties in dialogue informing each stakeholder about the purpose, goals, and possible outcomes of investing in a faith community nurse ministry. A precursor to the development of the vision and mission

P. A. Solari-Twadell (✉)
Marcella Niehoff School of Nursing, Loyola University Chicago, Chicago, IL, USA
e-mail: psolari@luc.edu

D. J. Ziebarth
Nursing Program Chair, Herzing University, Brookfield, WI, USA
e-mail: dziebarth@herzing.edu

© Springer Nature Switzerland AG 2020
P. A. Solari-Twadell, D. J. Ziebarth (eds.), *Faith Community Nursing*,
https://doi.org/10.1007/978-3-030-16126-2_20

statement is education. It is recommended that all involved in the planning for this professional Health Ministry role have a similar mindset or understanding of three concepts. These concepts are health, faith community, and nurse. Health is understood as being more than physical, including care of the body, mind, and spirit; a faith community as more than a place that one attends on Sunday to nourish their soul, but potentially being seen as the health place in the community. The faith community actively assists individuals of all ages to form beliefs, values, and actions consistent with being stewards of their personal health resources. The term "nurse" means more than an assistant to the doctor, a provider responsible for administering medications, administering medical treatments, and changing dressings. Nurse is understood in this context as a professional that can provide health promotion, disease prevention strategies and spiritual care while making assessments and referrals to appropriate agencies within and external to the faith community. Once a stakeholder has this understanding, then participation in the development of the faith community nursing ministry will proceed with creation of the vision and mission statements providing the beginnings of a solid foundation for a faith community nurse program.

A vision statement consists of one or two brief sentences that first informs about the future aspirations and second, is to motivate and inspire stakeholders to act on those aspirations (Free, 2014, p. 2). This vision statement is recommended to be related to the mission and vision statements for the faith community. An example of a vision statement for a faith community nurse ministry, whether that program be a solo faith community or a collaboration between a faith community and health care system could be, "Create the environment for all members of the faith community and community at large to 'live life abundantly' as God intended" or "Be the health place in the community providing whole person preventive care assisting all to be better stewards of personal and communal health resources." The vision statement is futuristic and should challenge all, stimulating thinking, encouraging values clarification and behavior change.

The mission statement is present-based, rather than future looking. The role of the mission statement is to answer, "Why does this program exist? What is it that it does?" (Free, 2014, p. 2). It is usually longer and may have more than one stipulation or goal. For example, "The faith Community of_____through the Faith Community Nursing Ministry intends to (a) support each member of the faith community to be a good steward of their personal health resources, (b) live out the Gospel proclamation of "loving your neighbor as yourself" and (c) support the faith community in striving to be health place in the community from a whole person perspective." Or another mission statement might be, "Seeing health from a whole person perspective—body, mind and spirit, we at _____ strive through the Faith Community Nursing Ministry to: (a) form beliefs and values consistent with making better decisions regarding our health on a daily basis in order to live life abundantly as God intended, (b) understand the needs of our neighbors and create time and resources to address those needs, and (c) reach out and partner with others in the community to sustain a healthy environment for the community at large." Both the mission and vision statements should be reviewed on a regular basis for currency and endorsement by faith community members.

The time and effort along with the continual reinforcement of the vision and mission statements is a reminder of the ongoing commitment the faith community is making to the sustainability of the faith community nurse program as well as a stimulus to educate new members on the purpose, commitment, and resources needed to continue this ministry as a priority for the faith community. The process of developing these statements is also an excellent time for engaging faith community members in the process and providing needed education. Inviting members to review and endorse these statements can support further buy in with implanting and sustaining the ministry.

20.3   Implementation of Organizational Structures

Creating a Health Ministry Committee or Cabinet that reports into the faith community council is helpful in communication, planning, and integration of the faith community nurse ministry into the life of the faith community (Westberg, 2006). The Health Cabinet can be made up of six to ten members. A mix of lay and health professionals often creates a good balance to the work of the committee. The Health Committee/Cabinet brings legitimacy to the faith community nurse ministry, allows for integration into the faith community, and provides excellent consultation resources for the faith community nurse. Meetings of the Health Ministry Committee/Cabinet should be held minimally on a quarterly basis, but may be held more frequently depending on the projects, programs, and service being provided by the faith community nurse. Change of membership on the committee/cabinet is recommended to occur on the cycle of other leadership in the faith community or at least every 3 years. Staggering the membership with a small portion of the membership leaving and entering positions each year brings new investment, ideas, and support for the faith community nurse.

20.4   Factors Important to Fulfilling the Faith Community Nurse's Functions

Research reports faith community nurses identified that "the three most important factors related to fulfilling their functions were attendance at a basic preparation course in parish nursing, their personal religious beliefs and support of their pastor" (Solari-Twadell, 2002, p. 127). These three factors were among 28 factors that were identified through review of parish nursing literature as important to supporting them in their ministry of faith community nurse practice (Burkhart & Solari-Twadell, 2006, p. 229). Respondents also noted that the support of their family was significant to their success as a faith community nurse when asked to write in any factor that appeared to be missing from the choices offered to them as part of this research. There can be times when faith community nurses are drawn away from their family to respond to the needs of their constituents or other responsibilities related to their position as faith community nurse. Having the support of family is very important as the patience and understanding of the family is necessary at times for the faith community nurse to focus on the emerging issues related to ministry related responsibilities.

The other top ten factors from this research that were identified as significant to a faith community nurse fulfilling their functions are as follows: networking, spiritual direction, their length of time in nursing, continuing education opportunities, the volunteers they work with in their faith community, the current person to whom they report, and the Health Cabinet. None of these top ten support factors need much discussion as their presence in the life and work of the faith community nurse clearly would be intended to be supportive to the faith community nurse, ministry, and practice.

The next 12 supportive factors, however important, were not perceived to be as significant to the faith community nurse work and ministry. These factors are: additional staff, the religious denomination served, length of time in parish nursing, regular reports, length of time in the present faith community nurse role, inclusion of the faith community nurse ministry as a line item in the budget of the faith community, written policies and procedures, written job description, being paid, current position title, documentation system, and access to a nursing supervisor. Although many of these factors are not identified in the top ten list, they remain important to supporting long-term viability of a faith community nurse program. Written policies and procedures, job descriptions, title, payment for service and established documentation system that can generate data reflective of the work, and value of the faith community nurse are significant to the establishment and longevity of this role, along with integration into the ministry of the faith community.

The least important factors identified as important to faith community nurses in fulfilling their functions were: professional certification, size of the congregation, geographic location, orientation to the faith community nurse role and faith community, and relationship with a health care system. Again, although apparently not identified as important, these factors also can contribute to longevity and sustainability of a faith community nurse ministry. For example, a small faith community in a rural area not proximate to a health care system may engage a nurse to fill the role of faith community nurse. However, given the size of the congregation and location the faith community nurse role may look very different from a faith community nurse in a large suburban faith community located near a health care system. The rural faith community nurse may have difficulty in succession management when the nurse faces retirement or relocation, whereas the large urban congregation may have established guidelines on recruitment, interviewing and hiring as well as more opportunities to attract another nurse to fill the faith community nurse role when the present faith community nurse is planning on relocating or retiring.

Further findings from early research noted that "the presence or absence of these factors differentiates the nursing practice. For example, faith community nurses who are paid are more likely to serve higher income families, work in larger congregations, located in larger cities, have more support from their pastors, and have a Health Cabinet in place. Faith community nurses in paid models also tend to have a relationship with a health care system, have policies and procedures in place, participate in an evaluation process and have access to nursing supervision. These faith community nurses also tend to be more interested in participating in a certification process in faith community nursing. Conversely, those not in paid positions worked fewer hours and had less structure and support" (Solari-Twadell, 2002, p. 104).

These findings, although probably not a surprise to many, have implications for not only sustainability of a faith community nurse ministry, but also for the engagement of the faith community nurse as part of the solution for access to care, increasing health care costs, lack of prevention services, and engagement with individuals in their episodes of wellness as well as their episodes of illness. If a faith community nurse is perceived primarily as "a nice service" that is offered by a faith community with few policies, procedures, evaluation mechanisms, documentation system, accountability and recorded outcomes, faith community nursing will remain in limbo. Faith communities may be concerned in initiating such a ministry and offering this service to members with the likelihood of not being able to sustain these services over time. This raises the question of how does the faith community retrieve its mission in health and healing, contribute to the solution of the reorganization of health care, and live out the gospel mandate of being counter to the culture while supporting its people to be good stewards, not only of their personal health resources, but health resources overall? This is a challenging question for challenging times, but essential to address if the trajectory of providing health resources, not just acute care, is going to be made accessible to all.

This is where the significance of advocating with influential parties becomes essential. Advocating with faith community leaders, key stakeholders, people in the pew, Chief Executive Officers of health care systems, and political leaders is important. Unfortunately, it is very difficult to draw the attention of media, popular press, and people in general as most do not really focus on health, until they are sick! When one is sick, of course, it is not the time to expect individuals to invest energy and attention on change in the delivery of health services. But an episode of illness may be the stimulus for individuals to experience the difference faith community nurses can make in referral, support, ongoing relationship development, and health surveillance along the continuum of care.

Faith community nursing has always been a local or "grass roots" endeavor. At some point it reached a "tipping point" with being designated a specialty nursing practice. The faith community nurse movement needs another "shove" to move it forward. *The Tipping Point: How Little Things Can Make a Big difference* is a "biography of an idea, and the idea is very simple" (Gladwell, 2002, p. 7). The author goes on to note that "Social epidemics… are driven by the efforts of a handful of exceptional people" (p. 21). His first rule of the *Tipping Point* is the "Law of the Few" where he describes that the "success of any kind of social movement," and it is believed faith community nursing is a social movement, "is heavily dependent on the involvement of people with a particular rare set of social gifts" (p. 33). As the book progresses, there are three particular types of individuals identified "the Connectors, Mavens and Salesmen" (p. 34). "Connectors know lots of people and they remember them" (p. 38), while "Mavens are information brokers and teachers." For a "social epidemic to start persuaders are needed"—enter the "Salesmen"

(p. 69). In summary, "the Connectors are social glue—they spread it, Mavens are data banks-they provide the message and the Salesmen are the persuaders who can move someone's thinking when they are unconvinced" (p. 70). All are needed to move an idea to a social epidemic.

Reverend Granger Westberg took an idea. He worked with others who implemented the idea. Westberg then took the data which he accumulated from all who followed and implemented his idea. He sold the concept of "parish nursing" over and over and over again. He did not do this by himself. "Connectors", "Mavens," and "Salesmen" have been a part of the development of the faith community nurse movement to this day.

Faith community nurses are very "exceptional" nursing professionals. They work with what they have, to create the best outcomes for the people they serve, undergirded by a strong belief system, prayer, and the support of a community of faith and in some instances health care systems. It is only through the sustaining of the faith community nurse ministry that changes in the understanding of health, creation of whole person health promotion strategies can be supported in the community. Looking to the future, the question remains what it will take, what is the "tipping point" for the sustaining and integration of a faith community nurse into the mainstream of health care services. It is clear it will take all dedicated to this professional model of Health Ministry to use all their individual gifts to reach out, carry the message, and not only sell the value of faith community nursing, but demonstrate how the investment in faith community nursing pays back in increased productivity of individuals, decreased expenditure for care, decrease in recidivism for chronic illness and better health outcomes over time. Establishing the systems, taking the time to do the documentation, to create the data that can effectively tell the story of the outcomes generated by the interventions employed by faith community nurse is foundational. Once this information is available, the "ultimate salesmen" in us all must be employed to continue to tell the story in the most convincing manner to anyone who will listen. Sustainability is not just a goal, but the lifeblood of the future of faith community nurse program.

20.5 Faith Community Nurse Termination

Recently there was a survey which addressed faith community nursing termination (Ziebarth, 2018). Although the study was not generalizable due to the convenience sample, out of 264 faith community nurses who responded to the survey, 23.69% (59) of these respondents lost a position as a faith community nurse and 12.73% (28) lost a position as a faith community nurse coordinator. Again, the total number of respondents was a small percentage of the total faith community projected population, of these respondents, a total of 46.58% ($N = 41$) who had been terminated (voluntarily or involuntarily) were in paid positions and 53.42% ($N = 46$) were in unpaid positions. The survey results indicate that of the 87 faith community nurse respondents who were terminated, more were unpaid (7%, $N = 5$) than paid, which is consistent with there being more unpaid, than paid faith community nurses. These results do raise the interesting issue that a faith community nurse in a non-paid position could be

Table 20.1 Reasons for faith community nurse termination—participants responses regarding why they were terminated as a faith community nurse

Reasons for faith community nurse termination
Change in leadership 29.11% ($N = 25$)
Not a strategic priority to leadership 26.58% ($N = 24$)
Organization restructuring 25.32% ($N = 22$)
Not a financial priority to hospital or health care organization 24.05% ($N = 21$)
Not a financial priority to the faith community 21.52% ($N = 19$)
Personal reasons 20.25% ($N = 18$)
Startup was grant driven and funds ran out 11.39% ($N = 10$)
Retirement 11.39% ($N = 10$)
Health related 8.86% ($N = 8$)
Not the best fit 7.59% ($N = 7$)

insulated from termination. That may not be the case. Table 20.1 lists participants' response as to why they believe they lost their position as a faith community nurse. Today in the business minded atmosphere of health care, programs operating with a mission focus and are non-revenue producing can be at "most at-risk for elimination when margin is threatened" (Ziebarth, 2015, p. 89). Revenue-producing activities are considered to be the core business of hospitals. Margin means having excess money to do missional activities such as faith community nursing. Whatever the model, termination is a loss of a faith community nurse in the community.

The top three reasons for termination as reported were "leadership change," "not a strategic priority to hospital or faith community leadership," and "organization restructuring or elimination of the program." In this study, the term "involuntary-termination" was synonymous with program closure. Leadership change suggests that site leadership had a positive impact on the program, but when leadership changed, there was an adverse effect. The 4th, 5th, and 7th reasons for termination were financial in nature: The results of this informal survey highlighted some issues related to termination, which are unique to faith community nursing within the discipline of nursing. They are: (a) the high percentage of involuntary faith community nurse terminations due to program closure (both hospital and faith community-based models); (b) the faith community nurses search for both a new job and new faith community post involuntary termination; (c) the high percentage of faith community nurses returning to unpaid positions after termination; and (d) the lack of resources for faith community nurses experiencing termination. With awareness being the first step, there may be some preventive measures to ensure that termination is less likely to occur.

20.6 Recommendations for Sustaining a Successful Faith Community Nurse Program

Actions in sustaining a successful faith community nurse program, regardless of model are: (a) have a clear and concise communication plan; (b) encourage the inclusion of "health of the congregation" as part of the mission and vision of the faith community; (c) create a job description in collaboration with leadership and have annual evaluations; (d) create an organizational structure; (e) create policies and procedures; (f) use evidenced-based resources and tools; (g) document, collect data, and communicate regularly regarding the altruistic and economic value of the program; (h) work hard to build a respectful and collegial relationship with leadership, stakeholders, and other health care providers; (i) nurture your volunteers; and, (j) pray, pray, pray!

Have a Clear and Concise Communication Plan Being able to communicate a clear vision of the faith community as a health place in the community, a broad whole person understanding of health and what a faith community nurse does as well as the value of the program is important to stakeholders. The faith community attenders are stakeholders. Ziebarth and Miller (2010) found that some nurses expressed frustration in transitioning into their faith community nurse role when the faith community expressed a lack of knowledge and understanding about the program. With that in mind, a faith community nurse may benefit from having a well-rehearsed response when asked about the value of the faith community nurse program within the faith community. Make sure that your Health Ministry/Cabinet members have the "elevator speech" memorized too. Remember that Health Ministry/Cabinet members are the program's representatives and should be able to effectively explain the faith community nursing program when asked.

Encourage the Inclusion of the Concept of "Health" as Part of the Mission and Vision of the Faith Community When you align the mission and vision of the program to that of the faith community, both are strengthened. The faith community nurse program is embedded and supported with budgetary dollars because the "health of the congregation and the community" is important to the faith community. In addition, when there is alignment with the mission and vision of the faith community nursing program to that of the faith community it raises the profile of the faith community to that of a "health place" in the community.

Create a Job Description in Collaboration with Leadership and Plan for Annual Evaluations for the Faith Community Nurse When the faith community nurse collaborates with faith community leadership, synergy and shared visioning occurs. The nurse has the knowledge of what a register nurse does. For specialty specific information, the *Scope and Standards of Faith Community Nursing (American Nurses Association and Health Ministries Association, 2017)*, the *Westberg Institute's Faith Community Nurse Foundation's Course* (Jacob, 2014), materials and *Position Statements* are available. There are also a great number of books that describe the practice of faith community nursing. The faith community leadership knows the faith community and how they believe a nurse can function within it. Creating the job description together ensures that all have a clear understanding regarding expectations for the faith community nurse role. The job description also guides the annual evaluation. Annual evaluations provide a time to discuss performance issues and expectations, which is important whether the position is paid or unpaid.

Create an Organizational Structure with Clear Reporting Relationships   As part of the job description, an organizational structure identifies reporting and working relationships for the faith community nurse and others in the faith community. A visual drawing of an organizational structure clarifies relationships and the chain of command as well as how the ministerial team will function. The faith community nurse should work within the boundaries as identified by the structure. The faith community nurse needs to be seen as a team-member that is a team-player.

Create Policies and Procedures   Policies and procedures conceptualize the practice, laying the foundation for a quality faith community nursing program (Ziebarth, 2006). They can also be used in annual evaluations as they describe the faith community nurse's practice and state competencies and program outcomes to be satisfied. A policy is a statement that sets forth an expectation and establishes a program's position on a particular issue. They set boundaries in which to act when performing activities and making decisions. There are six areas where policies are recommended for faith community nurses.

1. Areas in where there is confusion about the nurse's responsibilities that might result in neglect. These are necessary for a client's welfare. (Blood pressure screening, transportation, abuse and neglect, medical emergencies, etc.)
2. Areas pertaining to protection of the client rights. (Referrals to, referrals from, documentation records, etc.)
3. Areas defining relationships. (Relationships between the faith community, faith community nurse, and health care organization; collegiality, etc.)
4. Areas involving personnel management. (Annual evaluation, mileage, family leave, supervision, termination, etc.)
5. Areas involving the work environment and safety. (Visitation in a home, visitation at various health care institutions, personal safety, etc.)
6. Areas pertaining to professional and administrative expectations. (Preceptorship, continuing education, documentation, etc.)

The faith community may have policies that are related to personnel management, work environment, and safety. The nurse should be familiar with all policies and procedures that may affect the scope of their professional practice.

A procedure defines a series of steps and can provide direction on how a policy is to be carried out. Procedures show the protocol to be taken to complete an intervention or task.

There are three types of guidelines for faith community nursing:

1. Operational guidelines are suggested to aid in operational decision-making (e.g., How to set up a community-based blood pressure screening).
2. Practice guidelines are clinical practice statements based on research to assist the nurse and client with decisions about appropriate health care decisions. (e.g., American Heart Blood Pressure Standards).

3. Administrative guidelines are written statements that help organizational supported programs that have several faith community nurse perform more effectively. (e.g., Guidelines for signing out education equipment, such as a heart
model).

A policy and procedure can appear together in one document with the policy
statement first and the procedure protocol following the policy statement. Many
formats exist for policy and procedure development, but the final product should
include the following:

• Policy statement with a clear definition and purpose (what, when, who, and
  where may be included).

20.7 Procedure Statement Is the Protocol of How the Policy Is to Be Completed

• Who is responsible for implementing the procedure.
• The target audience to receive or to be impacted by the procedure.
• The steps necessary to carry out the procedure.
• The expected outcomes from the procedure.
• The method of documenting and communicating the results of the procedure.
• Supporting documentation and regulations are always included for reference to
  the user.

Use Evidenced-Based Resources and Tools Participants who attend the
Foundations Course in Faith Community Nursing through the *Westerberg Institute*
are supplied with many resources that have been tested by others. Whether the
resources needed are for the faith community nurse provider, or patient, health
resources should come from reputable sites and authors. Such resources can often
be recommended by faith community coordinators, the *Westberg Institute,* or any of
the membership organizations associated with faith community nursing. Chapter 6
in this text may also include information that addresses this suggestion.

**Document, Collect Data, and Communicate Regularly Regarding the Altruistic
and Economic Value of the Program** Documentation is necessary as a registered
nurse and all faith community nurses are registered nurses. Every *State Practice Act*
consists of legal responsibilities regarding documentation. Several formats are suggested in Chapter 19 of this text.

**Create Respectful and Collegial Relationship with Site Leadership,
Stakeholders, and Other Health Care Providers and Clients** More important
than defining individual responsibility, is how the whole faith community organization can serve and fulfill the health needs according to the mission statement. Mutual
respect through sharing, knowledge, and problem solving will enable trust among

colleagues in any environment. Initiating a dialogue with colleagues on subjects that matter to them can be a great start towards developing open communication. Conflicts can arise at times. Conflict can be constructive and may contribute to innovation and achievement (Jankowska & Marshall, 2004). Constructive conflict is non-emotional disagreement among those working towards a common goal. The facilitative process can only begin with the realization that there is an interrelatedness of one's actions or decisions. Collegiality also mitigates potential power struggles and protects professional boundaries. Many health care professionals work collaboratively to provide whole person care to patients. This inter-professional group may include the faith community nurse, faith community leadership, physicians, therapist, and other medical specialists. In addition, some of the clients served by the faith community nurse may be the biggest supporters, sales people, and financial sponsors. It is important to nurture all and any relationships as you never know where support for the faith community nurse may come from if the program is threatened.

Nurture Your Volunteers Faith community nursing programs provide an array of volunteer opportunities. It's a common mistake to think of volunteering as just something nice that people do. Volunteers have an enormous impact on the health and well-being of individuals assisted by their services. Volunteers can support meal programs, cards/calls of concern, transportation, and hospital or home visits. Each faith community nurse program that utilizes lay volunteers will have a different look based on the needs of attendees or their community. The hospitalized, elder house bound, and young families all benefit from a well-organized volunteer programs in a faith community.

Pray, Pray, Pray! Prayer is powerful. In addition to finding solace, prayer can bring people together. Make prayer a regular at Health Ministry/Cabinet meetings, faith community staff meetings, and during visits with patients. Networking with other faith community nurses is an excellent opportunity to pray for concerns related to faith community nursing ministry. It is important for a faith community nurse to consider having resources such as a spiritual director. Through regular meetings with the spiritual director, the faith community nurse can ensure a solid resource of spiritual care to support self.

20.8 Conclusion

Essential to the contribution of changing the understanding of health, creating new ways of supporting people in their wellness, providing more cost-effective community-based care and increasing access to health promotion and prevention programming, faith community nurse programs must be planned early in their development for long-term sustainability. It is only over time, with increase in numbers of faith community nurse providers that the landscape of health outcomes will be altered. It is like painting a house. If care is not taken at the beginning of the project, the new paint will not be able to adhere sufficiently and the time, money, and effort to complete the project will be impacted by less than desirable results. The new paint will peal sooner and the original painting project will not have achieved the longevity expected. It may take longer at the beginning, but hopefully, the work of educating, re-educating, and moving through the necessary planning stages will result in long-term sustainability of the faith community nurse and program.

References

American Nurses Association and Health Ministries Association. (2017). *Faith community nursing: Scope and standards of practice* (2nd ed.). Silver Spring, MD: American Nurses Association. nursesbooks.org

Burkhart, L., & Solari-Twadell, P. A. (2006). Quality of the ministry of parish nursing practice in an outcomes environment. In P. A. Solari-Twadell & M. A. McDermott (Eds.), *Parish nursing: Development, education and administration* (pp. 227–240). St Louis, MO: Elsevier.

Free, M. (2014). Vision, mission, purpose? *Production Machining, 14*(11), 17–19.

Gladwell, M. (2002). *The tipping point: How little things can make a big difference*. New York, NY: Back Bay Books.

Jacob, S. (Ed.). (2014). *Foundations of faith community nursing* (3rd ed.). Memphis, TN: Church Health Center.

Jankowska, M. A., & Marshall, L. (2004). Why social interaction and good communication. *The Reference Librarian, 40*(83–84), 131–144.

Solari-Twadell, P. A. (2002). The differentiation of the ministry of parish nursing practice within a congregation. *Dissertation Abstracts International, 63*(06), 569A. UMI No 3056442.

Westberg, J. (2006). *Health and wellness: What your faith community can do*. Cleveland, OH: Pilgrim Press.

Ziebarth, D. (2006). Policies and procedures for the parish nursing practice. In P. Solari-Twadell & M. McDermott (Eds.), *Parish nursing: Development, education, and administration* (pp. 257–282). St. Louis, MO: Elsevier.

Ziebarth, D. (2015). *Documentation position statement*. Westberg Institute. Church Health.

Ziebarth, D. (2018). Job termination survey: FCN. *International Journal of Faith Community Nursing, 4*(1), 34.

Ziebarth, D., & Miller, C. (2010). Exploring parish nurses' perceptions of parish nurse training. *Journal of Continuing Education in Nursing, 41*(6), 273–280.

Promoting Inner Strength in Faith Community Nurses and Faith Communities

Gayle Roux and Catherine Dingley

21.1   Inner Strength in Faith Community Nurses and Their Ministry Communities

Sustainability of a faith community nurse program is dependent on the sustainability of the faith community nurse. Why should faith community nurses be interested in building Inner Strength in their own lives and those of the community they interact with? Faith community nurses embody the spiritual mission to explore relationships between faith and health in their lives and their ministry communities. Rooted in inner strength flowing from a personal relationship with God or a Spiritual Power, faith community nurses sustain belief in a better way of caring for people. Inherent in their philosophy of patient care is that of caring for the whole person. At the same time, faith community nurses are facing unprecedented changes. Contemporary social and mental health issues, violence, changes in demographics resulting in more elderly populations aging at home, families that are dispersed across the country or internationally, and increases in the incidence of people living with chronic health conditions and cancer have created challenges for health professionals. In addition to ministering to others, the faith community nurse needs to address how to best minister to and care for themselves. While faith community nurses are very familiar with the spiritual mission to "Love thy neighbor as thyself," they are not usually thinking in terms of the spiritual mission of "Loving thyself as thy neighbor."

As faith community nurses focus on caring for their ministry communities and for themselves, having a framework that provides a perspective from a positive psychology point of view is valuable. One means of understanding the experiences of

G. Roux (✉)
Department of Nursing, University of North Dakota, Grand Forks, ND, USA
e-mail: gayle.roux@und.edu

C. Dingley
Department of Nursing, University of Nevada, Las Vegas, Las Vegas, NV, USA
e-mail: Catherine.Dingley@unlv.edu

© Springer Nature Switzerland AG 2020   287
P. A. Solari-Twadell, D. J. Ziebarth (eds.), *Faith Community Nursing*,
https://doi.org/10.1007/978-3-030-16126-2_21

individuals and families as they navigate today's society involves the use of an inter-pretive framework that can assist faith community nurses to identify existing strengths and foster health and healing. The middle-range theory of Inner Strength in Women (TIS-W) (Roux et al., 2002) provides such a framework for understand-ing the experiences faced by individuals and families with a challenging life situa-tion or chronic health condition. This chapter will review the concepts of the Theory of Inner Strength and discuss strategies to assess and expand strength-based inter-ventions for the faith community nurse and their faith community.

Developing *inner strength* is a potential human response when an individual is confronted, with a difficult and challenging life circumstance. While individuals possess the capacity for inner strength, it is often the challenge of life events that acts as a catalyst to build inner strength. Based on research study findings, a defini-tion of inner strength was devised: inner strength is having capacity to build the self through a developmental process that positively moves the individual through chal-lenging life events such as living with cancer or other chronic conditions (Dingley and Roux, 2014). As a universal concept, enhancement of inner strength provides a potential benefit to both men and women. While the authors' theory development has primarily focused on the gender-specific needs of women, a recent study exam-ined Inner Strength in men (Smith, 2017; Smith et al., 2019). The TIS-W addresses the human response when confronted with a difficult circumstance and describes a process that is dynamic with fluctuating patterns. The theory provides a basis for the instrument, the Inner Strength Questionnaire (ISQ) (Lewis and Roux, 2011) (Appendix) which has the potential to be used as a measure to predict relationships and test nursing interventions. The realization and growth of inner strength have been demonstrated in research to result in positive health outcomes of improved quality of life (QOL) and self-management (Dingley and Roux, 2014). The TIS-W with the outcomes that were demonstrated in this research are illustrated in Fig. 21.1.

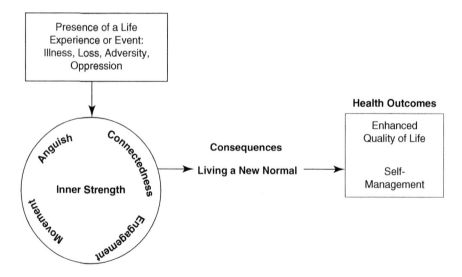

Fig. 21.1 Model of the Theory of Inner Strength in Women (Roux & Dingley)

Growing in Inner Strength is a dynamic process and involves multiple dimensions. The concepts and corresponding definitions of the theory of inner strength are (a) *anguish and searching* describes the fear, vulnerability, and search for meaning to process the challenging life event; (b) *connectedness* describes the nurturing of supportive relationships with self, family, friends, and a spiritual power; (c) *engagement* describes self-determinism, reframing, and engaging in possibilities; and (d) *movement* describes the dimension of movement, rest, activity, honest self-appraisal, and balance (see Fig. 21.1). The four dimensions of inner strength are not necessarily linear and involves a process that is fluid over time that moves individuals to "living a new normal." The new normal is expressed through finding new meaning and sense of purpose and can involve a renewed faith in God or Higher Power. The "new normal" is expressed through stories of new activities, relationships, understanding, sense of purpose, and a renewed faith in God or a Greater Source of Strength. Analysis revealed that *living a new normal* was determined to be a consequence or outcome of inner strength. The major four concepts comprising inner strength and their definitions are given below. Quotations given by individuals in research studies on inner strength provide exemplar statements of their experiences.

21.1.1 The Four Concepts and Definitions for the Theory of Inner Strength

Concepts	Definitions	Research participant statements
Anguish and searching	The fear, vulnerability, and search for meaning	I worry about my health I am scared about the future
Connectedness	The nurturing of supportive relationships	I have at least one person close to me I express my fears to my God or a Greater Source of Strength
Engagement	Self-determinism, reframing, and engaging in possibilities	I tell myself I can do this I believe I have inner strength
Movement	Balance of rest, activity, and honest self-appraisal	I take time for myself I try to rest my mind periodically

The TIS-W provides description and insight into human responses to challenging life experiences. The theory can serve as a framework for assessment of client needs and tailored interventions as well as self-care behaviors. The theory exemplifies the metaparadigm related to health, person, environment, and nursing. It also supports the view of health as a process and experience, encompassing opportunities for physical, emotional, and spiritual healing. Chronic illness, stress, and spiritual distress are conceptualized as a meaningful component of the whole and may serve as a facilitator of building strength and reaching the "new normal."

The focus on inner strength across the lifespan delineates an element of human experience from a positive, strengths-based perspective. The theory of inner strength provides an alternative perspective on processes and outcomes from the typical focus on "health problems," "dysfunction," and "negative outcomes." Currently, healthcare and nursing sensitive outcomes focus on prevention of untoward events or unwanted clinical outcomes, such as complications of treatment. As such, understanding ways to facilitate inner strength is valuable for faith community nurses and their ministry as they move through various complexities of life. The inner strength theory applied by the faith community nurse reinforces the need to focus on individual and community strengths and the relationship to positive outcomes such as healing, comfort, spiritual peace, and QOL. As an example, the interventions suggested in Table 21.1 were developed within the dimensions of the theory. The interventions were based on the descriptions of the concepts for facilitating inner strength using the items from the ISQ for assessment questions. For example, within the Anguish and Searching subscale, interventions initiated by faith community nurses could include assessment of clients as they move through the experience of distress and fear to searching and finding acceptance and meaning (see Fig. 21.1).

The question "How can the care by Faith Community Nurses foster inner strength for themselves?" is addressed in the unique aspects of the role as well as the interventions they minister (Table 21.1). Faith Community Nurses are an ideal role model for strength-based care as the model of care is very congregational and healing based. The faith community nurses' role is based on care of the whole person with an emphasis on spiritual care. Faith community nurses' care is unique in building a relationship with the individual and faith community that supports physical care, psychological care, spiritual care, well-being of the family, access to health care, and health of the entire faith community. Faith community nurses are practicing in all major religious denominations and states as well as internationally. The role of the faith community nurse as a trusted member of the community makes this community-based nursing role ideal to represent nursing for strength-based practice. Faith community nurses frequently employ strength-based interventions on a daily basis across cultures, races, age groups, and gender.

Pope Francis (2015), in his encyclical *Laudato Si*, On Care of our Common Home, stated, "Human Beings deserve a right to … happiness and dignity." The encyclical is full of both hope and candor on the obstacles of the human condition. He addressed the negative effects on human dignity as "The throw-away life." This has resulted in the breakdown of society, environmental deterioration, increased violence, racial intolerance, and religious oppression. Pope Francis stated the world is in the "silent rupture of the bonds of integration and social cohesion." He provided hope by encouraging a counter reaction to data overload by focusing on deep relationships, essential dialogue and generous encounters, and relationships between human beings.

Within the environment of obstacles described by Pope Francis, the faith community nurse must allocate daily attention and energy to self-care interventions. Faith community nurses must minister to themselves with the same commitment they have to their community. Faith community nurses should make space in their lives to appreciate and reflect on how to give themselves the "permission" to practice self-care and in doing so, promote inner strength. A little self-care can go a long

Table 21.1 Theoretically based strength needs and FCN practice interventions

Concepts and definitions	Item examples From inner strength questionnaire: assessment parameters	Theoretically based interventions
Anguish and Searching	There are many times when I am afraid of dying	Discuss what the client knows about their stressful event or illness
Point of shock and fear to one of accepting	I am scared about the future	Provide client-centered education Explore fears and worries regarding the future
Establishing meaning	I dwell on my situation or illness	Discuss potential meanings Discuss spiritual meanings Make appropriate ancillary referrals
Connectedness	I have at least one person close to me	Determine the client's possible sources of support
Sense of support and nurturance from self, family, friends, and a spiritual power	I feel the presence of God or a Greater Source of Strength	Assess nurturing support, including social and spiritual support
Nurturing of relationships resulting in a deeper connectedness	I have at least one person close to me	Assist the client to develop insight related to needing and asking for help. Refer for supportive services as needed
Movement	I can live with my physical limitations	Discuss balance of lifestyle
Movement, harmonizing, and facilitating desired change	I try to balance work and play	Daily patterns should include time for both reflection, quiet, and physical activity
Composure of the body achieved through both silent reflection and actualizing the athletic and creative self	I take time for myself	Encourage activities to promote physical and emotional strength Set activity goals Discuss changes in function, and assess fatigue and sleep
Engagement	I can change my attitude when I need to	Assist in reframing circumstance and refocusing thoughts and attitude
Having a positive attitude, refocusing thoughts, reframing circumstances, and engaging with life's possibilities	I believe I have inner strength	Encourage humor when appropriate Assess for anxiety and depression Make appropriate referrals Recommend support groups if client is amenable

way. It does not mean you have to go to spas or have expensive massages—although these are nice rewards if they are within your budget. The "connectedness" concept of inner strength is defined as nourishing and connecting with yourself as well as others. Faith community nurses should take time out of each day to assess the health and strength of their body, soul, and mind. When something is missing or there are personal worries, special attention needs to be placed on that strength-building domain. Research has demonstrated these strategies can improve quality of life and assist an individual to manage their own health (Dingley and Roux, 2014). Every faith community nurse should gift themselves with planned down time, supportive friendships, time for quiet and prayer, and nourishing food. Physical exercise and sleep are non-negotiable. As faith community nurses you want to prevent caregiver fatigue or burnout. It is critical to recognize patterns of exhaustion and burnout very early to restore balance. Self-care activities that foster inner strength and well-being will look different for everyone. While some enjoy yoga class, others are replenished by a quiet cup of tea. The American Nurses Association developed an extensive system of self-care resources in 2017 titled, "Healthy Nurse Healthy Nation" which is available at https://www.nursingworld.org/practice-policy/work-environment/health-safety/healthy-nurse-healthy-nation/.

Based on the TIS-W and research results, the plan you develop to care for yourself to grow in inner strength will be individualized but contain these universal characteristics:

1. *Realistic and Intentional.* Make a realistic plan and be intentional about your selected nourishing activities. Be very mindful that the first concept of inner strength is "Anguish and Searching". When you are performing the daily reality of your job as a faith community nurse, it is physically and emotionally demanding. Be a good barometer for your energy levels and feelings. Growing in inner strength does not mean that the responsibilities of your faith community nursing work are always fun or predictable. Having the energy field to face the unexpected when things go wrong is strength building. Expressing your frustrations and the reality of a difficult challenge with a trusted friend or loved one is the first step to building inner strength in the long run.

2. *Investment in Enjoyment.* A full life means investing in what you enjoy across your lifespan. True inner strength strategies are fostered over your entire career. Investing in yourself to live fully ensures you have water in your well to continue to share with others to drink. There are many proverbs and references to the "living water" in faith literature and the Bible. There are also references in music lyrics that you "never miss your water until your well is dry." These references remind us that faith community nurses should assess their own inner strength daily and nourish themselves beyond the daily to the "long haul of your personal life and professional career." The roles and responsibilities of faith community nurses are very rewarding, but also demanding. Nursing is hard work. Faith com-

munity nursing encompasses full body, mind, and spirit energies that require having your own strategic investment in the sources of your "living water."

3. *Nonlinear Movement.* Both professional nursing and our personal lives within family and the community are "nonlinear." While daily assessment and nourishing activities are needed for our own "living water," it is equally important to be flexible and tolerant of ourselves and the healthcare system. Nurses are engaged in dynamic, ever-changing roles. It is therapeutic to admit to yourself that being a faith community nurse is challenging. We experience multiple interruptions not only each day, but each hour of the day. Faith community nurses should not become discouraged or disheartened over variations caused with a difficult day or demanding time of their lives. Inner Strength is a developmental theory. Investment over a lifespan will give strength and energy for difficult challenges. As well, you may need to reevaluate and do something a little different during this situation. Varying prayer, quiet reflection time, physical activity, hobbies, having a difficult conversation to discuss the situation, and making time to spend with different friends can provide the nonlinear movement that is needed for replenishing your "living water."

4. *Communicating Value of Faith Community Nursing.* With every life you touch and with every personal and professional contact, communicate the message of the value of what faith community nurses do. Personal energy as a faith community nurse is fostered with acknowledgment and respect for your work and the personal presence you provide within your faith community. Inner strength is within the individual and has the potential to affect organizational strength. Organizational strength is derived from functioning as a faith community nursing professional within a system that values your contributions. As a professional organization of faith community nurses, it's important you communicate and role model the impact of your contributions. The value of faith-based nursing is not always acknowledged and understood by the public, insurance companies, and other inter-professional members of the healthcare system. Marketing, messaging, and relationship building for the good of the profession is strength-building for the good of the individual faith community nurse and their respective faith community ministries.

Table 21.2 highlights recommended suggestions for self-care interventions. While the role of faith community nurses is to help others and facilitate spiritual growth, a systematic plan needs to be incorporated into your hectic daily life for your own spiritual growth. Faith community nurses must have external support people you can call upon for help and for debriefing of your feelings. Embedded within the culture of nursing and faith community nursing is a reluctance to ask for help and express vulnerabilities. To grow in inner strength the faith community nurse needs a safe place and safe support people where you can express vulnerabilities and worries.

Table 21.2 Strength-based self-care interventions by faith community nurses

Strength-based practice	Self-care interventions by FCNs
Strategies to search and connect	
• Have a colleague or mentor listen to you	• Seek perspective and guidance from a trusted person
• Ask for help when needed	• Honest appraisal of self-care needs for social support
• Spiritual growth facilitation	• Acknowledge whole person integration (body, mind, spirit)
• Prayer	• Recognize God or a Higher Power and envision a favorable outcome
• Hope instillation	• Practice daily appreciation exercises
Strategies to engage and move	
• Validation of your situation or stresses	• Seek decision-making support and solution-focused strategies
• Learning facilitation from other FCNs	• Practice positive thinking patterns
• Journaling of feelings	• Manage emotional energy and focus on internal strengths
• Allow yourself to be nurtured rather than nurturing others	• Find a balance between caring for and being cared for. Encourage fun activities, physical and relaxation and exercises
	• Aerobic exercise

21.2 Conclusion

In summary, faith community nurses, nurse practitioners, researchers, and other community members need an open dialogue on strategies to address the social health determinants in today's society. Health vulnerabilities and whole person health have been the focus of faith community nurses. Organizations of faith community nurses of all faiths can create a momentum to develop a plan for shaping the inner capacity for individuals and families. The difficulties in today's society distressfully cry out in need for a way to cope with vulnerabilities and grow in inner strength. Currently, there is an interest in nursing to develop a full understanding of the complexities of inner strength. Nurses can play a key role in interventions using inner strength as a personal capacity for health improvements, spiritual growth, and healing over a lifetime. The ministry of inner strength for the self as well as the faith community holds promise to repair the bonds of social cohesion.

Appendix

Inner Strength Questionnaire

Instructions:
Circle one of the choices (5, 4, 3, 2, or 1) that corresponds with strongly agree, agree, slightly agree, disagree or strongly disagree.

Answer how you feel TODAY about YOUR HEALTH....

	Strongly Agree	Agree	Slightly Agree	Disagree	Strongly Disagree
1. I tell myself I can do this.	5	4	3	2	1
2. I can change my attitude when I need to.	5	4	3	2	1
3. I believe I am a strong person.	5	4	3	2	1
4. I am determined to get well.	5	4	3	2	1
5. I believe I have inner strength.	5	4	3	2	1
6. I can decide what to do.	5	4	3	2	1
7. I have at least one person close to me.	5	4	3	2	1
8. I feel the presence of God or a Greater Source of Strength.	5	4	3	2	1
9. I put control of my life in God's or a Greater Power's hand.	5	4	3	2	1
10. I feel close to God or a Greater Source of Strength.	5	4	3	2	1
11. I pray for strength.	5	4	3	2	1
12. I express my fears to my God or a Greater Source of Strength.	5	4	3	2	1
13. I pray for others.	5	4	3	2	1
14. I worry about my health.	5	4	3	2	1
15. I am scared about the future.	5	4	3	2	1
16. When I first learned about my health problem, I was afraid of dying.	5	4	3	2	1
17. There are many times when I am afraid of dying.	5	4	3	2	1
18. I feel my situation is out of control.	5	4	3	2	1
19. I dwell on my illness.	5	4	3	2	1
20. When I first learned about my health problem, I felt afraid.	5	4	3	2	1
21. I can live with my physical limitations.	5	4	3	2	1
22. I stay active.	5	4	3	2	1

(continued)

(continued)

	Strongly Agree	Agree	Slightly Agree	Disagree	Strongly Disagree
23. I spend time with my friends or family.	5	4	3	2	1
24. I try to balance work an d play.	5	4	3	2	1
25. I take time for myself.	5	4	3	2	1
26. I try to rest my mind periodically.	5	4	3	2	1
27. I set aside time to relax.	5	4	3	2	1

Copyright 2003, Roux, G. Lewis, K., & Dingley, C.

References

American Nurses Association. (2017). *Health nurse healthy nation*. Retrieved from https://www.nursingworld.org/practice-policy/work-environment/health-safety/healthy-nurse-healthy-nation/

Dingley, C., & Roux, G. (2014). The role of inner strength in quality of life and self-management in women survivors of cancer. *Research in Nursing & Health, 37*, 32–41. https://doi.org/10.1002/nur.21579

Francis, P. (2015). *Laudato Si. On care for our common home*. Rome: Libertia Editrice Vaticana.

Lewis, K., & Roux, G. (2011). Psychometric testing of the inner strength questionnaire: Women living with chronic health conditions. *Applied Nursing Research, 24*, 153–160. https://doi.org/10.1016/j.apnr.2009.06.003

Roux, G., Dingley, C. A., & Bush, H. A. (2002). Inner strength in women: Metasynthesis of qualitative findings in theory development. *Journal of Theory Construction & Testing, 6*(1), 86–93.

Smith, C. (2017). *Inner strength in men-a descriptive phenomenology*. Available from ProQuest Dissertations and Theses @ University of North Dakota. (1969130498).

Smith, C., Dingley, C., & Roux, G. (2019). Inner strength—State of the science. *The Canadian Journal of Nursing Research, 51*(1), 38–48. https://doi.org/10.1177/0844562118790714

Transitional Care

22

Deborah Ziebarth

22.1 Significance of Transitional Care

The provision of transitional care is an important determinant in health care outcomes of seniors discharged from hospitals in this nation. Preventable readmissions occur most often with at-risk Medicare patients. One out of five Medicare recipients are readmitted within 30 days of a hospital discharge (James, 2013), and many readmissions are prevented. When patients transfer from hospital to home a gap in the continuity of care often exists. This transitional period, if not well supported, can lead to poor health outcomes and ultimate readmissions, as well as causing increased demands on untrained caregivers in coordinating complex care.

Hospitals have a shared responsibility to Medicare patients to explore ways to keep them safe after discharge in their homes. One of the strategies to decrease Medicare spending outlined in the Patient Protection and Affordable Care Act (PPACA) is the reduction in hospital readmissions (Cauchi, 2012; Centers for Medicare and Medicaid Services, 2015; Cutler, Davis, & Stremikis, 2010). The *Independent Payment Advisory Board* (IPAB) created the *Continuity Assessment Record and Evaluation Medicare Tool* to measure the health and functional status of Medicare patients at acute discharge and determines payment reimbursement for hospital readmissions of less than 60 days (Centers for Medicare and Medicaid Services, 2015; Gage et al. 2012). The *Independent Payment Advisory Board* requires hospitals to take on more of the financial burden by decreasing payment reimbursements. Payment penalties began in October, 2012 for hospitals subject to the *Inpatient Prospective Payment System* (IPPS). Hospitals in the U.S.A. are financially penalized with a 3% loss on every Medicare payment if the hospital has an excessive 30-day readmission for three specific diagnosis: acute myocardium infraction, congestive heart failure, and pneumonia for 2014 readmissions. In 2015

D. Ziebarth (✉)
Department of Nursing Program Chair, Herzing University, Brookfield, WI, USA
e-mail: dziebarth@herzing.edu

© Springer Nature Switzerland AG 2020
P. A. Solari-Twadell, D. J. Ziebarth (eds.), *Faith Community Nursing*,
https://doi.org/10.1007/978-3-030-16126-2_22

exacerbation of chronic obstructive pulmonary disease, total hip and knee arthro-plasty were added as additional diagnosis to measure hospital performance. In 2017, coronary artery bypass surgery was added (Centers for Medicare and Medicaid Services, 2015; Nakazawa, Egorova, Power, Faries, & Vouyouka, 2017). These changes in Medicare reimbursements are forcing hospitals to look for alternative ways to decrease avoidable readmissions. The rate of avoidable readmission can be reduced by improving transitional care for patients from hospital to homes.

22.2   Transitional Care Research

Factors that lead to hospital readmissions and interventions that reduce them were explored through a review of literature (Ziebarth, 2015). Key findings of 62 articles were collected, compared, and combined into three distinct groupings: Factors that lead to hospital readmissions, interventions that decreased readmissions prior to hospital discharge, and interventions that decreased readmissions post discharge or after hospitalization.

Factors that Lead to Hospital Readmissions   Predictive factors of hospital readmis-sions give direction in identifying those patients most at-risk so that they may receive additional services in the hospital. Predictive factors were identified as follows:

- Elderly patients with complex medical, social, and financial needs.
- Patients living alone, absence of a formal or informal care giver.
- Patients with syndrome of frailty with associated symptoms of weakness, decreased energy, and weight loss.
- Diseases such as congestive heart failure, chronic obstructive pulmonary disease, pneumonia, diabetes, stroke, cancer.
- Major hip or knee surgery, vascular surgery, and major bowel surgery.
- Serious mental illnesses including psychosis and depression.
- Patients living with a disability.
- Patients with poor health literacy.
- The number of medications and the use of certain medications.

It was found that certain medications increased the possibility of adverse events after discharge. Patients using warfarin, insulin, digoxin, and aspirin when used in combination with clopidogrel were identified as having increased risk, as well as patients using narcotics. In addition, patients on five or more scheduled medications were found to be at increased risk due to decreased adherence (Budnitz, Shehab, Kegler, & Richards, 2007; Frank, 2008; Sehgal et al., 2013).

Additionally, some hospital characteristics were found to be associated with readmissions of patients with congestive heart failure. Hospital characteristics included: (a) publically owned hospital in a county with low median income; (b) a hospital lacking cardiac services; (c) small hospitals; and (d) units with lower nurs-ing staffing. Hospitals with higher nurse staffing had lower odds of readmissions penalties than hospitals with lower staffing (Joynt, Orav, & Jha, 2011; McHugh, Berez, & Small, 2013).

Interventions that Decreased Readmissions *Prior* to Hospital Discharge Interventions that decreased readmissions *prior* to hospital discharge included the following:

- Preparation for discharge early in the hospitalization.
- Patient and caregiver education (disease management).
- Patient tools (booklet, pictorial patient care plan, etc.).
- Check-off list used by hospitalist prior to discharge to ensure readiness for discharge.
- Collaboration between attending physician and hospital staff as in cross-site communication.
- Designated staff dedicated to case management/transitional care.

The particular needs of diverse communities in inner-city safety-net hospitals are often overlooked (Jack et al., 2009; Lipstein & Dunagan, 2014). Sociodemographic factors may impact readmission rates. Discharge advocates, who assist patient discharge preparation, medication reconciliation, national guideline adherence, and aftercare appointments, are dedicated to patients residing in specific zip codes.

Interventions that Decreased Readmissions Post Discharge or After Hospitalization Interventions that decreased readmissions post discharge or after hospitalization were:

- Follow-up phone calls
- Follow-up clinic visit
- Remote monitoring with telehealth technology
- Care management—Community-based nurses doing follow-up home visits.

Nurses in the community coach patients through transition. Chronically ill patients that were coached had more primary care visits, but significantly less specialty care and emergency room visits (Black et al., 2014; Linden & Butterworth, 2014; Morales-Asencio et al., 2010).

22.3 Nurses Role in Providing Transitional Care

Transitional care is defined as providing patients care that is, time sensitive to ensure continuity, avoid preventable complications, and promote a safe transfer from one physical setting to another or from one level of care to another (Naylor, Aiken, Kurtzman, Olds, & Hirschman, 2011). Time sensitive interventions including **educating patients and family caregivers, medication reconciliation and management, and supportive services for self-management** are key components of nearly all nurse-led transitional care models. Nurses are a trusted front-line health care members in the community and are used to manage patients through transitions. Being present with patients and their caregivers, providing transitional care ensures that discharge education is revisited, and needs are met, which reduces the rates of subsequent hospital readmissions (Carthon, Lasater, Sloane, & Kutney-Lee, 2015; Hennessey, Suter, & Harrison, 2010; Manderson, Mcmurray, Piraino, & Stolee, 2012; Marek, Adams, Stetzer, Popejoy, & Rantz, 2010; Piraino, Heckman, Glenny, & Stolee, 2012).

22.4 Why Use the Faith Community Nurse in Providing Transitional Care

Faith community nurses are community based and are familiar with local resources. They can provide coordination of care to ensure resources are used appropriately, decreasing fragmentation. This is especially true for the resources within the faith community where transportation, food, and social supports may be accessed, which can impact health outcomes of discharged patients. Faith community nurses also tend to come from the same community and have the same cultural context. This knowledge can be leveraged to motivate the patient and caregiver to engage in self-care or self efficacy.

In addition to formal nursing education, the *American Nurses Association* and *Health Ministries Association* in the *Faith Community Nursing: Scope and Standards of Practice* (American Nurses Association and Health Ministries Association, 2017) recommends additional training for the nurses in the faith community nursing specialty. Many faith community nurses choose to attend the *Faith Community Nurse Foundation's Course*, which is designed to introduce and prepare registered nurses (Jacob, 2014). This training provides additional knowledge of whole person health, spiritual care, and community nursing. Faith community nurses who attend this educational program may implement transitional care interventions differently. Because of this, patients may experience a range of assessments and interventions that considers wholistic health needs. The faith community nurse may ask questions like "What sustains you during difficult times?" or "Does your religious or spiritual beliefs influence the way you look at your disease and the way you think about your health?" (Ziebarth, 2017). The faith community nurse may use presence or prayer in providing transitional care.

The theoretical model of *Faith Community Nursing* (Ziebarth, 2014) may help to clarify the practice (Fig. 22.1). The practice of Faith Community Nursing is described theoretically as:

> …a method of healthcare delivery that is centered in a relationship between the nurse and client (client as person, family, group, or community). The relationship occurs in an iterative motion over time when the client seeks or is targeted for wholistic health care with the goal of optimal wholistic health functioning. Faith integrating is a continuous occurring attribute. Health promoting, disease managing, coordinating, empowering, and accessing

health care are other essential attributes. All essential attributes occur with intentionality in a faith community, home, health institution, and other community settings with fluidity as part of a community, national, or global health initiative (Ziebarth, 2014), p 1829].

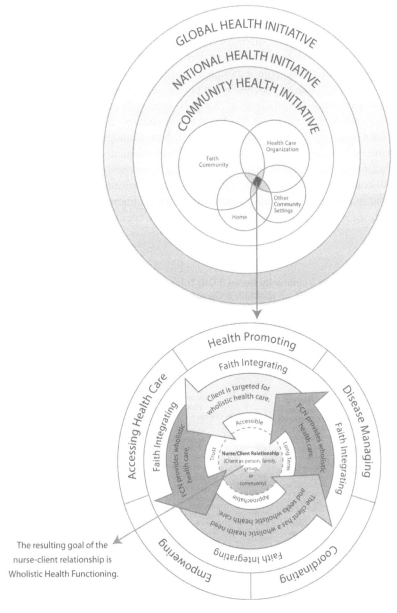

Fig. 22.1 Theoretical model, faith community nursing, a method of wholistic health care delivery (Ziebarth, 2014)

Faith integrating, health promoting, disease managing, coordinating, empowering, and accessing health care are essential attributes that operationalize the concept of faith community nursing.

Research states that the faith community nurse provides emotional and spiritual support for anxious and isolated elders and effectively assists them to obtain needed health care often preventing need for acute care or readmissions. They also help older persons link to community long-term care services, and to access resources such as free prescription medications for low-income individuals. Through hospital and faith community collaborations whole person health care is addressed and may improve the patient's discharge experience, ensure post-discharge support, and reduce re-hospitalization of patients. Faith community nursing is a cost-effective method of decreasing hospitalization (King & Pappas-Rogich, 2011; Rydholm, 1997; Rydholm & Thornquist, 2005; Yeaworth & Sailors, 2014; Ziebarth, 2016; Ziebarth & Campbell, 2017; Ziebarth, Campbell, Ahn, Munning, & Owens, 2018).

Ziebarth and Campbell (2016), created the *Faith Community Nurse Transitional Care Model* to provide clarity regarding how faith community nurses could work with faith communities in providing care to patients transitioning from hospital to home. The model has been tested several times. In addition, a *Faith Community Nurse Transitional Care Course* was created and has been taught throughout the U.S.A.

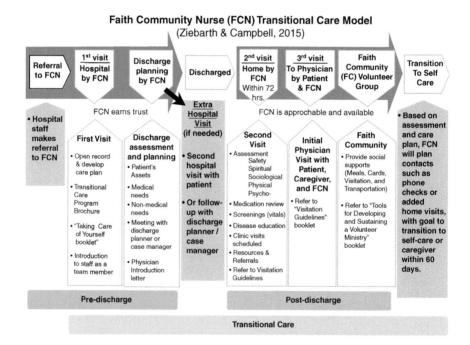

Fig. 22.2 Faith community nurse transitional care model (Ziebarth and Campbell, 2015)

22.5 Faith Community Nurse Transitional Care Model

In the *Faith Community Nurse Transitional Care Model*, there are two phases when time-specific interventions occur (Fig. 22.2). The two phases are pre-hospital discharge and post-hospital discharge (Ziebarth & Campbell, 2016). The model's aim is to transition to self-care within 30–60 days, based on the faith community nurses' assessment. Transitional care can be terminated when (a) access is established to primary care provider [medical home], (b) transportation issues are resolved, (c) there is competent and safe management of medications and other disease self-care activities, (e) the caregiver is prepared and engaged, (f) community resources are accessible and reliable, (g) there is effective demonstration of knowing what to do, who to call, and what to report, and, (h) patient and caregiver have in writing all instructions.

Pre-discharge In the pre-discharge phase, the **first visit** is made with the patient in the hospital. The faith community nurse goal in this phase is to earn the trust of the patient, caregiver, hospital staff/case manager, and doctor. This is done by introduction, information sharing, and plan development. The faith community nurse identifies the patient's assets and strengths, along with medical and nonmedical needs. The patient, caregiver, hospital staff, and doctor are oriented to the role of the faith community nurse in transitioning from hospital to home. The role of the faith community nurse is to avert unnecessary re-hospitalization by increasing contact between the patient and doctor and by making frequent home visits to offer time specific and wholistic nursing interventions. These interventions include: (a) whole person assessment, which include spiritual; (b) appropriate referrals; (c) screening (vitals); (d) disease education; (e) medication reconciliation; (f) self-care training; and (g) safety assessments. The faith community nurse should also contact the physician's office/clinic to introduce their role and let them know that the faith community nurse may accompany the patient and caregiver to the first doctor's visit post discharge.

A booklet entitled *Taking Care of Myself: A Guide for When I Leave the Hospital* (https://www.ahrq.gov/patients-consumers/diagnosis-treatment/hospitals-clinics/goinghome/index.html) can be used by the faith community nurse and patient to collect information such as discharge medications, important telephone numbers, doctors' appointment dates/times, and to develop a plan for emergencies, such as pain or anxiety. Another available tool is from the *Pittsburgh Mercy Parish Nurse & Health Ministry* (www.pmhs.org/parish-nurseprogram/educationand-resources.aspx).

An extra hospital visit with the patient or case manager may occur if: (a) the patient, caregiver, and case manager were not available during the initial visit; (b) a visit was requested by the patient, caregiver, or case manager; or (c) the patient has had complications necessitating a longer hospitalization. The faith community nurse's goal is to develop a working relationship with patient, caregiver, and hospital staff/case manager prior to discharge and to educate all regarding their role.

Post discharge The faith community nurse's goal in this phase is to be approachable and available. Soon after discharge (24–72 hours), **a second visit** is made in the patient's home setting. The visit includes (a) whole person assessment, which includes spiritual; (b) appropriate referrals; (c) screening (vitals); (d) disease education; (e) medication reconciliation; (f) self-care training; and (g) safety assessments. Based on the assessment, the faith community nurse will plan contacts and home visits with the goal to transition the patient to self-care or caregiver within 30–60 days.

In addition to the role of the faith community nurse, faith community volunteers can provide services in the post discharge phase. The faith community nurse and the faith community develop a team of volunteers and a plan focused on the needs of the patient. The use of volunteers extends the care being provided by the faith community nurse. The types of support that can be provided by faith community volunteers are:

- Friendly visits (in person or by phone)
- Cards or notes of encouragement
- Light yard work or minor repairs
- Transportation*
- Meals*.

*The author suggests that services such as transportation and meals are an important resource right after discharge. The faith community nurse should look for sustainable county support for patients. Information regarding the tools for developing and sustaining a volunteer ministry can be purchased through Amazon.

The third visit is made when the faith community nurse accompanies the patient and caregiver to their first post-hospitalization visit to the doctor. The faith community nurse attends the first visit with the patient to the doctor for the purpose of: (a) ensuring that the visit occurs; (b) introducing self and the faith community nurse role to the doctor and clinic staff; (c) facilitating information exchange between patient, caregiver(s), and healthcare provider; and (d) making sure that the patient and caregiver are fully engaged and participate in healthcare decisions. Visitation guidelines can be purchased through Amazon.

Additional home visits with the patient and caregiver may occur to continue the nursing plan of care, or are based on assessment and patient's need. In addition, telephone check-ins may occur. The faith community nurse may need to provide care coordination and advocate on behalf of the patient to set up services, change medications, access care, and so forth. The duration of transitional services generally will not exceed 60 days.

22.6   Faith Community Nurse Transitional Care Course

The aim of the *Faith Community Nurse Transitional Care Course* is to provide practical education and resources that will equip faith community for transitional care practice (Ziebarth & Campbell, 2014). The goals of the course are to: (a) use faith community nurses and faith communities together to provide transitional care; (b) enhance patient discharge experience from hospital to home; (c) engage patients in their care; therefore, increasing self-efficacy and positive health outcomes; (d) eliminate unnecessary hospital admissions; and (e) encourage collaboration and shared visioning between health care institutions and faith communities. In the course, the *Faith Community Nurse Transitional Care Model* (Ziebarth & Campbell, 2016) is used to describe a systematic approach to transitional care. Four standards from the *Faith Community Nursing: Scope and Standards of Practice* (American Nurses Association and Health Ministries Association, 2017) are reviewed. The standards reviewed in the course are: (a) Leadership Standard 12; (b) Communication Standard 11; (c) Collaboration Standard 13; and (d) Coordination of Care Standard 5A. These four standards (Leadership, Communication, Collaboration, and Coordination of Care) represent characteristics and skills necessary to perform transitional care interventions.

22.7 Transitional Care Research Using Faith Community Nurses

There are four studies that have tested the *Faith Community Nurse Transitional Care Model* and more are planned. Qualitative descriptive design was used in three of the four studies to collect and analyze nursing interventions from faith community nursing documentation (Ziebarth, 2016; Ziebarth et al., 2018). A qualitative descriptive design is often used first in order to provide evidence that certain variables exist and that there is construct validity (agreement). A construct must first be defined before it can be controlled, practiced, or taught (Clark & Lang, 1992). Naming transitional care interventions performed by faith community nurses was the first step towards understanding the impact and implications. The fourth study used a quantitative method. Ahn, Lee, Munning, Ziebarth, and Campbell (2017) used a propensity score matching analysis.

A fifth study employed a mixed method is planned using an experimental design with randomized assignment and a correlational design between the treatments of the faith community nurse to that of another transitional care intervention, *Boost* (Joynt & Jha, 2013). This study is designed to collect dependent variables of hospital readmissions and emergency department visits. Even though this study is not complete, the preliminary results look promising in regard to using faith community nursing as a transitional care intervention.

Study One: Transitional Care Interventions as Implemented by Faith Community Nurses (Ziebarth, 2016)
The setting of the first study was an acute care hospital located in central Florida that employed three faith community nurses practicing in local faith communities. Each faith community nurse attended both the *Faith Community Nurse Foundation's Course* and the *Faith Community Nurse Transitional Care Course*. The faith community nurses were prepared to use the Henry Ford Macomb's electronic documentation tool (Girard, 2013) to capture nursing interventions using the *Nursing Intervention Classification* format. The NIC has been tested in all nursing

specialties including acute care, intensive care units, home care, hospice care, long-term care, and primary care. It has also been tested in the specialty area of faith community nursing (Burkhart & Androwich, 2004; Burkhart, Konicek, Moorhead, & Androwich, 2005; Solari-Twadell & Hackbarth, 2010; Weis, Schank, Coenen, & Matheus, 2002; Ziebarth, 2016).

The 554 interventions in Nursing Intervention Classification System (6th ed.) are grouped into 30 classes and 7 domains for ease of use. A NIC Class contains a standardized group of interventions representing various nursing activities. A few interventions are located in more than one Class but each has a unique numeric code that represents the primary Class.

Church Health, which houses the *Westberg Institute* created a "business associate" contract with the employing hospital for this study to collect faith community nursing documentation. The *Privacy Rule* portion of the *Health Insurance Portability and Accountability Act* (HIPAA) of 1996 defines a "business associate" as a person or entity that performs certain functions or activities that involve the use or disclosure of protected health information on behalf of, or provides services to, a covered entity (Blackstone, 2015; US Department of Health and Human Services, 2006). The rule requires that a covered entity obtain satisfactory assurance in writing in the form of a contract from their business associates of their commitment to appropriately safeguard Protected Health Information. The documentation had no patient identifiers.

This study consisted of two phases:

- Phase 1 consisted of the collection of transitional care interventions documented by faith community nurses using the Nursing Intervention Classification System. In addition, nominal categorical analysis presented frequencies of the most often used nursing interventions in Nursing Intervention Classification System.
- Phase 2 consisted of the qualitative analysis of a focus group conducted with study participants (three faith community nurses) to ensure that the description of transitional care is comprehensive, well-developed, and validated.

To analyze the NIC interventions, the researcher worked with a computer programmer to develop a Microsoft Excel® software program, currently referred to as the *Nursing Intervention Classification Analysis Program* (Lane, 2015). This data management program was created specifically for the collection of NIC at the Domain, Class, and Intervention levels. The *Nursing Intervention Classification Analysis Program* provided the capacity to collect and organize large numbers of nursing interventions as coded by the NIC into a manageable database. In preparation for intervention collection, analysis, and translation, 554 non-duplicated nursing interventions (Bulechek, Butcher, Dochterman, & Wagner, 2013) and 91 duplications ($n = 645$) were manually entered into the *Nursing Intervention Classification Analysis Program*. Duplications occur in the NIC when interventions are repeated in more than one Class. Each nursing intervention in NIC entered had its own identifying numerical code ($n = 645$) and definition ($n = 554$). In addition, the 30 Classes and 7 Domains of nursing interventions were entered, along with definitions, and programed to align to nursing interventions. Even though the development was very time consuming, it proved useful in all three transitional care studies. All interventions that were documented electronically or by hand were entered into the *Nursing Intervention Classification Analysis Program*.

Results. A total of 73 nursing documentation records were collected representing 73 faith community nursing patient visits over a 3 month period. This represented faith community nurse visits either in person or by phone. Each visit averaged three nursing interventions. Each standardized nursing intervention represented up to 100 possible activities (Bulechek et al., 2013). Only standardized nursing interventions, Classes and Domains were used to describe transitional care as provided by faith community nurses. Out of the 554 possible nursing interventions in the NIC, 52 (10.6%) were reported to have been used at least once with a total of 210 interventions documented over a 3 month period.

The 26 most frequently recorded interventions by faith community nurses were Emotional Support, Spiritual Support, Active Listening, Medication Management, Health Education, Fall Prevention, Listening Visits, Telephone Follow-up, Coping Enhancement, Decision-Making Support, Learning Facilitation, Teaching: Individual, Caregiver Support, Family Support, Telephone Consultation, Pain Management, Environmental Management: Comfort, Socialization Enhancement, Anticipatory Guidance, Hope Instillation, Listening Visits. In phase two of the study, a focus group of participants confirmed these interventions to be core, important, and intentional to providing transitional care. Focusing on the most frequent *Nursing Intervention Classification System* interventions is consistent with recommendations from the Iowa Intervention Project Research Team and suggests a list of core interventions of any specialty be less than 30 (Tripp-Reimer, Woodworth, McCloskey, & Bulechek, 1996).

Eight of the nursing interventions represented 73% (*n* = 155) of the 210 interventions documented by faith community nurses. The eight interventions were Emotional Support, Spiritual Support, Active Listening, Medication Management, Health Education, and Fall Prevention. The researcher found this frequency pattern of interventions to be of interest since many nursing interventions recorded by faith community nurses represented those recorded by advanced practice registered nurses in the previous studies (Naylor et al., 2004, 2011, 2012; Naylor & McCauley, 1999). In addition to these advanced practice registered nurse interventions, emotional and spiritual support interventions were also recorded by faith community nurses. The faith community nurses in the focus group stated that emotional and spiritual support interventions are "intentionally" performed at each visit.

This finding is important because the *Joint Commission on Accreditation of Healthcare Organizations* (2010), states that patients have specific characteristics and nonclinical needs that can affect the way they view, receive, and participate in health care. In addition, supporting patient's spiritual needs may help patients to cope with illness better (Paloutzian & Park, 2014).

This study initially only analyzed three months of faith community nursing transitional care interventions, but the researcher went on to collect and analyze an additional 15 months of documentation in the same setting and sample. The process was identical in that nominal categorical analysis presented frequencies of most often used nursing interventions in the NIC. The datum extraction yielded a mirrored and exhaustive frequency pattern of nursing interventions and description of the faith community nursing transitional care.

Study Two: Describing Transitional Care as Initiated by Faith Community Nurses: Using the Intervention Classification (Jasper Indiana) (Ziebarth et al., 2018; Ziebarth & Campbell, 2017, 2019)

This project was supported by both the *Church Health Congregational Care Transitions Project Grant* (2013–2018), and the *University of Memphis Fogelman College of Business and Economics* (Methodist Le Bonheur Center for Healthcare Economics) *Summer Healthcare Research Grant* (2017). The setting for this study was a community hospital in Jasper, Indiana. Just as in the first study, the faith community nurses who participated attended both the *Faith Community Nurse Foundation's Course* and the *Faith Community Nurse Transitional Care Course* and were trained to use the Henry Ford Macomb's electronic documentation tool to capture nursing interventions using the NIC format. The faith community nurses were hired through grant funding to provide transitional care. *Church Health* again had a "business associate" relationship with the hospital, and thus, was able to collect and de-identify all documents collected over a 2-year period prior to the researcher's analyses.

A total of 986 nurse documentation records were analyzed. The faith community nurses documented an average of 6.4 interventions for each patient visit. Occasionally, the visits included more than one person at a time ($n = 43$). A total of 1556 nursing interventions were documented.

Out of the 554 possible nursing interventions, 40 were reported to have been used with some frequency. Out of the 1556 interventions documented, a list of the 32 nursing interventions described the bulk of transitional care interventions provided. The most frequent Classes of interventions were Coping Assistance, Communication Enhancement, Patient Education, Information Management, Health System Mediation, Physical Comfort Promotion, Lifespan Care, Behavioral Therapy, Activity and Exercise Management, Cognitive Therapy, Tissue Perfusion Management, Self-Care Facilitation, Drug Management, Nutrition Support, and Community Health Promotion. The three Classes containing the most frequently reported interventions were Coping Assistance, Communication Enhancement, and Patient Education.

The NIC Domains contain the Classes in which nursing interventions are aligned. The interventions documented by faith community nurses were found in all seven Domains, although there was only one intervention documented in the Community Health Promotion Domain as expected. The majority of interventions used while the faith community nurses provided transitional care, belonged to the Behavioral Domain (1376) as had occurred in study one.

The Behavioral Domain is defined as care supporting psychosocial functioning and facilitates life-style changes. The Behavioral Domain includes Classes of interventions such as Coping Assistance, Communication Enhancement, and Patient

Education. The Class of Communication Enhancement was most often used with Patient Education and Coping Assistance also frequently used.

The second most prominent Domain represented by faith community nurses transitional care interventions was that of Health System, which is defined as care that supports effective use of the health care delivery system. The third domain identified as significant was Safety. The Safety Domain is care that supports protection against harm. The fourth prominent Domain was Physiological: Basic. Physiological: Basic is care that supports physical functioning. It contains the Classes of Physical Comfort Promotion and Nutrition Support. The Domain of Family was fifth and the Domain of Physiological: Complex was sixth.

Study Three: Transitional Care Provided by a Faith Community Nurse (DeSoto, Mississippi)
This research study is supported by both the Church Health Congregational Care Transitions Project Grant (2015–2018) and the Baptist Memorial Hospital—DeSoto Foundation Grant. Data has been collected and analyzed. The plan is to publish the results with permission from the funders.

Study Four: A Faith-Based Community Nurse Care Transition Pilot Program: A Propensity Score Matching Analysis Results (Jasper, Indiana) (Ahn et al., 2017)
This project was supported by *Church Health*, the Congregational Care Transitions Project Grant (2013–2018), and the University of Memphis Fogelman College of Business and Economics (Methodist Le Bonheur Center for Healthcare Economics) Summer Healthcare Research Grant (2017). The goal statement in this project was to measure the effectiveness of faith community nurses on the likelihood of hospital readmission and length of stay in 30, 90, and 180 days after discharge compared to a non-faith community nursing group. The method used was two groups (faith community nurses vs. non-faith community nurses) with a pre-and multiple post-tests design. The results yielded a propensity score 0.1% reduction in Length of Stay from 19.3% to 19.2%. Assuming an average hospital stay as $2000 per day in Indiana, the results are significant. It can be estimated that the treatment provided by the faith community nurse saved the hospital more than $120,000 without considering any benefit from Emergency Department visit reduction. This study is the first quantitative study to evaluate the effectiveness of faith community nursing on hospital utilization and was considered to be a pilot. The next qualitative study planned will address scalability to a larger hospital and population, while blindly randomizing to two treatments (faith community nurse and Boost). The data will be collected over a two year period. The hope is that faith community nursing will be cataloged as one of the effective care transition programs and that there will be clear documentation of how it can be developed, implemented, and evaluated when collaborating with local organizations such as a hospital and a faith community.

22.8   Conclusion

Transitional care is provided by faith community nurses. A faith community nurse model has been developed. Faith community nurse's documentation while providing transitional care has been collected, defined using and compared using the NIC. The model has been tested with the results showing that patients benefit and financial savings have been achieved for a health care organization. Testing of the model continues.

References

Ahn, S., Lee, J., Munning, S., Ziebarth, D., & Campbell, K. (2017). *A faith community nurse (FCN) care transition pilot program: A propensity score matching analysis*. Poster session presented at the APHA international conference, Atlanta.

American Nurses Association and Health Ministries Association. (2017). *Faith community nursing: Scope and standards of practice*. Silver Spring, MD: Nursesbooks.

Black, J. T., Romano, P. S., Sadeghi, B., Auerbach, A. D., Ganiats, T. G., Greenfield, S., et al. (2014). A remote monitoring and telephone nurse coaching intervention to reduce readmissions among patients with heart failure: study protocol for the Better Effectiveness After Transition-Heart Failure (BEAT-HF) randomized controlled trial. *Trials, 15*(1), 124.

Blackstone, S. W. (2015). *Issues and challenges in advancing effective patient-provider communication*. Patient provider communication: Roles for speech-language pathologists and other health care professionals (pp. 9–35).

Budnitz, D. S., Shehab, N., Kegler, S. R., & Richards, C. L. (2007). Medication use leading to emergency department visits for adverse drug events in older adults. *Annals of Internal Medicine, 147*(11), 755–765.

Bulechek, G. M., Butcher, H. K., Dochterman, J. M. M., & Wagner, C. (2013). *Nursing interventions classification (NIC)*. St. Louis, MO: Elsevier.

Burkhart, L., & Androwich, I. (2004). Measuring the domain completeness of the nursing interventions classification in parish nurse documentation. *Computers, Informatics, Nursing, 22,* 72–82.

Burkhart, L., Konicek, D., Moorhead, S., & Androwich, I. (2005). Mapping parish nurse documentation into the nursing interventions classifications: A research method. *Computers, Informatics, Nursing, 23,* 220–229.

Carthon, J. M. B., Lasater, K. B., Sloane, D. M., & Kutney-Lee, A. (2015). The quality of hospital work environments and missed nursing care is linked to heart failure readmissions: a cross-sectional study of US hospitals. *BMJ Quality & Safety, 24*(4), 255–263.

Cauchi, R. (2012). State health insurance mandates and the PPACA essential benefits provisions.

Centers for Medicare & Medicaid Services. (2015). *Readmissions reduction program*, November 16, 2015 update. https://www.cms.gov/Medicare/Medicare-Fee-for-Service-Payment/AcuteInpatientPPS/Readmissions-Reduction-Program.html

Clark, J., & Lang, N. (1992). Nursing's next advance: An internal classification for nursing practice. *International Nursing Review, 39*(4), 109–111.

Cutler, D. M., Davis, K., & Stremikis, K. (2010). The impact of health reform on health system spending. *Issue Brief (Common Wealth Fund), 88,* 1–14.

Frank, M. G. (2008). Medication use leading to emergency department visits for adverse drug events in older adults. *The Journal of Emergency Medicine, 35*(2), 229.

Gage, B., Ingber, M., Smith, L., Deutsch, A., Kline, T., Dever, J., et al. (2012). Post-acute care payment reform demonstration: Final report volume 4 of 4.

Girard, S. (2013). Henry Ford Macomb's faith community health program is in the national spotlight. *Macomb News*.

Hennessey, B., Suter, P., & Harrison, G. (2010). The home-based chronic care model: A platform for partnership for the provision of a patient-centered medical home. *Caring: National Association for Home Care Magazine, 29*(2), 18–24.

Jack, B. W., Chetty, V. K., Anthony, D., Greenwald, J. L., Sanchez, G. M., Johnson, A. E., et al. (2009). A reengineered hospital discharge program to decrease rehospitalization. *Internal Medicine, 150*(3), 178–187.

Jacob, S. (Ed.). (2014). *Foundations of faith community nursing* (3rd ed.). Memphis, TN: Church Health Center.

James, J. (2013). Medicare hospital readmissions reduction program. *Health Affairs, 34*(2), 1–5.

Joynt, K. E., & Jha, A. K. (2013). Characteristics of hospitals receiving penalties under the Hospital Readmissions Reduction Program. *JAMA, 309*(4), 342–343.

Joynt, K. E., Orav, E. J., & Jha, A. K. (2011). Thirty-day readmission rates for Medicare beneficiaries by race and site of care. *Journal of the American Medical Association, 305*(7), 675–681.

King, M. A., & Pappas-Rogich, M. (2011). Faith community nurses: Implementing healthy people standards to promote the health of elderly clients. *Geriatric Nursing, 32*(6), 459–464.

Lane, M. (2015). Nursing intervention classification analysis program. In D. Ziebarth, *Transitional care interventions as implemented by faith community nurses* (Doctoral dissertation, The University of Wisconsin-Milwaukee).

Linden, A., & Butterworth, S. W. (2014). A comprehensive hospital-based intervention to reduce readmissions for chronically ill patients: A randomized controlled trial. *The American Journal of Managed Care, 20*(10), 783–792.

Lipstein, S. H., & Dunagan, W. C. (2014). The risks of not adjusting performance measures for sociodemographic factors. *Annals of Internal Medicine, 161*(8), 594–596.

Manderson, B., Mcmurray, J., Piraino, E., & Stolee, P. (2012). Navigation roles support chronically ill older adults through healthcare transitions: A systematic review of the literature. *Health & Social Care in the Community, 20*(2), 113–127.

Marek, K. D., Adams, S. J., Stetzer, F., Popejoy, L., & Rantz, M. (2010). The relationship of community-based nurse care coordination to costs in the Medicare and Medicaid programs. *Research in Nursing & Health, 33*(3), 235–242.

McHugh, M. D., Berez, J., & Small, D. S. (2013). Hospitals with higher nurse staffing had lower odds of readmissions penalties than hospitals with lower staffing. *Health Affairs, 32*(10), 1740–1747.

Morales-Asencio, J. M., Martin-Santos, F. J., Morilla-Herrera, J. C., Fernández-Gallego, M. C., Celdrán-Mañas, M., Navarro-Moya, F. J., et al. (2010). Design of a case management model for people with chronic disease (Heart Failure and COPD). Phase I: Modeling and identification of the main components of the intervention through their actors: Patients and professionals (DELTA-icE-PRO Study). *BMC Health Services Research, 10*(1), 324.

Nakazawa, K. R., Egorova, N. N., Power, J. R., Faries, P. L., & Vouyouka, A. G. (2017). The impact of Surgical Care Improvement Project measures on in-hospital outcomes following elective vascular procedures. *Annals of Vascular Surgery, 38*, 17–28.

Naylor, M., Brooten, D., Campbell, R., Maislin, G., McCauley, M., & Schwartz, S. (2004). Transitional care of older adults hospitalized with heart failure: A randomized, controlled trial. *Journal of the American Geriatrics Society, 52*, 675–684.

Naylor, M. D., Aiken, L. H., Kurtzman, E. T., Olds, D. M., & Hirschman, K. B. (2011). The importance of transitional care in achieving health reform. *Health Affairs, 30*(4), 746754.

Naylor, M. D., Kurtzman, E. T., Grabowski, D. C., Harrington, C., McClellan, M., & Reinhard, S. C. (2012). Unintended consequences of steps to cut readmissions and reform payment may threaten care of vulnerable older adults. *Health Affairs, 31*(7), 1623–1632.

Naylor, M. D., & McCauley, K. M. (1999). The effects of a discharge planning and home follow-up intervention on elders hospitalized with common medical and surgical cardiac conditions. *The Journal of Cardiovascular Nursing, 14*(1), 44–54.

Paloutzian, R. F., & Park, C. L. (Eds.). (2014). *Handbook of the psychology of religion and spirituality*. New York, NY: Guilford Publications.

Piraino, E., Heckman, G., Glenny, C., & Stolee, P. (2012). Transitional care programs: Who is left behind? A systematic review. *International Journal of Integrated Care, 12*.

Rydholm, L. (1997). Patient-focused care in parish nursing. *Holistic Nursing Practice, 11*(3), 47–60.

Rydholm, L., & Thornquist, L. (2005). *Supporting seniors across systems: effectiveness of parish nurse interventions*.

Sehgal, V., Bajwa, S. J. S., Sehgal, R., Bajaj, A., Khaira, U., & Kresse, V. (2013). Polypharmacy and potentially inappropriate medication use as the precipitating factor in readmissions to the hospital. *Journal of Family Medicine and Primary Care, 2*(2), 194.

Solari-Twadell, P. A., & Hackbarth, D. P. (2010). Evidence for a new paradigm of the ministry of parish nursing practice using the nursing intervention classification system. *Nursing Outlook, 58*(2), 69–75.

Tripp-Reimer, T., Woodworth, G., McCloskey, J. C., & Bulechek, G. (1996). The dimensional structure of nursing interventions. *Nursing Research, 45*(1), 10–17.

US Department of Health and Human Services. (2006). Office for civil rights. 2003. HIPAA administrative simplification: Regulation text: 45 CFR Parts 160, 162, and 164 (Unofficial version, as amended through February 16, 2006).

Weis, D. M., Schank, M. J., Coenen, A., & Matheus, R. (2002). Parish nurse practice with client aggregates. *Journal of Community Health Nursing, 19*(2), 105–113.

Yeaworth, R. C., & Sailors, R. (2014). Faith community nursing: Real care, real cost savings. *Journal of Christian Nursing, 31*(3), 178–183.

Ziebarth, D. (2014). Evolutionary conceptual analysis: Faith community nursing. *Journal of Religion and Health, 53*(6), 1817–1835.

Ziebarth, D. (2015). Factors that lead to hospital readmissions and interventions that reduce them: Moving toward a faith community nursing intervention. *Journal of Faith Community Nursing 1*(1), 1. http://digitalcommons.wku.edu/ijfcn/vol1/iss1/1

Ziebarth, D. (2016). *Transitional care interventions as implemented by faith community nurses* (Doctoral dissertation, The University of Wisconsin-Milwaukee).

Ziebarth, D. (2017). *Visitation guidelines for faith community nurses*. https://www.amazon.com/Visitation-Guidelines-Faith-Community-Nurses/dp/1546311459

Ziebarth, D., & Campbell, K. (2014). *Faith community nurse transitional care curriculum*. Memphis, TN: Church Health Center.

Ziebarth, D., & Campbell, K. (2015). *Faith community nursing transitional care model in Faith community nurse transitional care curriculum*. Memphis, TN: Church Health Center.

Ziebarth, D., Campbell, K., Ahn, S., Munning, S., & Owens, L. (2018). *FCN transitional care*. In Poster session presented at the Westberg conference, Memphis.

Ziebarth, D., & Campbell, K. P. (2016). A transitional care model using faith community nurses. *Journal of Christian Nursing, 33*(2), 112–118.

Ziebarth, D., & Campbell, K. P. (2017). FCN transitional care. In *APHA international conference*, Atlanta.

Ziebarth, D. J., & Campbell, K. (2019). Describing transitional care using the nursing intervention classification: Faith community nursing. *International Journal of Faith Community Nursing, 5*(1), 20.

Integration of Faith Community Nursing into Health Care Systems: Stimulating Community-Based Quality Care Strategies

23

P. Ann Solari-Twadell and Ameldia R. Brown

23.1 Faith Community Nursing and Health Care Reform

The topic of health care reform can seem nebulous and beyond the reach of faith community nurses. Often, it is not clear exactly what "health care reform" really means or entails. The subject seems to be the work of policy makers, elected officials, Chief Executive Officers of health systems, and health care organizations. These are individuals and groups that also seem to be far away from the faith community-based health promotion, disease prevention spiritual care offerings of a faith community nurse. Yet the core values of faith community nursing include "Community: fostering new and creative responses to health and wellness in partnership with other community health resources" (American Nurses Association and Health Ministry Association, 2017, p. 4). Going further into the *Faith Community Nursing Scope and Standards of Practice,* Provision 7: "The nurse in all roles and settings, advances the profession through research and scholarly inquiry, professional standard development and the generation of both nursing and health policy" (p. 21); Provision 8: "The nurse collaborates with other professionals and the public to protect and promote human rights, health diplomacy and health initiatives" (p. 22); and Provision 9: The profession of nursing collectively through its professional organizations must articulate nursing values, maintain the

The authors appreciate the contribution of Ronette Sailors, Alegent Health, and Barbara Williams, Henry Ford Health System, Macomb in contributing to the content of this chapter.

P. A. Solari-Twadell (✉)
Marcella Niehoff School of Nursing, Loyola University Chicago, Chicago, IL, USA
e-mail: psolari@luc.edu

A. R. Brown
Department of Faith & Community Health, Henry Ford Macomb Hospitals, Henry Ford Health System, Clinton, MI, USA
e-mail: abrown1@hfhs.org

© Springer Nature Switzerland AG 2020
P. A. Solari-Twadell, D. J. Ziebarth (eds.), *Faith Community Nursing*,
https://doi.org/10.1007/978-3-030-16126-2_23

integrity of the profession, and integrate principles of social justice into nursing and health policy (p. 23). There clearly is a "call" for the faith community nurse to expand the boundaries of the faith community and engage in creative solutions. Working through professional organizations, promoting changes, and engaging in the development of health policy will support constructive change in the delivery of health care.

National research completed in 2002 using a convenience sample of 2330 faith community nurses who had completed the basic preparation course yielded a 54% return rate of 1161 faith community nurse respondents. The results of this study reflected that only 17% (*n* = 198) of respondents were members of the *American Nurses Association* and State nursing Organizations while a smaller percent [13% (*n* = 151)] were members of the *Health Ministry Association*; the results of this research demonstrated that most respondents had no affiliation with any professional nursing organizations (Solari-Twadell, 2002). However, in reviewing the work of the *Health Ministry Association* and the *Faith Community Nurses International*, neither organization appears to have a committee or platform that would engage faith community nurses in political advocacy. In some respects, lack of membership in a professional organization is understandable as many faith community nurses are not being paid and belonging to a professional nursing organization costs money. However, there is a stronger sense that the majority of faith community nurses are not "joiners." Faith community nurses are focused on their work at a local level. Their time is filled with establishing relationships in their congregations and collaborations with other agencies in the community. There seems little time or energy to consider the broader picture of health care or the nuances of health care reform. Yet, the commitment to the profession "calls" each faith community nurse to reflect on the larger picture. What does the work at the local level have to do with the larger scheme of health care or health care reform? In the view of the authors, work being done in faith communities by faith community nurses is a definite part of the solution in the work of health care reform.

23.2 Steps to Engaging in Health Care Reform

Sustainability of Faith Community Nursing Programs This subject is discussed in depth in Chapter 20 of this book. However, just to reiterate, the time, attention, and dedication to keeping abreast of health care reform is not a likely possibility if all the time and attention of the faith community nurse are needed to ensure the sustainability of the faith community nursing program. If the identified stakeholders of the program have little recognition of the value, contribution and outcomes of the program, there is less likelihood that it will maintain continued ongoing integration, meaningful collaboration and funding. The faith community nurse then spends valuable energy in trying to ensure that others understand and that the program will be continued. Long-term sustainability, support, and strategic partnerships are significant to engaging in creative thinking, financing, integration, and attention to advocacy as well as health care policy related to the integration of faith community nursing. If the value of faith community nursing is recognized externally through national organizations, statewide initiatives, and local community organizations, there may then be more effort put into nurturing and sustaining this community-based service offered through faith communities.

Translating Value from Faith Community Nursing Language to Outcomes and Cost Language Understood by Health Care The most important ingredient in communicating value is documentation as noted in Chapter 19 and reiterated throughout this book. More specifically, standardized documentation that is managed through an electronic data system, that make outcomes easily accessible to health care systems, and uses language to which stakeholders are accustomed is essential to communicating the effectiveness of faith community nurses. This process is most successful when a standardized language such a *North American Nursing Diagnosis Association* (NANDA), *Nursing Intervention Classification* (NIC) and *Nursing Outcome Classification* (NOC) are used by faith community nurses in documenting patient care and outcomes. Additionally, it is important that this information is not only provided to the health system, but also published in journals and presented at national conferences such as those sponsored by the American Hospital Association, Catholic Hospital Association, and other organizations invested in cost-effective health care reform that engage various health providers and health care administrators. If you are saying that this ability to report effective outcomes requires collaboration and support, you are correct. Thus, basic to this strategy is the faith community nurse being connected through a structured partnership with a health care system or well-supported faith community nursing regional network.

As **Health Care Systems identify value in faith community nursing, all departments of the health care system become integrated with faith community nursing services and the faith community nursing network grows**. Once the value of faith community nursing is established within a health care system, the faith community nursing network becomes an important strategy for prevention of hospital readmission, reducing key lab values which indicate ongoing pathology, reduction in weight, fewer hospital admissions, and increased quality of life. These outcomes and measures provide impetus for all departments in the health system and member hospitals to understand the imperative to support this program. Faith community nursing has the potential to be a value-added collaboration for the Chaplains and cancer care departments, advance care planning, community outreach, and other disease-specific initiatives of the organization. Once this integration occurs, its successes communicate a very strong message of its power, cost effectiveness to health policy officials locally and nationally. However, foundational to this strategy is an astute, well-prepared *Faith Community Nurse Coordinator* position that is salaried by the health care system. The *Faith Community Nurse Coordinator* has a unique set of skills. The skillset includes, in addition to other leadership skills, knowledge and experience that understands the nature of the work of the faith community nurse, support necessary to the success of the faith community nurse, and the sustaining of the faith community nurse program through the faith community. This is a nurse who has a unique skill set, experience bank, and strong ongoing faith experience.

Spread the Message Boldly. That was one characteristic that Rev Granger Westberg did very well. In the early days of parish nursing where there were six nurses working in six congregations, he told the story as though this innovative strategy was well integrated and the most important ingredient to linking not only faith and health, but to resurrect the faith communities role in health and create "uncanny" community-based partnerships that had the potential to impact the delivery of health care service no matter what denomination, location, or resources. Westberg carried the message with vigor, spirit, certainty, and conviction that attracted those who felt "called" to blend their faith and work life, make a difference in the health and well-being of their constituents and create a new paradigm for the delivery of health promotion, disease prevention. One, Westberg had a clear vision, and two, he acted as though it was already a reality. "Act as if" was a strong mantra in his everyday life.

More exemplars exist today that can relate powerful stories of how lives are being changed, health improved, and disease curbed. The following are but a few.

Exemplar 1. Bridging Faith Community Nursing and Ambulatory Care Services Through an Evidence-Based Education Program—Diabetes Prevention Program (DPP)

The Henry Ford Macomb Hospital (HFMH) Faith Community Nursing Network (FCNN) of Henry Ford Health System (HFHS) is a part of its Faith and Community Health (F&CH) department. Established in November 1994, it has had many opportunities to collaborate with the community partners to promote and improve the health of the community. Integrating this work with the acute side of health care and across the health care continuum has been difficult over the past decades. The most penetrating strategy incorporated into the work of the HFMH FCNN has been the collaborative development and implementation of the Henry Ford Macomb Hospital (HFMH)/American Medical Association (AMA)/EPIC Prediabetes and Hypertension Registry. This one year project has made collegiality among faith community nurses, Ambulatory Clinicians, and the community an everyday experience in Macomb County Michigan. A major gap in services for patients with prediabetes has been filled by the connection of primary care providers with Center for Disease Control (CDC) sanctioned evidence-based classes [Diabetes Prevention Program (DPP) classes] in familiar, culturally sensitive community settings.

The registry identifies patients who meet risk test or lab test criteria for prediabetes. It alerts the medical providers to evaluate and refer appropriate patients to the Faith and Community Health Department for further information and registration of the patient in DPP classes. Patients with pending clinic visits are sent the American Diabetes Association prediabetes survey to complete and bring with them to the next visit. Clinic staff are alerted to assist patients who forget to bring the surveys or did not complete them and make them available to the provider in the exam room. HFMH employed physicians and providers were targeted for this pilot. With support from the Ambulatory Service Chief, the quality practice nurse, and the American Medical Association the registry was developed, 37 providers engaged and educated, 11 office staff groups oriented and tutored on registry use. The project was seen as quality improvement, rather than research. The HFM Internet Technology Department maintained communications with EPIC and American Medical Association staff as needed and remained flexible for changes and improvements after the initial "Go Live." Faith and Community Health Department staff had to learn to receive referrals and run reports in EPIC. Processes to assure timely responses to referrals and timely class enrollment were created and instituted.

As the work on the registry proceeded, the Center for Disease Control Diabetes Prevention Recognition Program (DPRP) was developed. The 20 plus year partnerships with faith communities in the community at large formed a strong base on which to build. Faith community nurses and their teams were recruited to participate as coaches, host sites, and help recruit class participants. Many of the faith community nurses and their health ministries had years of experience with extended "diabetes self-management" classes. Making the shift to the Center for Disease Control prediabetes classes was less daunting than if there had been no previous experiences with the management of this disease. Coaches were educated and trained according to Center for Disease Control standards. The extensive documentation requirements of the DPRP were added to the HFM existing community electronic health record (EHR) allowing all coaches and coach assistants to document individual encounters while meeting and expediting Center for Disease Control, registry pilot, and health system quality measurement reporting.

Referrals from medical providers mushroomed from a six month baseline of 20 (June to December 2016, all methods except the registry) to 476 from March 15, 2017 to March 28, 2018 (the registry alone). Numerous tweaks in the process of gathering referral data and reporting capabilities were made during the pilot year. The challenge became providing enough coaches and classes to meet the demand. As referrals from the registry continued to rise each month, it became clear that there was not enough capacity to meet the needs. More financial resources were secured to continue to expand the number of coaches and classes (see Table 23.1). Each class represented the potential for 20 participants. One hundred percent of referring providers were notified via Electronic Health Record when their participant was enrolled in class. Referring providers were also given the option to request monthly or quarterly client reports from the DPP class.

Table 23.1 Diabetes prevention program class numbers—capacity expansion

	2015	2016	2017	2018
No. classes	2	13	8	11
No. new locations	2	11	2	6
No. coaches trained	9	10	11	20

Each year class participant outcomes improved. The July 2016 to June 2017 Center for Disease Control Diabetes Prevention Recognition Program, Diabetes Prevention Program quality review for HFHS showed that all quality measures were met except the average of 5–7% weight loss requirement for the aggregate data of the cohort (it was 4.8%). The HFHS Diabetes Prevention Recognition Program received designation of preliminary status in January 2018. In July 2018, the quality review for July 2017 to June 2018, posted compliance with all quality measures needed for designation of "full recognition" status (average weight loss of 5.9%). For July 2017 to June 2018, 77 (37%) of 207 registry enrolled participants were reviewed. Fifty-seven percent of the 77 ($n = 57$) qualified for Center for Disease Control review. Forty-three of the 57 participants were age 65 or older and over, with weight loss of 5% or more. Medicare began allowing Diabetes Prevention Recognition Programs to apply for designation as "suppliers" of Medicare Diabetes Prevention Programs (MDPP) gaining the privilege to apply for reimbursement for class participation. With a $460.00 maximum reimbursement for the first year per qualified participant, and these participants having met Medicare reimbursement eligibility during this time period, the participant outcomes demonstrated the *potential* for:

- new revenue (approximately $19,000.00 the first year);
- a $2670.00 (Center for Disease Control calculation) health insurer cost avoidance per participant who does not convert to diabetes for the first year post Diabetes Prevention Program class equaling a savings of $114,810.00 ($n = 43$);
- The American Dietetic Association cites an average cost of $7900 per year for diabetes care. By avoiding conversion to diabetes, approximately $339,700.00 ($n = 43$) is saved.

These income dollars and financial enticements combined with operational dollars towards Diabetes Prevention Programs, grants, and other incomes, and the favorable review of primary care providers helped the Henry Ford Macomb, Faith and Community Health Department to be viewed as a more attractive asset to the health care system than prior to the implementation of the registry. Staff was provided to support expansion from 8 new classes in 2017 to 20 new classes in 2018 and a goal of 26–30 new classes in 2019.

Using a care team model established the faith community nurse as an essential component for successful patient outcomes for ambulatory services, insurers, patients, and the community. Thirty-seven providers were targeted for engagement to use the registry during the first year of the registry pilot. Great success was attained. Provider engagement went from 7 to 26. Even more impressive was the realization, although not targeted with publicity and clinic education, 26 non-pilot providers found and used the registry to refer patients, 3 of whom are among the top 10 referrers. A total of 66 physician/providers were engaged in this community/ health system effort! By broadening the community-based connections through faith communities and faith community nurses in partnership with the resources of the health system, the Diabetes Prevention Program classes in collaboration with the primary care providers and patient-centered medical homes resulted in ambulatory clinic patient care outcome measures achieving a significant improvement. Not only were the outcome measures improved, but the participants received ongoing information and support in a faith community where they are more familiar with the context, more likely to attend regularly, and work on managing their diabetes with a person who is known—the faith community nurse.

In summary, faith community nurses, faith community nurse coordinators, and administrators value the partnership and ongoing collaboration in sustaining the ministry of faith community nursing. In order for others to value faith community nursing enough to finance, the services must be shown to benefit:

(a) community members,
(b) the health care institution,
(c) insurers,
(d) health care providers,

in multiple settings, and across the health care continuum from community through acute care, and back home to self-care; fully integrated. Exemplars like this one demonstrate faith community nursing to be "vital partners in advancing the nation's health initiatives" such as the fight against the prediabetes epidemic (ANA, 2012, p 17). The reform of health care must include culturally sensitive whole person elements that are found immersed in the scope and standards of practice exemplified by faith community nurse. Projects like the Diabetes Prevention Program can become vehicles and targets lessons for health care providers to identify and use the power of partnership and collaboration. Over time, partnering, collaborating, and leading in projects of this type will elevate the value of faith community nursing to health care administrators, policy makers, and the American public if the stories are told in language that is digestible to each party. There is great opportunity to enhance the potential for faith community nursing networks to substantially contribute to community and population health and thereby promote sustainability for this specialty practice through local endeavors.

Exemplar 2. Alegent Creighton Health Network, Faith Community Nursing Network, Omaha, Nebraska Community-Based Outcomes
Alegent Creighton Health initiated a Faith Community Nursing Network through a grant from Alelgent Health Community Benefit Trust in 2005. Beginning with only five nurses the current numbers of faith communities include 55, with 84 faith community nurses serving these faith communities (Yeaworth & Sailors, 2014, p 180). The following are two community-based programs where collaboration with faith communities and faith community nurses are aimed at prevention and ultimate cost avoidance for the health care system, clients, and other payers.

Through partnering with the American Cancer Society and the Great Plains Colon Cancer Task Force the Faith Community Nursing Network distributes Fecal Occult Blood Test kits to partnering congregations and the community at large. This program is aimed at the *Healthy People 2020* goal to increase the number of people who are appropriately screened for colon cancer. Evaluation of this effort resulted in 517 Fecal Occult Blood Testing kits being distributed by 36 faith communities. Out of the 517 Fecal Occult Blood Testing kits distributed 452 were returned for screening. This resulted in an 87% return rate for the Faith Community Nurse Network. In comparison, the average return rate is 45–50% when distributed to the general community. Through relationships faith community nurses have with their constituent faith community members, the faith community nurses were able to encourage a higher utilization of occult blood screening. A regional comparison reported a total of 918 screenings in this area. The number of screenings completed by faith community nurses was 56% of the total persons screened. This screening is significant to early detection of colon cancer. Because of the support of faith community (sponsorship) and faith community nursing (follow-through) more individuals were able to be good stewards of their health by insuring colon health through screening. This screening did not require a trip, other than to a place the participants go to regularly, their faith community.

Tai Chi is an ancient practice that is known for enhancing balance and reducing the risk of falls in up to 50% in those over age 60, if practiced regularly. *Supporting Tai Chi for Balance*, a local organization that trains tai chi instructors for teaching tai chi classes in the community, partnered with Alegent Health to address a priority that was identified through a Community Health Needs Assessment completed by the Alegent Health System in collaboration with the community. This opportunity for participation in the Tai Chi Classes was promoted through the Faith Community Nursing Network. In addition, referral pathways have been built into the Epic Electronic Medical Record so that care providers can refer clients who are identified at increased risk for falls. The results of this program included more than 80 class locations in Omaha and surrounding areas, with over 2500 participants. The pre-post balance assessments noted a 44.2% improvement in "Sit to Stand," 97.6% improvement in "Single Limb Stand," and 53.7% improvement in "Single Limb Stand Eyes Closed."

Exemplar 3. Faith Community Nurse Compliance as Provider of Diabetes Transitional Care Program

Another example from the state of Michigan which demonstrates the valuable role faith community nurses can provide in administering community-based programming complying with stated protocols addresses diabetes. Diabetes is a major health problem in Macomb County, MI. From 2011 to 2013 diabetes was the seventh leading cause of preventable hospitalizations, and 8.5% of the county's population was diagnosed with this disease. Nurses at a clinic in Macomb County developed and implemented a transitional care program to address this health concern. The clinic, which is nurse managed, is affiliated with a health system. Nurse practitioners developed the program and faith community nurses implemented it. The program, which was initiated in 2014 and had 30 participants, had not been evaluated formally. A process evaluation was conducted in 2016 to determine how well faith community nurses adhered to the program's protocol.

A provision of the Affordable Care Act mandated changes in the U.S. health system. These changes included using transitional care programs, which are interventions that promote coordination and continuity of care for patients (Centers for Medicare and Medicaid Services, 2014). The diabetes transitional care program at the nurse-managed clinic sought to improve clients' lives by using the science and art of nursing to teach them self-management of their disease.

Process evaluation, which is a subset of program evaluation, is concerned with the extent to which planned activities are implemented. This evaluation method helps to determine if the program is proceeding as planned, and includes procedures and other aspects of the implementation process. This method provides data about program fidelity, that is, the extent to which the program runs as it was intended to by its creators. When programs are not implemented with fidelity, it is difficult to determine if unexpected outcomes are due to the program design or to implementation. Linking measures to program outcomes can provide information to stakeholders and support the adoption of evidence-based programs (Centers for Disease Control and Prevention and Program Performance and Evaluation Office, 2012; Fink, 2015; Gifford, Wells, Bai, & Malone, 2015).

This process evaluation was conducted by collecting data through reviewing documentation in 30 clients' charts and by having the faith community nurses complete surveys. Charts were reviewed for 13 items. Documentation was found in 50% of the charts for one item, 11% of the charts for a second item, and 20% of the charts for a third item; however, for the remaining ten protocol items, documentation was found in 93.3–100% of the charts. Four nurses completed the surveys; three of them rated themselves as completing the steps of the protocol always or most of the time. The aim of the evaluation was to determine how well faith community nurses adhered to the diabetes transitional care program protocol. Prior to conducting the process evaluation the evaluator expected to discover that the nurses adhered to the protocol most of the time. The chart review and survey data revealed that the nurses did adhere to the protocol most of the time.

Limitations to the process evaluation was the number of clients served ($n = 30$ clients enrolled) and the limited number of faith community nurses ($n = 4$) implementing the program. In addition, clients were in the program for different lengths of time. The important facet of this evaluation process was to be able to document that the faith community nurse is conscientious in following the necessary directives to ensure that the intended process is followed ensuring better outcomes for the client being served. The process evaluation of the diabetes transitional care program at a nurse-managed clinic revealed that the faith community nurses adhered to the protocol most of the time. As with many programs, contextual issues impacted the results and, thus, support the necessity for a formal evaluation of these community-based programs. This evaluation data contributed to a summative evaluation and assisted the health system leaders in determining the sustainability of the program and the valued contribution of the faith community nurse.

23.3 Summary

The maturation of the faith community nurse role mandates inclusion of advocating for access to quality health care. All faith community nurses are urged to identify who are the policy makers that have a mindset consistent with faith community nursing, are open to being educated on the valuable contribution the faith community nurse can make in preventing and reducing health care costs. Once these, leaders, legislators, and policy makers are identified, make time to visit them. Bring to that visit pertinent literature that can be left for them to review at a later time. This literature should be current, address a difference that was made through partnership with a faith community nursing program, and reflect interdisciplinary collaboration with potential cost savings. Yes, this takes courage, time, and preparation. However, this effort could make a big difference long term in the thinking and contribution of that policy maker. Another lobbying effort is that of encouraging reimbursement systems to take notice and address creative ways in which faith community nurses can be included in current payment systems.

However ambitious this all sounds, it will not be possible until all faith community nurses, the faith communities they serve, and their collaborating health care systems systems, faith community professional organizations believe and invest in the vision of faith community nursing being part of the solution of making prevention and health care services more available ensuring quality outcomes. This is an important ingredient to faith community nursing being recognized as part of the solution to increased access to care, availability of prevention and health promotion activities for all, and ultimately a healthier community.

References

American Nurses Association and Health Ministries Association. (2012). *Faith community nursing: Scope and standards of practice* (2nd ed.). Silver Springs, MD: Nursebooks.org.

American Nurses Association and Health Ministry Association. (2017). *Faith community nursing: Scope and standards of practice* (3rd ed.). Silver Springs, MD: Nursebooks.org.

Centers for Disease Control and Prevention, Program Performance and Evaluation Office. (2012). *Introduction: What is program evaluation?* https://www.cdc.gov/eval/guide/introduction/

Centers for Medicare & Medicaid Services. (2014). *Readmissions reduction program.* www.cms.gov

Fink, A. (2015). *Program evaluation: A prelude. Evaluation Fundamentals, insights into program effectiveness, quality, and value.* Los Angeles, CA: Sage.

Gifford, E. J., Wells, R. S., Bai, Y., & Malone, P. S. (2015). Is implementation fidelity associated with improved access to care in a school-based child and family team model? *Evaluation and Program Planning, 49,* 41–49.

Solari-Twadell, P. A. (2002). The differentiation of the ministry of parish nursing practice within congregations. *Dissertation Abstracts International, 63*(06), 569A. UMI NO.3056442.

Yeaworth, R. C., & Sailors, R. (2014). Faith community nursing: real care, real cost savings. *Journal of Christian Nursing, 31*(3), 178–183.

Prevention and Faith Community Nursing

24

Angela E. Glaser and Dia D. Campbell-Detrixhe

24.1 The Role of the Faith Community in Health

Historically, the concepts of religion and health were understood as one and the same (Wiley & Solari-Twadell, 1999). No matter what the traditional readings or rituals, there was an emphasis on health, healing, and salvation understood from a whole person perspective. For example, in the Christian tradition the Gospels speak richly of what practices, rituals, and beliefs that are important to the well-being and salvation of the person; God's intention that all would "live life abundantly"; and the importance of whole person health for the purpose of serving one' neighbors. Healing is a central focus in many of the Gospel stories with health and salvation being tightly linked with faith and beliefs.

Today, however, all faith communities are not necessarily acknowledging or actualizing their mission of health, particularly physical health. Physical health is often seen as the work of the hospitals, health providers, and health clinics. Thus, the idea that the faith community is a health place in the community, intentional in encouraging prevention, self-care, and the importance of people of faith being good stewards of their personal health resources is lacking from the central mission and work of the faith community. The presence of a faith community nurse as part of the staff of a faith community can bring alive the faith communities mission of health and healing. Consistent with the purpose of faith community nursing is the focus on health promotion, disease prevention, and spiritual care reinforcing the significance of the role of the faith community in prevention of disease, stewardship of personal

A. E. Glaser (✉)
Department of Nursing Management, Ecumenical Home Care Nursing Service,
Schifferstadt, Germany
e-mail: angela@glaser5.de

D. D. Campbell-Detrixhe
Oklahoma City University, Kramer School of Nursing, Oklahoma, OK, USA
e-mail: ddcampbelldetrixhe@okcu.edu

© Springer Nature Switzerland AG 2020   323
P. A. Solari-Twadell, D. J. Ziebarth (eds.), *Faith Community Nursing*,
https://doi.org/10.1007/978-3-030-16126-2_24

health resources, and the importance of caring for ones health in order to be in service to others. Chase-Ziolek and Iris (2002), stated, "Congregations have been and will continue to be places where promoting health makes sense" (p. 184). The needs of the faith community will often prescribe the priorities of the faith community nurses' functions regarding engagement in prevention activities/interventions (Chase-Ziolek & Iris, 2002).

24.2   Faith Communities, Research, and Prevention

Odulana et al. (2014), quantitative research surveyed adult churchgoers ($n = 1204$) of 11 predominately African American churches in North Carolina using the Congregational Health Assessment (CHA) survey to examine the "relationship between African American congregant characteristics and their willingness to attend health promotion programs through their church. This study also assessed how members of the faith community wanted to receive their health information" (p. 130). Findings revealed that participants expected the faith community

1. To promote health
2. Use scripture to teach members of the faith community about healthy living.

Furthermore, these two findings were reported as strongly associated with the faith community members willingness to attend health promotion events through their church (p. 130).

Ayton, Manderson, Smith, and Carey's (2016), qualitative exploratory study, aimed to investigate health promotion activities of local churches in Victoria, Australia. Three different expressions of church (influenced by theological interpretations, understandings of church mission, and involvement with local community) were identified as *traditional, new modern, and emerging*. These expressions were found to "differentiate the levels and types of health promotion activity" (p. 728). Findings further revealed that the *traditional* churches were primarily involved in disease screening and health education activities with the older members of the faith community; *new modern* churches were involved in activities that were related to prevention and promotion health efforts; and *emerging* churches were involved in broad health-promoting activities (Ayton et al., 2016).

Holt-Woehl's (2010), qualitative exploratory study, on inclusive faith communities focused on how three different faith communities came to be inclusive and welcoming of all individuals. Data was collected on each faith community through key stakeholders consisting of an interview with the pastors and additional conversation with members through the use of a focus group. In addition, review of written histories of the faith communities, participation in a worship services, and review of the faith community websites provided additional information. Each interview utilized the same set of questions regarding history of the faith community and "how they think the congregation came to include people with developmental disabilities as full participants" (p. 144). Study findings from all three faith communities revealed two attitudes that formed an accepting, welcoming, and supportive environment toward all people. One attitude present in each of the faith communities was that every person is a child of God and respected as such. The other attitude/belief reported was that all people are gifted by God and therefore, have gifts to offer in service to God and the faith community (Holt-Woehl, 2010, p. 150).

Baruth, Bopp, Webb, and Peterson's (2015), qualitative study explored the impact of faith leaders on health-related issues within their church congregations in the Centre County, PA, and Kansas City, MO regions. Semi-structured interviews were conducted on 24 faith leaders' perceptions, attitudes, beliefs, and experiences with health asking the following questions: (1) In your opinion, what are some of the biggest health challenges facing your congregation currently; (2) What activities does your church do, if any, promoting the general health of the entire congregation? (3) What kind of a role do you play in any health-related activities at your church; (4) What kind of influences do you believe you have on your congregation for health- and wellness-related issues; and (5) Describe how your own personal health habits influence how you interact with your congregation members about health or wellness. Poor health behaviors and chronic conditions were identified as the top health challenges facing the faith leader's congregation. Most of the faith leaders mentioned health-related activities taking place at their church, as well as the majority believed they had influence on their congregation for health- and wellness-related issues. Finally, the majority of faith leaders talked about the significance of being a role model for their church congregations (Baruth et al., 2015).

24.3 Prevention and the Faith Community

A faith community is an ideal place to emphasize prevention for the people it serves. At a time when poor diet, lack of sleep, being overweight or obese, hypertension, chronic stress, and other lifestyle factors contribute over time to patterns of chronic illness which ultimately translates into very expensive, often long-term health care. Prevention is highlighted as contributing to individual productivity and well-being of an individual as well as a reduction in health care costs. Prevention often goes hand and hand with changing behavior and sustaining that change over time. So what does a faith community have to do with behavior change and resulting well-being of the individual?

24.4 Protective Factor and Participation in a Faith Community Over Time

Long-term participation in a faith community is known and documented as a possible factor in contributing to an individual's overall health. Early research documented this finding noting:

- Mormons in Utah have a 30% lower incidence of most cancers,
- Seventh-Day Adventists have from 10 to 40% fewer hospital admissions for epidermoid and nonepidermoid malignancies,

- Regular church-attenders in Washington County, Maryland have 40% less risk from arteriosclerotic heart disease (Vuax, 1976, p. 523).

By engaging regularly in a community of faith, people develop life long and life giving relationships. These relationships can be important in supporting the individual in maintaining an important lifestyle change that contributes to their health and well-being or in episodes of illness they can be a source of ongoing support. Martin Marty (1999), related this point best in writing:

> …when misfortune comes, it is important to be part of a community of care. A Congregation enfolds one in intercessory prayer-loving one's neighbors on one's knees. A good congregation provides care and casseroles, rides to clinics and cards for the bedside table. It represents a gathering of people who have heard and keep on hearing the word of the Healer, who are busy interpreting the message of wholeness in a world of brokenness. By their own stumbling words, halting actions and only sometimes of distracted thoughts, they help the person who is ill come to terms with some of his or her problems, to cope, and in some way transcend them on the pilgrimage to triumph (xx).

24.5   Moral Development

One of the key outcomes found in those who participate in a faith community over time, is that through studying the beliefs and participating in the rituals of a particular religion, sharing like beliefs with others in community, the individual develops a moral grounding that guides their everyday life. Consequently, a connection between behavior, deeper beliefs, and an attitude toward oneself as well as one's role in society is based on a strong belief system which professes a value-based life. Therefore, in making difficult changes in lifestyle, an individual tends to draw on these deeper beliefs to sustain behavior change. It is not just about engaging in more exercise, eating healthier, drinking less alcohol, or finding a moment to rest, this change is recognized as being accountable to self, leading an authentic life through living out deeper beliefs and values based on connection to a being greater than oneself. Difficult behavior change becomes easier to sustain when on a regular interval the individual is meeting others who are, on a daily basis, trying to make better decisions related to their health based on similar beliefs and values. In other words, participation in a faith community that has a focus on prevention and stewardship of personal health resources, applying teachings and rituals to reinforce positive personal choices, stewardship of health and accountability guided by the resources of a faith community nurse sustains and encourages better decisions based on deeper beliefs and values. Again, the other members of the faith community serve as a support in sustaining the needed change. Prayer with others also cannot be underestimated in supporting and sustaining ongoing behavior change.

For example, John, a 40-year-old man, who is overweight comes to church every Sunday morning. During one of his visits he decides to talk to the faith community nurse about his weight problems. John also suffers from diabetes and is aware of the importance of losing weight. John has already discussed different options with his personal physician. The faith community nurse takes time to talk to John about the deeper reasons for eating unhealthily and eating too much. During their talk, issues about a low self-esteem, early neglect by his father, and uncertainties for life are illuminated. Eating a lot is not only a habit for John, it is also a compensation for feeling neglected and unloved. So now, when his way of life is challenged through daily nutrition and food choices, it is not only about eating different, but also about "who loves me and takes care of me" and "where is my place in life." The faith community nurse suggests to John that God has always loved him. She also encourages participation in a small prayer group would provide additional support to John in his quest to change his eating pattern. In the prayer group, members of the church will pray for John and his plan to lose weight by his request, they will talk to him about the progress, and help him through rough times of failure. They will encourage him to be a better steward of his personal health resources. In this example, prevention and education go together. Through John, other members in the congregation develop a higher awareness for the risks of making poor dietary choices. As a result, this can lead over time to changes in the varieties of food being offered at meetings and more faith community members deciding to make better decisions regarding their dietary and lifestyle choices.

24.6   Self-care as a Foundation for Prevention

Foundational to health is self-care. Faith communities, no matter what denomination, hold up the "golden rule: love your neighbour as you love yourself." So it becomes important to take care of self, not just to look and feel good to meet one's own satisfaction, but to be in the best position to serve one's neighbor. Service is at the basis of a healthy spiritual life. Often in doing something for another, those who are serving, walk away feeling like they have received a gift. And indeed many times they have! Through reaching out and being present to someone in need, a deep call to ensure the well-being of "my neighbor" is satisfied through bringing personal energy, a joyful attitude and hope to another. In the midst of serving another however, what is perceived as personal problems and obstacles are put aside and a greater good is able to be addressed. Often what seemed problematic is adjusted to be a circumstance of life to be managed in comparison to being privy to experiencing the burdens of another. It is this capacity to be in "mutuality" with another that often humbles the server and allows them to see God working in their life and the lives of others.

24.7   Stress Prevention

In 1940, Hans Selye, an Austrian-Canadian doctor and biochemist, introduced the term "stress" to medicine. His research revealed the influence of physical and mental strains on health. Since then the development of stress and its influence on health has been thoroughly investigated. Surveys in Europe identified that every 3rd employee suffers from stress and almost 50–60% of lost working-days are because of stress related health problems (Kaluza, 2018).

Stressors include the situations and occurrences presenting themselves in our environment, how we react to these situations and finally, our ability to cope with the perceived stress (Kaluza, 2018). Kaluza (2018), further identifies five stress intensifiers: Be perfect! Be liked! Be independent! Keep control!, and Stick to it! Looking at these stress intensifiers we can see where a change of attitude is important.

Participation in a faith community worship service can produce a sense of relaxation through reflection and application of readings, music, and song which accompanies the service and through prayer that is integral to the service. Often this participation in a religious service can reinforce that there is something larger than oneself in charge. Through further participation in small groups offered by many faith communities, individuals can talk about their problems, the stress resulting from the problems and gain another way of thinking and approaching their management of stress. Following tragedies such as the attack on the twin towers on September 11, 2001, many people flocked to their faith communities seeking abatement of their fear, loss stress, and strength to go out and reengage with society following this sudden assault on the U.S.A.

Just taking the time to sit quietly in the environment of a faith community can often reduce an individual's stress, encourage a mind-set of prayerfulness, and reliance on a power greater than oneself. Having a faith community nurse available can further ameliorate stress through meeting and talking about identified problems. Through this therapeutic discussion based on the beliefs and traditions of a particular faith tradition, often stress can be reduced, new and successful strategies for stress reduction be identified and the individual leaves having new strategies for coping based on personal beliefs and rituals.

24.8   Education

Teaching about prevention is one thing a faith community can provide to assist in personal behavior change. For example, a German Lutheran Church developed a lesson about depression-prevention as part of preparation for confirmation to address young people aged 13 and 14 years old. At this age, feelings can be intense and coping skills to manage these feelings may not yet be developed. Pressure to perform is high, and pressure can lead to fears of failure. If these young people do not learn how to cope with their feelings, a depressive disorder can develop (Haussmann, 2014).

The educational program incorporated into the preparation for the confirmation classes in the faith community was based on a theme and called "Lust for Life with Lars and Lisa." This program was developed at the department for clinical psychology and psychotherapy at Tübingen University. The aims were to learn a strategy to check and reassess a situation (reality-check), to learn to recognize automated negative thoughts that encourage depressive thinking, and to encourage positive thoughts (Haussmann, 2014). The first lesson in the series emphasized the connection between feelings, thoughts, and behavior. The group of young people were encouraged to share times when they experienced negative feelings and how these feelings produced negative thoughts. In the following sessions, the participants were taught to differentiate between feelings and thoughts, and initiate strategies to replace automated negative thoughts in their everyday life (Haussmann, 2014). The faith community nurse is an excellent partner in the development, publicizing, and implementation of such programming. The faith community is an excellent place for this information to be offered as the faith beliefs, prayer, support and rituals of the faith community can be drawn on to reinforce the didactic information.

24.9   Embracing Change

"While all changes do not lead to improvement, all improvement requires change" (Institute for Healthcare Improvement, 2018, para 1).

Change is vital to progress. Change is one of the irreducible facts of life. Whether realized or not, each person's body is changing and adjusting each day to changing environments and aging. However, as individuals, often the person's goal is to keep everything in life the same or comfortable. If given a choice, most people would like things to stay the same. Of course that would be easy, but not realistic. Individuals often resist change, as well as faith communities, when understanding and practicing health prevention activities/interventions (DeSchepper, 2015; Geiger, 2016; McCallum, 2018; Rainer, 2016). Commonly, it is the faith community nurse who must lead this change of implementing inclusion of health promotion in the life of the faith community. Faith community nurses can be instrumental in transforming plans into action by being that agent of change.

While there are numerous ways of implementing change, the faith community nurse must fully understand the process of planned change. It was Kurt Lewin (1890–1947), also known as the father of social psychology, who theorized a three-stage model of change (Unfreezing-Moving-Refreezing) that requires prior learning to be rejected and replaced (Lewin, 1952; Mitchell, 2013; Morrison, 2014; Nursing Theories, 2011). The three stages include *unfreezing* (when change is needed), *moving* (when change is initiated), and *refreezing* (when equilibrium is established) (Morrison, 2014). Utilizing Lewin's change theory model gives the faith community nurse a framework to implement a change effort effectively and with sensitivity.

The process of change can be difficult for many; as "humanity tends to stick to things they are comfortable and familiar with rather than experimenting with change" (McCallum, 2018, para 1). Change is something faith community nurses and other leaders will encounter and need to be prepared in how to lead through it (Geiger, 2016). In Rainer's (2016), book entitled, *Who Moved My Pulpit: Leading Change in the Church,* an eight-stage roadmap for leading change in the faith community was developed with the purpose of creating a resource for pastors, faith community staff, and lay leaders who wanted add an education on the process of leading change in a faith community. The eight-stage roadmap for leading change in the church includes: (1) *Stop and pray*—realize that change takes time and seeking the power and strength of God through prayer is essential; (2) *Confront and Communicate a Sense of Urgency*—develop an open communication style with the faith community by sharing the important facts in a timely fashion; (3) *Build an Eager Coalition*—strategically select the right people with influence, expertise, position, and leadership is imperative for creating change; (4) *Become a Voice and Vision of Hope*—embrace hope within the faith community is critical for change to occur; (5) *Deal with People Issues*—have the courage to address people issues through building a team, loving each other, expecting opposition, leading change over time, working through difficult decisions in a timely fashion, realizing that some people will leave, and prayer; (6) *Move from an Inward Focus to an Outward Focus*—having the understanding that change will require purposely "outward focused movement"; (7) *Pick Low-Hanging Fruit*—realizing that small change achievements are necessary to maintain positive energy and to foster larger change to occur; and, (8) *Implement and Consolidate Change*—understanding change requires transparency, ongoing communication, and dealing with success, skepticism, and complacency (Geiger, 2016).

The functional roles that the faith community nurse provides to members of a congregation are multifaceted, providing faith and health through active engagement and discern-ability within the faith community setting (Cassimere, 2014). Cassimere (2014), further identified some of these functional roles of faith community nursing ministry to include: (1) building relationships within the congregation through presence; (2) promoting health not only as the absent of disease, but as spiritual, physical, social, and psychological well-being; (3) providing education by disseminating information that supports optimal health/well-being and minimizes health risks; (4) providing both formal and informal health teaching within a caring environment with follow-up teaching as needed; (5) promoting health through advocacy representing the individual, family, and congregation within the community's healthcare system and community at large; and (6) embracing the roles of advocate, coordinator, and referral agent to promote health by assisting individuals and their families to access various resources, agencies, and healthcare services within the community setting. Stanhope and Lancaster (2018), describe activities that the faith community nurse may provide to his/her faith community: offering to pray after an individual encounter or group gathering; providing blood pressure screenings monthly with an educational component discussing ways to reduce risk of high blood pressure; creating a bulletin board display on "whole-person health of body, mind, and spirit, including the connection between faith and health" (p. 520); referring an adult female to a gynecologist for preventative women's care issues; working with homeless individuals accessing congregational resources of food; planning an annual health fair; and organizing a bereavement/grief support group for older adults. All of this is foundational to bringing alive the mission of health and health promotion within a faith community.

24.10 The Role of the Faith Leader in Prevention

Faith leaders often are the "gate-keepers" regarding new initiatives, allocating necessary resources to sustain a ministry or program and actively supporting the integration of a new ministry into the life of the faith community. Faith leaders themselves may have their own struggle with weight, lack of sleep, stress, hypertension, and other health-related issues. The faith community nurse often finds herself providing support to the faith leader encouraging behavior change to improve personal health. After all, there is one clear thing that can alter the ability of a faith leader to minister to their congregation-loss of health. There is nothing stronger to draw attention to the significance of a health behavior change than to get the faith leader on board. For example, in one Lutheran Synod, the Bishop took health seriously. He proceeded to arrange for a health screening for all faith leaders in the synod so that each faith leader would be aware of their health risks. Faith community nurses assisted at the health screening to provide education to the faith leaders regarding faith community nursing. The Bishop took his own results to heart leading by example. He was overweight and lab values indicated some changes that did not support a healthy diet, exercise pattern, or level of stress. He not only began to change his lifestyle through making different dietary choices and incorporating more exercise, but he began to visibly lose weight. The fact that he was attending to his own health was very visible and a strong witness to his faith and health beliefs. Other clergy that followed the same pattern were visible billboards of the importance of being a good steward of personal health resources. Each Sunday when these pastors stood in the pulpit, they were visibly demonstrating to their faith community an important lesson in making changes to support health.

24.11 Faith Community Religious Seasons and Prevention

Through the seasons of faith community life, prevention can be integrated in order to support attention to the importance of making healthy lifestyle choices. Themes of sacrifice which are woven through faith traditions can be important to highlighting the significance of making new and better choices over time to support health and being a better steward of personal health resources. For example, two periods in the Christian liturgical year can be used for fostering preventive lifestyle changes: lent and advent. Lent, in many Christian traditions calls for fasting or a time to reduce food intake. This time period can be used to initiate healthier behavior and to practice health promoting behavior by making different choices.

Eating less chocolate and sweets, eliminating alcohol, and eating smaller portions are all strategies that are employed. Often faith communities will sponsor communal suppers gathering their members together for a meal. It is important that thought goes into what is served and how food is prepared so that those on restricted diets can comfortably participate. Adding recipes next to dishes is a good way for individuals to see if they can eat what is included in the buffet. This also allows members of the faith community to learn about a new healthy dish. In addition to providing a healthy communal supper, lent prayers, and worship times, churches can also add programs to help people learn ways of not only changing their lifestyle, making better choices, and making lifestyle change, but through working in groups to get to know other members and build in needed support to the desired change.

24.12   Faith community Health Promotion and Prevention Programs

Faith community-based health promotion and prevention programs can improve health outcomes for members within a faith community setting, as well as individuals living within the community at large. As stated by Baruth et al. (2015), "Churches may have the potential to reach many people, especially those who do not participate in traditional health programs" (p. 1748). A variety of church-based health promotion and prevention programs were identified in literature focusing on health screenings (Young, 2015), exercise/fall prevention (Notter, 2017), behavioral lifestyle changes (Schwingel & Gálvez, 2016), heart health (Tettey, Duran, Anderson, & Boutin-Foster, 2017; Tettey, Duran, Anderson, Washington, & Boutin-Foster, 2016), stroke prevention (Williamson & Kautz, 2009), diabetes prevention (Oakley & Hoebeke, 2014), injury prevention (Willis & Krichten, 2012), immunizations (Pappas-Rogich, 2012), and medication management (Shillam, Orton, Waring, & Madsen, 2013); thereby, demonstrating how the faith community nurse can be instrumental in implementing prevention activities/interventions within a faith community setting.

While research supports the faith community nurse's role in providing church-based health promotion and prevention program planning (Ayton et al., 2016; Maitlen, Bockstahler, & Belcher, 2012; Notter, 2017; Oakley & Hoebeke, 2014; Pappas-Rogich, 2012; Shillam et al., 2013; Williamson & Kautz, 2009; Willis & Krichten, 2012), barriers and challenges affecting church engagement in the participation of these programs remain (Ayton, Manderson, & Smith, 2017; Baruth et al., 2015).

Ayton et al.'s (2017), qualitative study explored underlying barriers and challenges affecting faith community engagement in health promotion to better understand the "potential for engaging Australian churches in health promotion programs and partnerships" (p. 53). Semi-structured face-to-face or telephone interviews with church leaders ($n = 30$) representing Anglican, Baptist, Catholic, Church of Christ, Uniting, and Salvation Army denominational groups and church-affiliated organization directors ($n = 5$) were conducted.

Ayton et al. (2017), identified two research questions that guided the analysis: "What barriers and challenges do local churches experience when undertaking health promotion activities? and how are these perceived by church leaders?" (p. 54). Two broad themes emerged: *The social context of churches* and *the attributes of congregations*. Furthermore, subthemes identified several factors that inhibit the engagement of faith communities in health promotion activities including: *perceptions of relevance, mistrust of churches, a contested agenda, discordant values, volunteers, and risk management*.

A qualitative research study, interviewing 24 faith leaders on health-related issues within their church congregations, the most common health challenges facing faith communities included: chronic health conditions (cancer, heart-related conditions, diabetes, overweight/obesity, arthritis, and mental conditions), an aging population, poor health behaviors, and failure to access healthcare services. Further, faith leaders mentioned a variety of health behavior challenges including: poor diet such as eating too much, lack of exercise, tobacco and drug usage, and alcohol consumption (Baruth et al., 2015). The Appendix to this chapter identifies sources of programs and content that could be used by faith community nurses in developing programs and initiatives focusing on prevention.

24.13 Collaboration: Networking for Prevention

As a faith community nurse, it is important to become familiar with what the community has/does not have in relation to planning prevention activities. Assessing the community is essential to better understand individual, family, and group needs, issues, and/or problems; to identify community strengths and health-related resources; and to learn about possible gaps in resources in community services.

One example of a simple community assessment that the faith community nurse can use is the windshield survey (Stanhope & Lancaster, 2018). A windshield survey is the "motorized equivalent of simple observations" (Stanhope & Lancaster, 2018, p. 213), conducted from a motor vehicle (e.g., car, truck, SUV) that provides a visual overview of a community. A windshield survey could also include walking through an area and making organized observations (Deres, 2014).

Stanhope and Lancaster (2018), identified elements that should be considered when conducting a windshield survey including: geographic boundaries, housing and zoning, open space, common green space, transportation, social service centers, stores, people living on the street, animals running loose, physical condition of streets, blocks, neighborhoods, race and ethnicity, religious institutions, health indicators, political advertisements, health care providers, business, and industry.

Important in this process is the understanding that a windshield survey may uncover information that could involve further investigation. To make the survey successful, leading it is helpful to develop questions that can guide the process. For example, where are the hospitals, healthcare providers, dental offices, drugstores, therapists, and health centers? How is the community infrastructure? Are there sidewalks and pedestrian crossings, ramps for wheelchairs, and are old or disabled people able to get where they want to go safely? Are there places dedicated to health promotion to improve well-being? Are there locations to rest and sit down?

In addition to driving and walking through the community to complete this survey, a faith community nurse can go on prayer-walks. Walking, observing, and praying for the community, for important observations to be made, and grace to use the gathered information to benefit the members of the faith community and community at large. The prayer-walks can be completed over time, designating particular geographic areas that will be observed.

24.13.1 One Example of Developing Prevention Programming

In Germany, parish nursing has a long tradition with the first deaconesses working with a local church starting in 1844 (Friedrich, 2010). Today the Catholic and Lutheran Church provide professional healthcare services, like hospitals, nursing homes, ambulant homecare, and counselling services. Many nurses work for the church in the community to provide medical treatment and care. As time is limited there is a lack for prevention and spiritual care. This is the gap where parish nursing fits in. Translating parish nursing or faith community nursing into German would lead to an already well-known term. To show that this is an innovative and an addition to what already exists, the decision was made to use a new term. The result was "Vis-à-vis," which is French and means "face to face." On the one side this means the faith community nurse and the parishioner meet face to face, and the second meaning is the local church and church-based (and other) healthcare organizations work together side by side, putting an emphasis on the importance of networking.

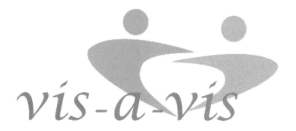

Christlicher Dienst an Kranken und Gesunden

This is expressed in the logo of the German faith community nursing project Vis-a-vis. Working with a congregation, a faith community/Vis-a-vis nurse would not be on her own, but together in a team. This interprofessional team includes other church members working in the healthcare system, like healthcare providers, social workers, therapists, and of course, other nurses. Bringing together professionals from different healthcare professions enlarges the perspective and helps to develop a broader program of prevention and counselling for the members of the faith community. Together, they plan what the congregation can offer as, for example, sportgroups, readings from books about health-issues, and seminars about preventive actions that can be taken. To get new ideas and reflect on prevention activities offered within the faith community, it is necessary for faith community nurses to meet other faith community nurses at least once a year to build partnerships. Attending faith community nursing workshops, seminars, conferences, and local, state, national, and/or internationally association meeting events can be an effective means of collaboration with ones' peers. For example, the Faith Community Nurses Association of Oklahoma (FCNA-OK) is a very active association offering quarterly membership meetings and continuing education offerings on various health prevention topics including diabetes prevention, human trafficking, mentorship, mental health prevention, and aging in place. This organization also offers an annual conference event held each spring focusing on thematic topics including: "Balancing Mind, Body & Spirit: Complete Health for Self & Community," "Transition to the Beyond: Being a Sacred Presence during End of Life Care," "Transitions to Transformation," "Weaving Presence into Nursing Ministry," and "Collecting the Wisdom: Harnessing the Power of Faith Community Nursing."

With today's technological advancements, faith community nurses can also connect with other faith community nurses via the internet. Participating in webinars, podcasts, and "zoom" conference calls are just a few of the many opportunities that the faith community nurse can have access to further their networking partnerships and learn of prevention programming offered by other colleagues.

24.13.2 Environment for Health Promotion for Faith Community Nurses and Their Faith Communities

Planning for health prevention programming is driven by the assessment a faith community nurse does of members of the faith community, staff members of the faith community, demographic information, and other assessments that may be completed by local health care agencies and systems. The following are some suggested formats and opportunities for faith community nurses actualizing prevention activities.

24.14 Preventive Home Visits for Older Adults

The purpose of preventive home-visits is to identify and support the resources and networks of older adults, to maintain their functional abilities, to improve life quality, to support safety, and to inform about activities and services of the community (Häkkinen, 2016). These visits can be undertaken as a recommendation provided by volunteers from the faith community that do home visitation or requests from faith community members to the faith community nurse. Or the faith community nurse can offer this to all older adults in the faith community.

Subjects addressed during visits may include: individual risk assessment such as fall prevention, the necessity of regular medication to prevent high blood pressure, and issues related to diet and physical, mental, social activities (Hurrelmann, Klotz, & Haisch, 2014). Preventive home visits with older adults will focus on prevention from the perspective of need for long-term care. The assessment of older adults in their home can also be the first step in preparing the elder for change in their living environment. The faith community nurse can help people to reflect on their own situation and assist the older adult to gain a new perspective. The primary aim of the prevention visit is to assist people to live at home as long as possible (Bundeszentrale für gesundheitliche Aufklärung, 2018). Preventive home visits carried out by the faith community nurse may also address spiritual issues ascertaining what provides meaning and purpose and connection to the larger community for the older adult. Preventive home visits are intended to connect the older adult more tangibly with the faith community and be proactive in what is needed for the older adult to be safe in their home for as long as possible.

24.15 Partnerships: Café for People with Dementia

Partnerships are important to supporting the health ministry of faith communities. One example of a partnership between a health care system and faith community nurse is the "Café Forget-Me-Not." Through this program the faith community nurse and the health-care system work together to provide support for people with dementia and their relatives. The faith community nurse having expertise and experience working with older adults with dementia can educate volunteers to assist with the programming. Additional resources and support are provided by the health care system in order for this programming to be made available in the faith community. The program consists of "memory workouts." An example of a "memory workout is to take a topic such as gardening, identify all the important parts of gardening." Then afterwards during coffee the participants will be asked to remember the items, how they are used and important to the gardening process. Often prayer and singing of hymns are part of the gathering as well. The singing of the songs and music along with prayer are also good exercises in memory work.

24.16 Educational Workshops

Health promotion and disease prevention involve educating members of the church faith community about healthy behaviors and helping members alter risky or unhealthy behaviors. There are many topics that could be helpful to members of a faith community in addressing prevention. Topics are chosen by age group and need assessment. Some topics for infants and children include: immunization guidelines, bullying, bicycle safety, sex education classes, sleep hygiene, good touch and bad touch, swimming safety, self-esteem classes, dental health, and spiritual practices for health and healing. Topics for adults can include: fitness, prenatal care and child-birth, conflict resolution, retirement planning, disaster preparation, marriage seminars, parenting classes, weight management, relaxation and stress management, healthy cooking on a budget, and spiritual practices for health and healing. Topics for the older adults may include: advance directives, importance of immunization for pneumonia and influenza, healthy cooking for one and two, finding health information on the Internet, fitness, and spiritual practices for health and healing (Cassimere, 2014, p. 11).

The advantage of a faith community offering these topics in the context of the faith community is that the beliefs, values, and behaviors inherent in the faith tradition can be integrated into the content to support values-based health decisions. In addition, faith communities span all age groups and socioeconomic groups.

24.16.1 Support Groups

Faith communities often use small groups in order to focus on particular health-related opportunities. It is important that before initiating a support group that an assessment is done to ensure that the faith community is not duplicating a service already available in the community. Or if there is the ability to collaborate with an organization that is offering a health promotion/prevention activity that will strengthen the participation in the activity. Partnerships can enhance attendance, viability, and participation and bring awareness of the faith community nurse role in the faith community.

The following are examples of additional group activities.

24.16.1.1 Athletic Groups

Prevention through physical activities is a good fit for the faith community, its members, and the community to come together for physical training. Sports clubs can serve to exercise the body, increase socialization, and encourage healthy competition. Different sports such as badminton, baseball, volleyball, walking hiking, dance, and yoga can all serve to bring faith community members together to have fun and enjoy healthy movement of their body. An example is a Caribbean dance and workout group that bring young and middle-aged church members and friends together. Families can join in and to build stronger relationships, understanding of cultural aspects of dance, and importance of movement to health. Dancing to Caribbean music is fun and makes it easy to join in for non-church-goers who do not like sports, but enjoy music.

24.17 Healthy Cooking Club

Offering a healthy cooking club group for members of the congregation can be a very fun, creative, and healthy way to teach members how to create healthier choices in the kitchen when preparing family meals. Suggested ideas for this group include inviting a nutritionist to be the guest speaker to talk about basic nutrition, sharing healthy recipes with the group, and organizing a healthy potluck event for all members of the congregation.

24.18 Conclusion

There could substantially be more ideas and practice added, all showing how many options a faith community nurse and the faith community can employ to highlight prevention as an important offering of the faith community. The faith community can provide all levels of prevention through the ministry of the faith community nurse, primary, secondary, and tertiary prevention. The faith community is a health place in the community where change can be addressed from a whole person perspective, and where self-care can be supported through the values, beliefs, and rituals of the faith community. Forgiveness, encouragement, and hope can be woven into addressing behavior change through support of the faith community. A faith community nurse working with a team in the faith community and collaborating or partnering with other health organizations in the community will build a solid network for prevention. And as we all know…prevention is the key!

Appendix

Healthy People 2020 The website: https://www.healthypeople.gov/ provides scientific-based, 10-year national objectives for improving the health of all Americans furnishing tools and resources for professionals
Centers for Disease Control and Prevention (CDC) The CDC is a federal agency identified as the "nation's leading public health agency, dedicated to saving lives and protecting the health of Americans." The website: https://www.cdc.gov/ provides informative resources and educational materials supporting health promotion, prevention, and preparedness activities
World Health Organization (WHO) WHO, established in 1948, is a specialized agency of the United Nations that is concerned with international public health. The multilingual website: http://www.who.int/ provides informative publications and resources ensuring that "health information reaches the people who need it, in the languages they can understand"
National Institutes of Health Office (NIH) The Office of Disease Prevention (ODP) is the "lead office at the National Institutes of Health (NIH) responsible for assessing, facilitating, and stimulating research in disease prevention and health promotion, and disseminating the results of this research to improve public health." The website: https://prevention.nih.gov/ serves the public by offering immediate access to clinical studies, health and wellness information, research/library resources, clinical studies, scientific program, policy and planning documents, and other informative resources
The Office of Disease Prevention and Health Promotion (ODPHP) In 1976, Congress established ODPHP to "lead disease prevention and health promotion efforts in the United States." ODPHP sets national goals and objectives, and supports programs, services, and educational activities The website: https://health.gov/ is the home of ODPHP and an indispensable resource for health information
Rural Health Information Hub (RHIhub) The website: https://www.ruralhealthinfo.org/toolkits/health-promotion/ provides resources and best practices for rural communities. The RHI hub offers a toolkit designed to help organizations identify and implement a health promotion program
National Prevention Strategy The U.S. Surgeon General is focused on improving the country's health by "communicating the best available scientific information to the public." The National Prevention Strategy found on the website: https://www.surgeongeneral.gov/priorities/prevention/index.html aims to "guide our nation in the most effective and achievable means for improving health and well-being" and "envisions a prevention-oriented society where all sectors recognize the value of health for individuals, families, and society and work together to achieve better health for all Americans"

References

Ayton, D., Manderson, L., & Smith, B. J. (2017). Barriers and challenges affecting the contemporary church's engagement in health promotion. *Health Promotion Journal of Australia, 28,* 52–58.

Ayton, D., Manderson, L., Smith, B. J., & Carey, G. (2016). Health promotion in local churches in Victoria: An exploratory study. *Health & Social Care in the Community, 24*(6), 728–738.

Baruth, M., Bopp, M., Webb, B. L., & Peterson, J. A. (2015). The role and influence of faith leaders on health-related issues and programs in their congregation. *Journal of Religion and Health, 54*, 1747–1759.

Bundeszentrale für gesundheitliche Aufklärung. (2018). *Präventive Hausbesuche.* https://www.gesund-aktiv-aelter-werden.de/projektdatenbank/angebot/praeventive-hausbesuche/

Cassimere, M. H. (2014). Unit III: Wholistic health: Health promotion. In The Church Health Ministry (Ed.), *Faith Community Nursing Education, Foundations of faith community nursing curriculum: Faculty. 2014 Revision* (pp. 1–42). Memphis, TN: International Parish Nurse Resource Center: A Ministry of the Church Health Center.

Chase-Ziolek, M., & Iris, M. (2002). Nurses' perspectives on the distinctive aspects of providing nursing care in a congregational setting. *Journal of Community Health Nursing, 19*(3), 173–186.

Deres, P. (2014). Unit IV: Assessment. In International Parish Nurse Resource Center, A Ministry of the Church Health Center (Ed.), *Faith Community Nursing Education, Foundations of faith community nursing curriculum: Faculty* (pp. 1–25). Memphis, TN: The Church Health Center.

DeSchepper, C. (2015). Leading congregations through change. *Perspectives.* http://elpna.org/docs/Leading%20Congregations%20through%20Change-Summer%202015.pdf

Friedrich, N. (2010). *Der Kaiserswerther. Wie Theodor Fliedner Frauen einen Beruf gab.* Berlin: Wichern-Verlag.

Geiger, E. (2016). *The 8 stages of leading good change in the church.* https://ericgeiger.com/2016/06/the-8-stages-of-leading-good-change-in-the-church/

Häkkinen, H. (2016). Präventive Praxis- und Politikansätze in Europa. In S. Pohlmann (Ed.), *Alter und Prävention* (pp. 301–310). Wiesbaden: Springer.

Haussmann, A. (2014). Konfirmandenarbeit und Depressionsprävention. In B. Weyel, A. Haussmann, B. Jakob, & S. Koch (Eds.), *Menschen mit Depression* (pp. 140–156). Gütersloh: GütersloherVerlagshaus.

Holt-Woehl, H. M. (2010). Education and inclusive congregations: A study of three congregations. *Journal of Religion, Disability & Health, 14*, 143–152.

Hurrelmann, K., Klotz, T., & Haisch, J. (2014). *Lehrbuch Prävention und Gesundheitsförderung* (pp. 96–97). Bern: Verlag Hans Huber.

Institute for Healthcare Improvement. (2018). *Using change concepts for improvement.* http://www.ihi.org/reources/Pages/Changes/UsingConceptsforImprovement.asp

Kaluza, G. (2018). *Gelassen und sicher im Stress. Das Stresskompetenz-Buch: Stress erkennen, verstehen, bewältigen* (pp. 4–82). Heidelberg: Springer.

Lewin, K. (1952). *Field theory in social science: Selected theoretical papers.* London: Tavistock Publications.

Maitlen, L. A., Bockstahler, A. M., & Belcher, A. E. (2012). Using community-based participatory research in parish nursing: A win-win situation! *Journal of Christian Nursing, 29*(4), 222–227.

McCallum, C. (2018). A review of Thom Rainer's "who moved my pulpit" by Rev. Charles McCallum, discipleship pastor, Old Fort Baptist Church. *Church and Gospel.* http://www.churchandgospel.com/2016/06/06/a-review-of-thom-rainers-who-moved-my-p

Mitchell, G. (2013). Selecting the best theory to implement planned change. *Nursing Management, 20*(1), 32–37.

Morrison, M. (2014). *Kurt Lewin change theory three step model – Unfreeze, change, freeze.* https://rapidbi.com/kurt-lewin-three-step-change-theory/

Notter, J. (2017). Balance and more out of the congregation setting: Creating a meaningful class for older adults. *Perspectives, 6*–7.

Nursing Theories. (2011). *Change theory: Kurt Lewin.* http://currentnursing.com/nursing_theory/change_theory.html

Oakley, J., & Hoebeke, R. (2014). I choose health (elijo salud): Impacting youth through parish nursing. *Journal of Christian Nursing, 31*(4), 252–257.

Odulana, A. A., Kim, M. M., Isler, M. R., Green, M. A., Taylor, Y. J., Howard, D. L., et al. (2014). Examining characteristics of congregation members willing to attend health promotion in African American churches. *Health Promotion Practice, 15*(1), 125–133. https://doi. org/10.1177/1524839913480799

Pappas-Rogich, M. (2012). Faith community nurses: Protecting our elders through immunizations. *Journal of Christian Nursing, 29*(4), 232–237.

Rainer, T. S. (2016). *Who moved my pulpit? Leading change in the church.* Nashville, TN: B&H Publishing.

Schwingel, A., & Gálvez, P. (2016). Divine interventions: Faith-based approaches to health promotion programs for Latinos. *Journal of Religion and Health, 55,* 1891–1906.

Shillam, C. R., Orton, V. J., Waring, D., & Madsen, S. (2013). Faith community nurses & brown bag events help older adults manage meds. *Journal of Christian Nursing, 30*(2), 90–96.

Stanhope, M., & Lancaster, J. (2018). *Foundations for population health in community/public health nursing* (5th ed.). St. Louis, MO: Elsevier.

Tettey, N.-S., Duran, P. A., Anderson, H. S., & Boutin-Foster, C. (2017). Evaluation of HeartSmarts, a faith-based cardiovascular health education program. *Journal of Religion and Health, 56,* 320–328.

Tettey, N.-S., Duran, P. A., Anderson, H. S., Washington, N., & Boutin-Foster, C. (2016). "It's like backing up science with scripture": Lessons learned from the implication of HeartSmarts, a faith-based cardiovascular disease health education program. *Journal of Religion and Health, 55,* 1078–1088.

Vuax, K. (1976). Religion and health. *Preventive Medicine, 5*(4), 522–536.

Wiley, L. J., & Solari-Twadell, P. A. (1999). Health and the congregation. In P. A. Solari-Twadell & M. A. McDermott (Eds.), *Parish nursing: Promoting whole person health within faith communities.* Thousand Oaks, CA: Sage.

Williamson, W., & Kautz, D. D. (2009). "Let's get moving: Let's get praising:" promoting health and hope in an African American church. *The ABNF Journal, 20,* 102–105.

Willis, R. E., & Krichten, A. E. (2012). Stopping the ouch of injury. *Journal of Trauma Nursing, 19*(1), 17–22.

Young, S. A. (2015). Urban parish nurses: A qualitative analysis of the organization of work in community-based practices. *Journal of Nursing Education and Practice, 6*(2), 19–27.

Research Agenda in Faith Community Nursing

25

P. Ann Solari-Twadell and Deborah Jean Ziebarth

25.1 Research and Faith Community Nursing

Faith community nurses engage with research as both consumers of research and producers of new knowledge that will contribute to the ongoing development of faith community nursing. Faith community nurses vary in their academic preparation and knowledge of developing research projects, but all faith community nurses can be discriminating consumers of research and participate in research projects developed by others. Nursing research in faith communities can have several purposes, such as description of practice, testing an intervention, or interpreting the human experience of spirituality in illness and health.

Research that applies to faith community nursing includes studies that are specifically conducted by or about faith community nursing, and other studies that can inform faith community nursing practice. For example, research on health promotion, grief, spiritual care, family development, and issues such as depression or addictions can be helpful to a faith community nurse in advancing practice. The next section will provide a simple overview of the construct for research articles. This overview is intended to inform faith community nurses interested in reviewing nursing research articles of the basic format and purpose of each section of the article. For the seasoned researcher you may want to fast forward to the next section of this chapter focused on "Establishing a Research Agenda for Faith Community Nursing."

P. A. Solari-Twadell (✉)
Marcella Niehoff School of Nursing, Loyola University Chicago, Chicago, IL, USA
e-mail: psolari@luc.edu

D. J. Ziebarth
Department of Nursing Program Chair, Herzing University, Brookfield, WI, USA
e-mail: dziebarth@herzing.edu

© Springer Nature Switzerland AG 2020
P. A. Solari-Twadell, D. J. Ziebarth (eds.), *Faith Community Nursing*,
https://doi.org/10.1007/978-3-030-16126-2_25

25.2   Basic Structure of a Research Article

25.2.1 Introduction

All research articles should have an "introduction" which addresses the "why" of the article. This section will include a stated purpose, which may be as direct as "to evaluate satisfaction and value of an educational program," to more complicated things like a "cost benefit analysis" for a program of ministry. The purpose or stated research question is what will drive the remainder of the study.

Reading and reflection on any research articles are best when the reader is informed by previously published reports, articles, or books on the subject. Research articles can be found by searching public databases such as Medline or Pubmed and Cinahl. Looking at these databases using specific search terms will help to focus what studies are related to different research topics. Access to journals may be a problem for the faith community nurse working independently, but public libraries or even local colleges, universities, and hospitals may grant access to their search resources with special permission. Partnering with a researcher at a college or school of nursing might also be a good strategy for searching, discussing, and conducting research. Sometimes a local faith community network that meets regularly is a good place to help develop ideas on future research article topics related to best practices, discussions, and possible future projects. Through the *Westberg Institute*, the *Faith Community Nursing Citation List* is accessible in the "Research Group" on Yammer (Yammer > Research Group > Files). This citation list is a 47-page compilation of research articles that are published in various journals and address faith community nursing.

25.2.2 Methods

This section addresses the "how." Included in this section may be the context setting of the research, design, population, sample information, intervention, study variable, data collection, and analysis. The research question and the context of the research purpose determine the design that will be used to collect and analyze data for a research project. The type of question being researched should lead to a logical choice of design for collecting data. There are different ways collection of data can be completed depending on the stated purpose or research question. For the purpose of this basic review, two ways of collecting data are described. They are "quantitative" and "qualitative" research design.

25.2.2.1   Quantitative Research Design
Quantitative research is used to quantify a stated problem by way of generating numerical data or data that can be transformed into usable statistics. It is used to quantify attitudes, opinions, behaviors, and other defined variables—and generalize results from a larger sample population. Quantitative research uses measurable data

to formulate facts and uncover patterns in research (DeFranzo, 2011). Many times this research design involves the use of paper and pencil surveys or electronic "Survey Monkey" strategies.

Probably the simplest and most frequent type of quantitative research is "descriptive" in nature. Descriptive research may count such data as the number of care activities, number of patient blood pressures, attendance at health fairs or programs, or faith community surveys to support program planning. Descriptive research often uses fairly simple statistics like totals, means, ranges, or full data display. Descriptive research is important to share through publication because it helps to explain the concepts that faith community nurses address. Also through sharing descriptive information examples of activities that faith community nurses' offer in support of the health or changing of the understanding of health for members of the faith community can be reported.

25.2.2.2   Qualitative Research Design

Qualitative research is used to gain an understanding of underlying reasons, opinions, and motivations. It provides insights into a problem or helps to develop ideas or hypotheses for potential quantitative research. Qualitative research is also used to uncover trends in thought and opinions, and dive deeper into a particular problem. Qualitative data collection methods vary using unstructured or semi-structured techniques. Some common methods include focus groups (group discussions), individual interviews, and participation/observations. The sample size is typically small, and respondents are selected to fulfill a given quota (DeFranzo, 2011). This research design is often more consistent with the depth of the work that faith community nurses engage in with their clients.

25.2.3   Results or Findings

Results or findings are the "what" and report information that addresses the research question and purpose of the paper. The results or findings of a research study may be *thought* to be the most important information by a faith community nurse. However, to comprehend more fully the nature of the study is important to understanding the applicability of the findings to a particular setting, population, or denomination.

"Conclusions" describe the meaning and usefulness of the findings or results of the research project.

25.2.4   Discussion

The "discussion" applies the research findings to previous research findings from other articles. This section may include information on the "strength and limitations" of the research project. All research has strengths that support the results such as a large sample size, use of a reliable and valid tool, or percent of response. At the same time, this research can have weaknesses such as a small sample size, little response rate, or unknown total number of a population. That is the case with studying faith community nursing. There is no definitive number of practicing faith community nurses known.

Some research articles may address "implications" of the study. Implications will present how the findings and results from this study could impact or modify the subject under discussion.

25.2.5 Conclusion

Not all research articles will include a separate section which describes the "implications" or significance of the research results or findings on practice, context, or environment. Often "implications" are included in the conclusion section of the research article. The conclusion usually addresses "What next?" So, given the work that has been accomplished in the research study under discussion, what recommendations are there for further research or modification in practice? This section of the article can be helpful in creating ideas for future research projects.

The purpose of this simple review is to stimulate the practicing faith community nurse to engage in reading the work of others invested in advancing faith community nursing. Through a regular discipline of setting aside time to read the current research in faith community nursing, the faith community nurse is better informed in their care of others, able to contribute to discussions on "best practices," engage in an informed manner in other faith community research projects, and contribute in the future to the progress of faith community scholarship and ongoing development of the research agenda for faith community nursing.

25.3   Establishing a Research Agenda for Faith Community Nursing

Research has always been a part of the development of faith community nursing through having professional nurse researchers invested in the development of the practice from its inception. *The Journal of Christian Nursing* published results of early survey research completed by Dr. MaryAnn McDermott, faculty Loyola University Chicago and a graduate student working with her Erin Mullins (McDermott & Mullins, 1989), titled, *Profile of a Young Movement*. This study relied on a convenience sample of 37 nurses who attended the first *Annual Westberg Symposium* in 1987. The article reported on demographic data, employment, recruitment and motivation, satisfaction and frustrations, personal and professional characteristics of the respondents, as well as their involvement in professional and program evaluation. Notable in the demographics is that there was one male respondent. Employment data noted two of the 37 respondents were in full time salaried positions, 27 held half time salaried positions, and 12 reported volunteer status (p. 29).

The first student research paper that surveyed parish nurses was titled *Personal Time and Innate Perceptions of the Parish Nurse Role*. This paper was completed for an independent nursing research study at St. Olaf, a Lutheran College in Minnesota (Reiter, 1987, Personal and innate perceptions of the paris nurse role, Unpublished Manuscript). The findings were not published, but used to develop educational and orientation programs for nurses. Research in faith community nursing has come a long way since 1987.

Almost each year, at the *Annual Westberg Symposium*, results of nursing research regarding faith community nursing or a related subjects have been presented. In addition, as a result of a three-year Kellogg funded grant, *Looking Back: the Parish Nurse Experience* (Djupe and Lloyd, 1992), reported on a study of an institutional based model of parish nursing involving Lutheran General Health System and United Medical Center in Moline, Illinois. This report was published as a paper bound book. The study which undergirded the report was a quantitative perspective on 40 parish nurse programs. This mixed method research reported on program structure, financial allocations, scope of services, impact of the services, environmental assessment, and program goals. The problem appeared, as with many nurses and research, that completing the research is one matter, presenting the findings at a conference is a natural, however bringing that research to publication is a whole other effort.

There are three aspects of faith community nursing that are notable in reviewing the history of scholarship, research, and publication in faith community nursing:

1. In 1997, 21 articles were published on parish nursing. *The Journal of Christian Nursing* dedicated one of their issues to parish nursing. Eight of the 21 articles in that issue were focused on parish nursing. Kuhn, (1997) wrote about a study completed on four organizational frameworks for parish nursing, while Whitney-Miller, (1997) authored an article on a Christian-based conceptual model for parish nursing practice. Zetterlund, (1997) and Zerson, (1994) focused on historical perspectives related to the deaconesses, while Schmidt, (1997) wrote about her "call" to parish nursing and Atkins, (1997) highlighted the functions of the parish nurse. Wilson, (1997) also wrote about another parish nurse model based on person, holistic health, and personal responsibility for health. Miles, (1997) emphasized the importance of a job description in assisting church members to understand the role of the parish nurse. This increase in publications on different topics pertinent to faith community nursing signaled a strong interest in studying and understanding this new nursing role, its historical roots, context, and the nurse practicing in that role more thoroughly.

2. The first international replication research titled *Global Perspectives on the Ministry of Parish Nursing Practice: Frequently Used Interventions by Parish Nurses in the United States, Swaziland, Africa, and the United Kingdom* was presented at the Westberg Symposium in 2010 and at a Sigma Theta Tau International Meeting in 2011 (Solari-Twadell et al., 2007, 2011) The research

projects in the United Kingdom and Swaziland, Africa replicated the 2002 study completed in the United States Practice (Solari-Twadell, 2002). The participant from each study could not be as the numbers of respondents were very different given the longevity of the role in each country and the size of each country. However, the findings were interesting in that the most frequently used interventions in the United Kingdom appeared more consistent with the United States than Swaziland, Africa where the people were at that time dying from HIV/AIDS. The work of the nurses in Swaziland, Africa at the time was more concerned with death and dying than health promotion.

3. Research was not identified as a chapter heading in any parish nursing/faith community nursing text until 2006. The chapter "Uncovering the Intricacies of the Ministry of Parish Nursing Practice through Research" reported largely in nationwide research on parish nursing using the *Nursing Intervention Classification System* to describe the differentiation of practice within parish nursing (Solari-Twadell, 2006). Faith Community nursing has, to date, many research articles published in various journals that discuss the specialty practice. However, the research efforts must be emphasized to continue to advance this specialty practice.

25.4   Ongoing Development of a Research Agenda

25.4.1 St Louis, 2008, Nursing Research Conference, International Parish Nurse Resource Center

In March, 2008, a Research conference was held in St. Louis resulting in approximately 30–35 nurses attending. At that meeting four themes were identified for future research efforts. These themes were (1) Practice Outcomes, (2) Curriculum Evaluation, (3) Spirituality, and (4) Roles of the Parish Nurse. There was follow-up on these themes following the meeting. For example, an evaluation of the educational curriculum for parish nursing was conducted with the educational partners attending the 2007 Faculty Retreat, sponsored by the *International Parish nurse Resource Center.* A survey of providers that utilized the 2004 parish nurse basic preparation curriculum was completed. The results from this evaluation were used as the basis for the 2009 curriculum revision. Another follow-up was a survey of faith community nurses in 2008 using "Survey Monkey." Demographic data was collected on 946 respondents; however, these results were never published. The 2008 research conference also stimulated a research pre-conference session at the 2009, 2010, and 2011 *Westberg Symposiums.* In addition, a Research Electronic Letter was sent out regularly to a list of persons, which included about 130 names. There was also an effort to identify the number of nurses interested in faith community nursing that had an advanced degree. At the time, it was estimated that there were about 180 individuals who were on that list (West and Solari-Twadell, 2012).

25.4.2 Chicago, 2012 Research Conference for Faith Community Nursing, Loyola University Chicago

Through a donation from the Westberg family, Loyola University Chicago, Niehoff School of Nursing, hosted a 2-day conference in downtown Chicago at the Water Tower Campus on August 7th through 8th, 2012. Dr. Fran Lewis, University of Seattle, Washington was the keynote speaker (Exhibit A). In her keynote address, Dr. Lewis noted the unique value that faith community nursing as a specialty practice can bring into nursing research and reasons for establishing a research agenda for the specialty practice of faith community nursing has as a specialty practice. Dr. Lewis's presentation provided the following reasons:

1. Faith Community nurses have access to diverse families, persons who are invisible or underserved;
2. The holistic model of nursing enables thinking outside the box and required in more traditional settings.
3. Core faith-based values can motivate new research directions and studies that otherwise might be underdeveloped;
4. New networks of collaboration could surface;
5. Population-based services can be directly linked to community members;
6. Ongoing contact with faith communities fosters deep trust enabling hard issues to be addressed;
7. Faith community nursing practice is not restricted to ill persons or provider-based agencies; and
8. Trust between the faith community nurse and the client can foster health-related changes in persons and SYSTEMS.

In closing, Dr. Lewis spoke about the importance of focusing research proposals on the mission and priorities of the funder being sought to provide financial support for a designated research project.

The remainder of the day the participants engaged in a three-round, Delphi exercise to elicit a prioritized list of research topics to guide future research efforts in faith community nursing. The following day the wording of the statements was reviewed and modified. The recommended results from this 2-day focused meeting are included in Exhibit B.

Subsequent to this 2-day meeting, groups of interested nurses gathered at the 2014, 2016 and 2018 *Westberg Symposium* Pre-conferences meetings for the purpose of reviewing, modifying, and updating the Research Agenda for Faith Community Nursing (Lewis, 2012).

25.4.2.1 Scholarship and Research Position Statement

The 2018 Westberg Symposium came on the heels of the publication of "National Nursing Science Priorities: Creating a Shared Vision" (Eckardt et al., 2017) which was published through the work of the *Council for the Advancement of Nursing Science.* This effort which was sponsored by the *American Academy of Nursing* "serves the nursing community and public by advancing health policy and clinical practice through synthesis, and dissemination of knowledge and research findings" (Eckardt et al., 2017, p. 727). The *Council for the Advancement of Nursing Science* (CANS) is an "open membership entity of the Academy and was established to foster better health through nursing science" (Eckardt et al., 2017, p. 727) The CANS Science Committee was asked by the Academy of Nursing to identify national nursing science priorities. These published results established the blue print for nursing science priorities to inform future collaborations, lines of scientific inquiry, and resource allocation.

What seemed like the first time, faith community nursing had an opportunity to align it's research priorities with national research priorities of nursing. However, for this national work to be considered by the faith community nurses' professional community, the faith community nurses would need to be educated on the national nursing research priorities. At the 2018, *Westberg Symposium*, a break out session was offered in addition to the post-conference. This break out session presented the blue print of nursing science priorities for the profession of nursing. This session preceded the work that was done post-conference on reviewing and updating the "Research Priorities for Faith Community Nursing." Those who were registered for the post-conference reviewed and updated the research priorities for faith community nursing were urged to attend this session on the national research priorities.

The outcome from the post-conference on the research priorities for faith community nursing was a position paper (Exhibit C). The essence of the position statement is a clear mandate supporting research in faith community nursing noting four priorities for research and scholarship, a framework for conceptualizing research and scholarship in faith community nursing, and action steps that can be taken by any faith community nurse. In addition, process issues were affirmed as significant to supporting future research efforts in faith community nursing.

25.5   Conclusion

Even though the professional faith community nursing specialty has been attending to the significance of research related to the growth and development of this practice, there is much more work to be done. As noted in Chapter 17, *Faith Community Nursing International* with a committee dedicated to faith community nursing research and the sponsorship of an annual research forum is in a position to foster an ongoing focus on nursing research in faith community nursing.

Faith community nurses must be supported in the very important work that each is doing in communities around the world. However, when given the opportunity to engage with other faith community nurses in the documenting of significant interventions and outcomes, there must also be recognition of the importance of this work to the future integration of faith community nursing into community-based systems of care. Thus research will remain an issue significant to the future of faith community nursing.

Appendix 1

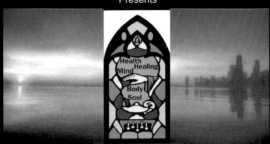

Loyola University Chicago
Marcella Niehoff School of Nursing
Presents

Research Conference on Faith Community Nursing

This conference is being underwritten by the Family of Reverend Granger Westberg.

August 7 - 8, 2012

Tuesday Aug 7, 12:30 – 7:00 pm
Wednesday Aug 8, 7:30 – 11:30 am

NEW VENUE
Beane Hall
Water Tower Campus
Loyola University Chicago
Chicago, Illinois

CONFERENCE OBJECTIVES

The purpose of the conference is to establish the research agenda for faith community nursing. In addition, this conference is intended to increase collaboration among researchers interested in the specialty practice in faith community nursing.

For more information, please contact:

Janet Campbell   Dr. Ann Solari-Twadell
(708) 216-3643   (773) 508-2909
jcampbell2@luc.edu   psolari@luc.edu

LOYOLA
UNIVERSITY CHICAGO

Preparing people to lead extraordinary lives

Keynote Speaker

Frances M. Lewis
PhD, RN, FAAN

Virginia & Prentice
Bloedel Professor
University of
Washington

Affiliate, Fred
Hutchinson Cancer
Research Center

"Setting Research Priorities: Policy, Funding and Other Considerations"

Speakers / Presenters

Dr. Andrea West, previous Director of Curriculum and Research International Parish Nurse Resource Center, St. Louis, Missouri

Dr. Gayle Roux, Associate Professor, Texas Women's University, College of Nursing

Dr. Roberta Schweitzer, Assistant Professor, Purdue University, School of Nursing

Dr. P. Ann Solari-Twadell, Associate Professor, Loyola University Chicago, Marcella Niehoff School of Nursing

Dr. Mary Ann McDermott, Professor Emerita, Loyola University Chicago, Marcella Niehoff School of Nursing

Conference Objectives

- Identify research priorities for the faith community nursing practice.
- Introduce examples of potential questions for study within faith community nursing consistent with the identified research priorities.
- Increase collaboration among researchers interested in the faith community nursing practice.
- Discuss funding sources to support research projects in faith community nursing.
- Set goals for publication of completed faith community nursing research.

Map and Directions
Campus Map (also attached as separate PDF)
Beane Hall located on 13th Floor in Building 6.
http://www.luc.edu/media/lucedu/wtc_map_020911.pdf

General Registration..............$125.00
Registration Website
www.luc.edu/nursing/faithconference.

Includes the cost of registration, materials, and meals. Refunds for the full amount will be made one week prior to conference.

IMPORTANT NOTICE: minimum number of attendees is required for this conference to take place. We will send a separate email confirming that it will be held to all who registered. Please do not make travel arrangements before July 6th or until you have received email confirmation that the conference will occur.

Accommodations

Wyndham Hotel -Anne Bahr Direct (312) 274-4438
The Talbott Hotel (312) 944-4970
Westin Michigan Ave. (312) 943-7200
Mariott Hotel Michigan Ave. (312) 836-0100

Special Needs
If you have a disability or need special accommodations to participate in this event, please let us know in advance to better serve you.

Attire

Business casual. For your comfort, we suggest that you dress in layers.

Accreditation

For this conference, 7.5 CEU's will be applied for through Loyola University Health System Department of Nursing Education. The evaluation that is prescribed by the Continuing Education Unit (CEU) application will be given to participants at the end of the conference as a means of evaluating the speakers, environment and content of the program. Certificates denoting the number of CEU's earned will also be given to participants at the end of the conference.

Chicago Information
http://www.choosechicago.com
http://www.explorechicago.org/city/en.html

Conference Agenda

Tuesday, August 7, 2012

12:30 PM   Arrival, Registration, Light Lunch

1:00 PM   Welcome and Invocation

1:30 PM   Introductions

2:00 PM   Presentation - *"Current State of Research in Faith Community Nursing"*
Dr. Andrea West and Dr. P. Ann Solari-Twadell

2:30 PM   **Keynote Presentation** - *"Setting Research Priorities: Policy, Funding and Other Considerations"*
Dr. Frances M. Lewis

3:15 PM   Break

3:45 PM   Directed Discussion and Questions, Research Prioritization

5:00 PM   Dinner and Informal Networking

6:00 PM   Reflections on Day One

7:00 PM   Adjournment

Wednesday, August, 8, 2012

7:30 - 8:30 AM Breakfast

8:30 AM   Morning Reflection

8:45 AM   Presentation - *"Collaborating with others: Demonstrating the Effectiveness of Faith Community Nurses"*
Dr. Frances M. Lewis, Dr. Gayle Roux and Dr. P. Ann Solari-Twadell

9:45 AM   Break

10:00 AM   Directed Discussion and Questions

11:00 AM   Recap: Report of Conference Proceedings - *"Recommendations for Moving Research Priorities and Setting a Research Agenda for the Specialty Practice of Parish Nursing"*
Dr. Andrea West, Dr. Roberta Schweitzer, Dr. Mary Ann McDermott and Dr. P. Ann Solari-Twadell

11:30 AM   Conference Evaluation and Conclusion

Loyola University Chicago Marcella Niehoff School of Nursing is grateful for the generous donation from the Family of Reverend Granger Westberg and its support of the Research Conference on Faith Community Nursing.

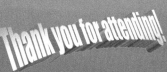

Appendix 2: Final Priorities 2012

Faith Community Nursing Research Conference

Priority #1: Outcomes research by an FCN with a multidisciplinary team:

1. Included: Hospital readmission, ER visits, falls
2. Spirituality is key piece of research—hallmark of FCN practice
3. Cost effective is an outcome of the intervention
4. Health policy development
5. Chronic illness
6. Health promotion

Priority #2: Develop a sustainable infrastructure for a faith community nursing national research program

1. Key stakeholders
2. Development of a national clearing house of foundation funding that will allow for seed grants for FCN research

Priority #3: Describe best practices that address sustainability of FCN practices Process issues:

- How to prepare FCNs to function in the process—skill level
- How to convince our colleagues that they should be involved in the process—monthly meetings, journal clubs
- Data collectors must see themselves as a part of the team
- Sustainability of a program within a faith community—infrastructure—key stakeholders
- FCN has to be educated to value the research process
- Preparing the members of the faith community to engage in the research process

Appendix 3: Research and Scholarship

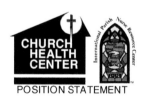

POSITION STATEMENT

Research and scholarship are important aspects of the profession of nursing that require clarification and actualization. Since 2008, FCN through a series of dedicated workshops and pre-conferences has engaged members of the FCN community in formulating how research should be addressed within this specialty nursing practice. Since 2012, where a conference dedicated to establishing research priorities was hosted by Loyola University Chicago, the research priorities for FCN have been reviewed, modified and disseminated. In 2018, the research priorities for Faith Community Nursing were reviewed considering the four research priorities established for the profession of nursing by The Council for the Advancement of Science (CANS). These priorities are: Precision Science, Big Data and Data Analytics, Determinants of Health and Global Health (Eckardt et al., 2017). FCN research and scholarship encompasses global FCN discovery (new knowledge research), integration, teaching, and practice/service/ministry. The purposes of developing research priorities for FCN specialty practice are to 1.) Demonstrate the contribution of Faith Community Nurse's (FCN's) to healthcare outcomes; 2.) Identify cost effect strategies for prevention and ongoing care across the continuum of care; 3.) Identify the faith community as a strategic partner in fostering health and wholeness; and, 4) Advance FCN as a specialty nursing practice. In order to meet these objectives, research and scholarship are essential (Dyess, Chase, & Newlin, 2010).

Faith Community Nurses Engagement in Research and scholarship

Researchers and scholars are all nursing professionals who demonstrate reflection, critical thinking, continuous learning, and engage in practice based on evidence as a means to enhance patient and family outcomes (Carter, Mastro, Vose, Rivera, & Larson, 2017). Carter et al also simplify and define the terms of evidence based practice (EBP), quality improvement (QI), and research to be: "EBP as the combination of scientific evidence, patient preferences, and clinician expertise when making decisions for patient care; QI as data-driven efforts that improve processes specific to an organization; and research as activities aimed at contributing to generalizable knowledge" (p. 266). FCN as professional nurses interested in providing excellent care are required to be continuous learners through ongoing reading of literature that will enhance their nursing practice, collaborating with those that can advance FCN practice through research and challenge themselves to be engaged in the larger mission of FCN –Health Care Reform.

At a recent Westberg Institute workshop, several FCN experts came together to determine the following four priorities for research and scholarship:

1. Engage in research & scholarship in accordance with skillset (from Associate Degree frontline FCN to Doctorally prepared FCN- all levels of education and practice)
2. Conduct outcomes research through intentional collaboration (of FCN's) with institutions such as Churches, Health Care Systems and Universities.
3. Utilize and disseminate evidence–based practices that sustain practice and influence policy
4. Align global FCN research& scholarship with current national and international nursing science priorities.

Importance of Research and Scholarship

Standard Thirteen of the *Faith Community Nursing Scope and Standards* states "The faith community nurse integrates evidence and research findings into practice" (American Nurses Association & Health Ministry Association, 2017). This standard continues by describing eight competencies for FCN's and an fourteen competencies for those FCN's prepared at the graduate level. In order for the FCN to successfully address the quadruple aim mandate, and achieve cost-effective, safe, quality patient and family outcomes engagement with the latest EBP and research initiatives is important. Community health outreach initiatives from formalized health care systems, and academic settings present options for achievable collaborative research and scholarship approaches for FCNs. The FCNs collaborative options are able to address population health challenges, determinants of health, spiritual distress and other dominant chronic illnesses. Linkages to before, during and after acute care health encounters impact altruistic and economic concerns as well as long-term patient quality of life (Dyess, Opalinski, Saiswick, & Fox, 2016; Ziebarth, 2016).

FCN Responsibility in Research and Scholarship?

All FCN's are responsible to engage in the continuum of clinical research and scholarship. The practice of research and scholarship is inclusive of the Scope and Standards of Practice that guide the specialty for FCN's (American Nurses Association & Health Ministry Association, 2017). More specifically, all aspects of the nursing process need to be accounted for within any encounter. All FCN's are responsible for assessment, nursing diagnoses, planning, implementation and evaluation with documentation capturing the encounter (Campbell, 2014; Solari-Twadell & Hackbarth, 2010).Wilkes, Mannix, and Jackson (2013), suggest that research and scholarship must be made public through dissemination networks, available for peer review, and be able to be further developed by other FCN practitioners and scholars. They offer a framework for conceptualizing research and scholarship; the image below is adapted for FCN's.

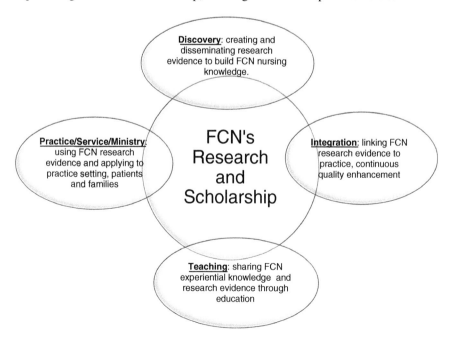

What actions can be taken and what are process issues for FCN research and scholarship?

Action Steps:

1. Document in a consistent format and thoroughly.
2. Develop a practice based inquiry and life-long learning.
3. Articulate common language by adopting the 4 themes from national priorities with international adaptation.
4. Identify appropriate activities associated with personal competencies and skillsets
5. Learn the trilingual nature of FCN practice, nursing, theology and healthcare systems
6. Foster universal documentation practices
7. Collaborate with others.

Process Issues:

1. Preparing FCN's, health care systems and faith communities to collaborate in the research and scholarship process.
2. Engaging all FCN'colleagues to be involved in interdisciplinary research and scholarship that includes multi-disciplinary initiatives
3. Encouraging FCN's and system partners to value the importance of common language and documentation systems.
4. Maintain a global perspective for FCN's research and scholarship

References

- American Nurses Association & Health Ministry Association (2017) Faith *Community Nursing: Scope and Standards of Practice* (3rd Ed).
- Campbell, K. (2014). Documenting Practice. in Jacob, S. (Ed.) 2014 *Foundations of Faith Community Nursing.*(3rd Ed.). Memphis, TN: Church Health Center.
- Carter, E., Mastro, K., Vose, C., Rivera, R & Larson, E. (2017). Clarifying the conundrum: Evidence-based practice, quality improvement, or research?: The clinical scholarship continuum. *Journal of Nursing Administration, 47*(5), 266–270.
- Dyess, S., Chase, S. K., & Newlin, K. (2010). State of research for faith community nursing 2009. *Journal of Religion and Health, 49* (2), 188–199.
- Dyess, S., Opalinski, A., Saiswick, K., & Fox, V. (2016) Caring across the healthcare continuum: A call to nurse leaders to manifest values through action with community outreach. *Nursing Administration Quarterly, 40* (2) 137-145.
- Eckardt, P., Culley, J.M., Corwin, E., Richmond, T., Dougherty, C., Piokler, R., Krause-Parello, C. Reye, C., Rainbow, J.G. and DeVon, H. (2017). National nursing science priorities: Creating a shared vision, 65(6), 726-736)
- Solari-Twadell, P. A., & Hackbarth, D. P. (2010). Evidence for a new paradigm of the ministry of parish nursing practice using the nursing intervention classification system. *Nursing Outlook, 58*(2), 69–75.

- Westberg Institute (2018). *FCN Research Forum.* April 12, 2018.
- Wilkes, L. Mannix, J., & Jackson, D. (2013). Practicing nurses perspectives of clinical scholarship: a qualitative study. *BMC Nursing, 12*(21), 1-7.
- Ziebarth, D. (2016). Altruistic and economic measurements used for prevention health services: Faith Community Nursing Program. Journal of Evaluation and Program Planning, 57 (c), 72-79.

References

Atkins, F. (1997). What should the church do about health? *Journal of Christian Nursing, 14,* 29–31.

Djupe, A. M., & Lloyd, R. C. (1992, July). *Looking back: The parish nurse experience.* Battle Creek, MI: National Parish Nurse Resource Center. Published with support from W.K. Kellogg Foundation. ISBN #0-9627625-2-0.

Eckardt, P., Culley, J. M., Corwin, E., Richmond, T., Dougherty, C., Piokler, R. H., et al. (2017). National nursing science priorities: Creating a shared vision. *Nursing Outlook, 65*(6), 726–736.

Kuhn, J. (1997). A profile of parish nurses. *Journal of Christian Nursing, 14,* 26–28.

Lewis, F. (2012). Keynote address: Setting research priorities: Policy, funding & other considerations. In *Faith community nursing research conference*, Loyola University Chicago, 7–8 August.

McDermott, M. A., & Mullins, E. E. (1989). Profile of a young movement. *Journal of Christian Nursing, 6,* 29–30.

Miles, L. (1997). Getting started: Parish nursing in a rural community. *Journal of Christian Nursing, 14,* 22–24.

DeFranzo, S. E. (2011). *What's the difference between qualitative and quantitative research?* Retrieved December, 2018, from https://www.snapsurveys.com/blog/qualitative-vs-quantitative-research/

Schmidt, K. (1997). Answering God's call. *Journal of Christian Nursing, 14,* 12–13.

Solari-Twadell, P. A. (2002). The differentiation of the ministry of parish nursing practice within congregations. *Dissertation Abstracts International, 63*(06), 569A. UMI No. 3056442.

Solari-Twadell, P. A. (2006). Uncovering the intricacies of the ministry of parish nursing practice through research. In P. A. Solari-Twadell & M. A. McDermott (Eds.), *Parish nursing: Development, education and administration* (pp. 17–35). St. Louis, MO: Elsevier.

Solari-Twadell, P. A., Gustafson, C., Wordsworth, H., & Dlamini, T. (2007). Differentiating the ministry of parish nursing practice: International perspectives. In *21st annual Westberg Parish nurse symposium*, St Louis, MO, 29 September, 2007.

Solari-Twadell, P. A., Gustafson, C., Wordsworth, H., & Dlamini, T. (2011). Global perspectives on the ministry of parish nursing practice: Frequently used interventions by Parish nurses in Swaziland Africa, United Kingdom and United States people and knowledge: Connecting for global health. In *41st Biennial convention*, Grapevine Texas, 1 November, 2011.

West, A., & Solari-Twadell, P. A. (2012). Current state of research in faith community nursing. In *Faith community nursing research conference*, Loyola University Chicago, 7–8 August.

Whitney-Miller, L. (1997). Nursing through the lens of faith: A conceptual model. *Journal of Christian Nursing, 14,* 17–21.

Wilson, R. (1997). What does a parish nurse do? *Journal of Christian Nursing, 14,* 13–16.

Zerson, D. (1994). Parish nursing a 20th century fad? *Journal of Christian Nursing, 11*(2), 19–22.

Zetterlund, J. (1997). Putting care back into health care. *Journal of Christian Nursing, 14*(2), 10–13.

Epilogue

Envision that it is 2030. What do you think faith community nursing will look like then? Although an ideal scenario, let's go for what could be the most hopeful scenario and consistent with Reverend Granger Westberg's vision—a faith community nurse in each faith community!

2040 Envisioned

Faith community nursing is now over 50 years old. Faith communities, no matter what denomination, are recognized as central to the health and well-being of people in all communities. Nurses are drawn to this specialty practice as this nursing role is one which is consistently recognized for patient-centered care which addresses the whole person—body, mind, and spirit. Faith community nurses are integrated into their local health-care system working in full-time roles for larger faith communities and half-time roles in smaller faith communities. The cost for nursing services in the acute care setting is now a separate charge from the cost of a bed. These faith community nurses are part of the local health system network and now are reimbursed for coded interventions, such as transitional care, in working with local medical homes. The faith community nurses meet regularly for continuing education, spiritual direction, and information sharing. Each nurse has a contract with the faith community served and the health-care system. Each faith community has a contract with the nurse and health-care system.

Each nurse has the latest digital documentation app that allows voice recognition of the nurse and simultaneously summarizes all nursing diagnosis made, interventions employed, and lifestyle changes sustained by the client. The client is recognized through the relationship with the nurse for sustaining any lifestyle changes or healthy decisions. This recognition is noted by the health-care system and payer. The results of the faith community nurses' visits are programmed into the data systems of the health-care system, and there are logarithms that have been established that give the faith community nurse feedback as to which clients will benefit from return phone calls and visits by the nurse and/or other volunteers in the faith community. In addition, interventions that are employed by faith community nurses and most significant to the reduction of active symptoms are noted as creating patterns

© Springer Nature Switzerland AG 2020
P. A. Solari-Twadell, D. J. Ziebarth (eds.), *Faith Community Nursing*,
https://doi.org/10.1007/978-3-030-16126-2

of wellness at all stages of chronic illness. With data being automatically generated, nursing research is focused on "big data" to report on outcomes. These outcomes are utilized along with other health system data regionally to allocate health-care resources. In addition, certain clients are contacted to tell their health story in order to grapple more deeply with some phenomena.

Faith community nursing as a specialty practice is understood throughout health care internationally as significant to sustaining care that has made a significant change in the understanding of health and the delivery of health care. Through persistent listening to a greater "call," faith community nurses see nursing as a "calling" that is intended to counter the culture of the medical model of care. Each faith community nurse has a focus on nurturing their inner strength that is bolstered by an active spiritual life. The faith community nurse believes and lives out that the client is best cared for through the community in which they live and participate in a faith community. The fostering of health is seen as significant to being able to live out "the call" to serve others in the community with each person's unique gifts being used for the betterment of the whole.

The option remains for some individuals to choose a health insurance package that excludes participation in a faith community. For these individuals, prevention may not be the focus of their care. They will run the risk of paying for a more expensive health-care package as data will now reflect faith community nursing as a "best practice" for quality of life.

The reality is that without the faith community nurses and pastors who work tirelessly with their teams and volunteers in their faith communities, sustaining their effort to support their members in their episodes of wellness along with their episodes of illness the reality of the faith community nurse, the faith community as a whole-person health place in the community and health being more than the absence of disease falls flat.

So for us who are dreamers, let us continue to pray that there will be recognition, change, and better care of God's people over time through faith community nursing.

Index

© Springer Nature Switzerland AG 2020
P. A. Solari-Twadell, D. J. Ziebarth (eds.), *Faith Community Nursing*,
https://doi.org/10.1007/978-3-030-16126-2

9783030161286